OXFORD MEDICAL PUBLICATIONS

Oxford Handbook of
Clinical and Laboratory Investigation

Oxford Handbook of
Clinical and Laboratory Investigation

Drew Provan

Senior Lecturer in Haematology,
St Bartholomew's and The Royal London Hospital
School of Medicine & Dentistry, London, UK

Andrew Krentz

Honorary Senior Lecturer in Medicine,
Southampton University Hospitals NHS Trust,
Southampton, UK

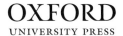

OXFORD
UNIVERSITY PRESS

OXFORD
UNIVERSITY PRESS

Great Clarendon Street, Oxford OX2 6DP

Oxford   New York

Auckland Bangkok Buenos Aires
Cape Town Chennai Dar es Salaam Delhi Hong Kong Istanbul
Karachi Kolkata Kuala Lumpur Madrid Melbourne Mexico City Mumbai
Nairobi Paris São Paolo Singapore Taipei Tokyo Toronto

Oxford is a trade mark of Oxford University Press

Published in the United States
by Oxford University Press, Inc., New York

© Oxford University Press 2002
The moral rights of the author have been asserted
Servier edn. printed 2003

First published 2002

British Library Cataloguing in Publication Data

Data available

Library of Congress Cataloging in Publication Data

3 5 7 9 10 8 6 4 2

ISBN 0 19 263283 3
ISBN 0 19 853082 X (Servier edn.)

Typeset by Drew Provan and EXPO Holdings, Malaysia
Printed in Italy by LegoPrint S.p.A.

Contents

Contributors

John Axford
Reader in Medicine, Academic Unit for Musculoskeletal Disease, Department of Immunology, St George's Hospital Medical School, London SW17 0RE
Immunology & rheumatology

Martyn Bracewell
Lecturer in Neurology, Department of Neurology, The Queen Elizabeth Hospital, Birmingham B15 2TH
Neurology

Joanna Brown
Clinical Research Fellow, University of Southampton, School of Medicine, RCMB Division, Southampton SO16 6YD
Respiratory medicine

Tanya Chawla
Specialist Registrar in Radiology, Department of Radiology, Southampton University Hospitals NHS Trust, Southampton SO16 6YD
Radiology

Keith Dawkins
Consultant Cardiologist, Wessex Cardiology Unit, Southampton University Hospitals NHS Trust, Southampton SO16 6YD
Cardiology

Colin Dayan
Consultant Senior Lecturer in Medicine, Division of Medicine Laboratories, Bristol Royal Infirmary, Bristol BS2 8BX
Endocrinology & metabolism

Tony Frew
Professor of Medicine, University of Southampton, School of Medicine, RCMB Division, Southampton SO16 6YD
Respiratory medicine

Stephen T. Green
Consultant Physician and Honorary Senior Clinical Lecturer, Department of Infection & Tropical Medicine, Royal Hallamshire Hospital, Sheffield S10 2JF
Infectious & tropical diseases

Alison Jones
Consultant Physician and Clinical Toxicologist, Medical Toxicology Unit, Guy's & St Thomas' Hospital, London SE14 5ER.
Poisoning & overdose

Andrew Krentz
Consultant in Diabetes & Endocrinology and Honorary Senior Lecturer in Medicine, Department of Medicine, Southampton University Hospitals NHS Trust, Southampton SO16 6YD
Endocrinology & metabolism

Val Lewington
Consultant in Nuclear Medicine, Department of Nuclear Medicine, Southampton University Hospitals NHS Trust, Southampton SO16 6YD
Nuclear medicine

Contributors

Praful Patel
Consultant Gastroenterologist, Department of Gastroenterology, Southampton University Hospitals NHS Trust, Southampton SO16 6YD
Gastroenterology

Drew Provan
Senior Lecturer, Department of Haematology, St Bartholomew's & The Royal London School of Medicine & Dentistry, London E1 1BB
Haematology, transfusion & cytogenetics

Rommel Ravanan
Specialist Registrar, The Richard Bright Renal Unit, Southmead Hospital, Westbury-on-Trym, Bristol BS10 5NB
Renal medicine

Charlie Tomson
Consultant Nephrologist, The Richard Bright Renal Unit, Southmead Hospital, Westbury-on-Trym, Bristol BS10 5NB
Renal medicine

Ken Tung
Consultant Radiologist, Department of Radiology, Southampton University Hospitals NHS Trust, Southampton SO16 6YD
Radiology

Adrian Williams
Professor of Neurology, Department of Neurology, The Queen Elizabeth Hospital, Birmingham B15 2TH
Neurology

Lorraine Wilson
Senior Registrar, Department of Nuclear Medicine, Southampton University Hospitals NHS Trust, Southampton SO16 6YD
Nuclear medicine

Dr Tanay Sheth
Specialist Registrar in Gastroenterology, Southampton University Hospitals NHS Trust, UK

Our registrars
We are indebted to our juniors for writing and checking various sections, in particular *Symptoms & signs.*

Southampton University Hospitals: *Martin Taylor, Michael Masding, Mayank Patel, Ruth Poole and Catherine Talbot.*

St Bartholomew's & The Royal London School of Medicine & Dentistry: *Simon Stanworth, Jude Gaffan, Leon Clark and Nikki Curry.*

Foreword

This book fills an obvious gap in the Handbook series and indeed a major lacuna in the medical literature. Too often investigations of a particular condition are lost in the welter of other text. Alternatively, they appear as specialist books in pathology and radiology. One unique feature of this book is the inclusion of all clinical investigative techniques, i.e. both truly clinical tests in the shape of symptoms and signs and then laboratory-based investigations. This stops what is often an artificial separation. Each section is clearly put together with the intent of easing rapid reference. This is essential if the book is to have (and I believe it does have) real use-fulness for bedside medicine. There are many other useful aspects of the text. These include a comprehensive list of abbreviations—the bugbear of medicine, as well as reference ranges which some laboratories still do not append to results. Overall, the Handbook should be of benefit to not just clinical students and junior doctors in training, but all who have patient contact. With this in one pocket, and Longmore in the other, there should be little excuse for errors in diagnosis and investigation, with the added benefit that the balance between the two will allow the upright posture to be maintained.

Professor Sir George Alberti
President of The Royal College of Physicians of London
July 2002

Preface

With the increasing complexity of modern medicine, we now have literally thousands of possible investigative techniques at our disposal. We are able to examine our patient's serum and every other body fluid down to the level of individual nucleotides, as well as being able to perform precise imaging through CT, MRI and other imaging technologies. The problem we have all faced, especially as senior medical students or junior doctors is: which test should we use in a given setting? What hazards are associated with the tests? Are there any situations where specific tests should not be used or are likely to produce erroneous results? As medical complexity increases so too does cost; many assays available today are highly expensive and wherever possible we would ideally like to use a test which is cheap, reliable, reproducible and right for a given situation.

Such knowledge takes many years to acquire and it is a fact of life that senior doctors (who have attained such knowledge) are not usually those who request the investigations. In this small volume, we have attempted to distil all that is known about modern tests, from blood, urine and other body fluids, along with imaging and molecular tests. The book is divided into two principal parts: the first deals with symptoms and signs in **The patient** section, because that is how patients present. We have tried to cover as many topics as possible, discussing these in some detail and have provided differential diagnoses where possible. We also try to suggest tests that might be of value in determining the cause of the patient's symptom or sign. The second part of the book, **Investigations**, is specialty-specific, and is more relevant once you know roughly what type of disease the patient might have. For example, if the symptom section suggests a likely respiratory cause for the patient's symptoms, then the reader should look to the *Respiratory investigations* chapter in order to determine which tests to carry out, or how to interpret the results.

The entire book is written by active clinicians, rather than scientists, since we wanted to provide a strong clinical approach to investigation. We have tried, wherever possible, to cross-refer to the *Oxford Handbook of Clinical Medicine*, 5th edition, Oxford University Press, which provides the clinical detail omitted from this handbook. The symbol 📖 is used to highlight a cross-reference to OHCM, in addition to cross-referencing within this book.

We would value feedback from readers since there will doubtless be tests omitted, errors in the text and many other improvements we could, and will, make in future editions. All contributors will be acknowledged individually in the next edition. We would suggest you e-mail us directly: *a.provan@virgin.net*.

Drew Provan
Andrew Krentz
2002

Acknowledgements

Even small books such as this rely on the input of many people, besides the main editors and we are indebted to many of our colleagues for providing helpful suggestions and for proofreading the text. Dr Barbara Bain, St Mary's Hospital, London, kindly allowed us to peruse the proofs of *Practical Haematology*, 9th edition (Churchill Livingstone) to help make sure the haematology section was up to date. Dr Debbie Lillington, Department of Cytogenetics, Barts & The London NHS Trust, London, provided invaluable cytogenetic advice. Our registrars have had input into many sections and we thank the London registrars: Simon Stanworth, Jude Gaffan, Leon Clark and Nikki Curry, and the Southampton registrars: Fiona Clark, Michael Masding, Mayank Patel, Ruth Poole and Catherine Talbot.

Dr Murray Longmore, the undisputed Oxford Handbook king, has provided invaluable wisdom and has very kindly allowed us to use his specially designed OHCM typeface (OUP) for many of the symbols in our text. Murray also provided page proofs of the OHCM, 5th edition, which was invaluable for cross-referencing this handbook.

Warm thanks are also extended to Oxford University Press, and in particular Esther (Browning) who first commissioned the book. Very special thanks must go to Catherine (Barnes), commissioning editor for medicine, who has stuck with the project, and most likely has aged 10 years as a result of it! She has provided constant encouragement and helped keep us sane throughout the entire process (well, almost sane). Katherine Sugg and Victoria Oddie relentlessly chased up missing artwork, text and generally kept the project moving.

Symbols & abbreviations

📖	cross-reference to OHCM 5th edition, or section of this book
▶	important
▶▶	very important
↓	decreased
↑	increased
↔	normal
♂ : ♀	male : female ratio
1°	primary
2°	secondary
A&E	accident & emergency
AAFB	acid and alcohol fast bacilli
Ab	antibody
ABGs	arterial blood gases
ACD	anaemia of chronic disease
ACE	angiotensin converting enzyme
ACh	acetylcholine
ACL	anticardiolipin antibody
ACR	acetylcholine receptor
ACS	acute coronary syndrome
ADA	American Diabetes Association
ADH	antidiuretic hormone
ADP	adenosine 5-diphosphate
AECG	ambulatory ECG
AF	atrial fibrillation
Ag	antigen
AIDS	acquired immunodeficiency syndrome
AIHA	autoimmune haemolytic anaemia
AKA	alcoholic ketoacidosis
ALL	acute lymphoblastic leukaemia
ALP	alkaline phosphatase
ALT	alanine aminotransferase
AMI	acute myocardial infarction
AML	acute myeloid leukaemia
ANA	antinuclear antibodies

ANAE	alpha naphthyl acetate esterase
ANCA	antineutrophil cytoplasmic antibody
ANF	antinuclear factor
APCR	activated protein C resistance
APL	antiphospholipid antibody
APML	acute promyelocytic leukaemia
APS	antiphospholipid syndrome
APTR	activated partial thromboplastin time ratio
APTT	activated partial thromboplastin time
ARF	acute renal failure
AT (ATIII)	antithrombin III
ATLL	adult T cell leukaemia/lymphoma
ATP	adenosine triphosphate
AXR	abdominal x-ray
BBB	blood–brain barrier
B-CLL	B-cell chronic lymphocytic leukaemia
bd	*bis die* (twice daily)
BJP	Bence-Jones protein
BM	bone marrow
BMJ	*British Medical Journal*
BMT	bone marrow transplant(ation)
BP	blood pressure
Bx	biopsy
C1 INH	C1 esterase inhibitor
C3Nef	complement C3 nephritic factor
C&S	culture & sensitivity
Ca	carcinoma
Ca^{2+}	calcium
CABG	coronary artery bypass graft
CAH	congenital adrenal hyperplasia
cALL	common acute lymphoblastic leukaemia
CBC	complete blood count (American term for FBC)
CCF	congestive cardiac failure
CCK	cholecystokinin
CCU	coronary care unit
CD	cluster designation
cDNA	complementary DNA
CEA	carcinoembryonic antigen
CF	cystic fibrosis *or* complement fixation
cfu	colony-forming units
CGL	chronic granulocytic leukaemia
CHAD	cold haemagglutinin disease

Symbols & abbreviations

CHD	coronary heart disease
CJD	Creutzfeldt-Jacob disease (v = new variant)
CK	creatine kinase
CL$^-$	chloride
CLL	chronic lymphocytic ('lymphatic') leukaemia
CLO test	*Campylobacter*-like organism
CML	chronic myeloid leukaemia
CMML	chronic myelomonocytic leukaemia
CMV	cytomegalovirus
CNS	central nervous system
CO$_2$	carbon dioxide
COPD	chronic obstructive pulmonary disease
CPAP	continuous positive airways pressure
CREST	calcinosis, Raynaud's syndrome, (o)esophageal motility dysfunction, sclerodactyly and telangiectasia
CRF	chronic renal failure
CRP	C-reactive protein
CSF	cerebrospinal fluid
CT	computed tomography
CTLp	cytotoxic T lymphocyte precursor assay
CVA	cerebrovascular accident (stroke)
CVD	cardiovascular disease
CVS	cardiovascular system *or* chorionic villus sampling
CXR	chest x-ray
DAT	direct antiglobulin test
dATP	deoxy ATP
DCCT	Diabetes Control and Complications Trial
DCT	direct Coombs' test
DDAVP	desamino D-arginyl vasopressin
DE	evoked potential
DIC	disseminated intravascular coagulation
DIDMOAD	diabetes insipidus, diabetes mellitus, optic atrophy and deafness
DKA	diabetic ketoacidosis
dL	decilitre
DM	diabetes mellitus
DNA	deoxyribonucleic acid
2,3-DPG	2,3-diphosphoglycerate
dRVVT	dilute Russell's viper venom test

DTT	dilute thromboplastin time
DU	duodenal ulcer
DVT	deep vein thrombosis
DXT	radiotherapy
EBV	Epstein-Barr virus
ECG	electrocardiograph
EDH	extradural haemorrhage
EDTA	ethylenediamine tetraacetic acid
EEG	electroencephalogram
ELISA	enzyme-linked immunosorbent assay
EMG	electromyogram
Epo	erythropoietin
ERCP	endoscopic retrograde cholangiopancreatography
ESR	erythrocyte sedimentation rate
ESREF	end-stage renal failure
ET	essential thrombocythaemia
etOH	ethanol
FAB	French–American–British
FACS	fluorescence-activated cell sorter
FBC	full blood count (*aka* complete blood count, CBC)
FDPs	fibrin degradation products
Fe	iron
FeSO$_4$	ferrous sulphate
FISH	fluorescence *in situ* hybridisation
FIX	factor IX
fL	femtolitres
FMRI	functional MRI
FOB	faecal occult blood
FPG	fasting plasma glucose
FUO	fever of unknown origin (like PUO)
FVIII	factor VIII
FVL	factor V Leiden
g	gram
G&S	group & save serum
GAD	glutamic acid decarboxylase
γGT	γ-glutamyl transpeptidase
GBM	glomerular basement membrane
GIT	gastrointestinal tract
GPC	gastric parietal cell
G6PD	glucose-6-phosphate dehydrogenase
GPI	general paralysis of the insane
GTN	glyceryl trinitrate
GU	gastric ulcer

GvHD	graft versus host disease
h	hour
HAV	hepatitis A virus
Hb	haemoglobin
HbA	haemoglobin A ($\alpha_2\beta_2$)
HbA$_{1c}$	haemoglobin A$_{1c}$
HbA$_2$	haemoglobin A$_2$ ($\alpha_2\delta_2$)
HbF	haemoglobin F (fetal Hb, $\alpha_2\gamma_2$)
HbH	haemoglobin H (β_4)
HBsAg	hepatitis B surface antigen
HBV	hepatitis B virus
hCG	human chorionic gonadotrophin
HCO$_3^-$	bicarbonate
Hct	haematocrit
HCV	hepatitis C virus
HDN	haemolytic disease of the newborn
HE	hereditary elliptocytosis
HELLP	haemolysis, elevated liver enzymes and low platelet count
HIV	human immunodeficiency virus
HLA	human leucocyte antigen
HNA	heparin neutralising activity
HONK	hyperosmolar non-ketotic syndrome
HPA	human platelet antigen
HPFH	hereditary persistence of fetal haemoglobin
HPLC	high-performance liquid chromatography
HPOA	hypertrophic pulmonary osteoarthropathy
HPP	hereditary pyropoikilocytosis
HTLV	human T-lymphotropic virus
IAGT or IAT	indirect antiglobulin test
IBS	irritable bowel syndrome
ICA	islet cell antibodies
ICH	intracranial haemorrhage
IDA	iron deficiency anaemia
IDDM	insulin dependent (type 1) diabetes mellitus
IEF	isoelectric focusing
IFG	impaired fasting glucose
IFN-α	interferon alpha
IGT	impaired glucose tolerance
IHD	ischaemic heart disease

Ig	immunoglobulin
IgA	immunoglobulin A
IgD	immunoglobulin D
IgE	immunoglobulin E
IgG	immunoglobulin G
IgM	immunoglobulin M
IIF	indirect immunofluorescence
IM	intramuscular
INR	international normalized ratio
ITP	idiopathic thrombocytopenic purpura
ITU	intensive therapy unit
iu/IU	international units
IV	intravenous
IVI	intravenous infusion
IVU	intravenous urogram
JCA	juvenile chronic arthritis
JVP	jugular venous pressure
K^+	potassium
KCCT	kaolin cephalin clotting time ($\equiv$ APTT)
kDa	kiloDaltons
kg	kilogram
KUB	kidney, ureter, bladder (x-ray)
L	litre or left
LA	lupus anticoagulant or lactic acidosis or local anaesthetic
LAP	leucocyte alkaline phosphatase (score)
LBBB	left bundle branch block
LCM	left costal margin
LDH	lactate dehydrogenase
LFTs	liver function tests
LIF	left iliac fossa
LKM	liver/kidney microsomal
LP	lumbar puncture
LUQ	left upper quadrant
LVF	left ventricular failure
LVH	left ventricular hypertrophy
MAG	myelin-associated glycoprotein
MAIPA	monoclonal antibody immobilisation of platelet antigens
MAOI	monoamine oxidase inhibitor
MC&S	microscopy, culture & sensitivity
MCH	mean cell haemoglobin
MCHC	mean corpuscular haemoglobin concentration
MCV	mean cell volume

MDS	myelodysplastic syndrome
MELAS	myelopathy, encephalopathy, lactic acidosis and stroke-like episodes
mg	milligram (10^{-3} gram)
MGUS	monoclonal gammopathy of undetermined significance
MHC	major histocompatibility complex
MI	myocardial infarction
min	minutes
MoAb	monoclonal antibody
MODY	maturity onset diabetes of the young
mOsm	milliosmole
MPD	myeloproliferative disease
MPV	mean platelet volume
MRI	magnetic resonance imaging
mRNA	messenger ribonucleic acid
MS	multiple sclerosis *or* mass spectroscopy
MSU	mid-stream urine
MTP	metatarsophalangeal
MUD	matched unrelated donor (transplant)
µg	microgram (10^{-6} gram)
Na^+	sodium
NaCl	sodium chloride
NADP	nicotinamide adenine diphosphate
NADPH	nicotinamide adenine diphosphate (reduced)
NAP	neutrophil alkaline phosphatase
NEJM	*New England Journal of Medicine*
NH_3	ammonia
NHL	non-Hodgkin's lymphoma
NRBC	nucleated red blood cells
NSAIDs	non-steroidal anti-inflammatory drugs
NSTEMI	non-ST-elevation myocardial infarction
OA	osteoarthritis
OCP	oral contraceptive pill
od	*omni die* (once daily)
OGD	oesophagogastroduodenoscopy
OGTT	oral glucose tolerance test
OHCH	*Oxford Handbook of Clinical Haematology*
OHCM	*Oxford Handbook of Clinical Medicine*
PA	posteroanterior *or* pernicious anaemia *or* pulmonary artery

PACWP	pulmonary artery capillary wedge pressure
PAD	peripheral arterial disease
PAN	polyarteritis nodosa
PaO_2	partial pressure of O_2 in arterial blood
PAS	periodic acid-Schiff
PB	peripheral blood
PBC	primary biliary cirrhosis
PC	protein C *or* provocation concentration
PCH	paroxysmal cold haemoglobinuria
PCI	percutaneous coronary intervention
PCL	plasma cell leukaemia
PCP	*Pneumocystis carinii* pneumonia
PCR	polymerase chain reaction
PCT	proximal convoluted tubule
PCV	packed cell volume
PDA	patent ductus arteriosus
PE	pulmonary embolism
PEFR	peak expiratory flow rate
PET	positron emission tomography
Ph	Philadelphia chromosome
PIFT	platelet immunofluorescence test
PK	pyruvate kinase
PO	*per os* (by mouth)
PO_4^{3-}	phosphate
PR	*per rectum*
PRL	prolactin
PRV	polycythaemia rubra vera
PS	protein S *or* Parkinson's syndrome
PSA	prostate-specific antigen
PT	prothrombin time
PV	plasma volume
qds	*quater die sumendus* (to be taken 4 times a day)
RA	refractory anaemia *or* rheumatoid arthritis
RAS	renal angiotensin system *or* renal artery stenosis
RBBB	right bundle branch block
RBCs	red blood cells
RCC	red blood cell count
RDW	red cell distribution width
Rh	Rhesus
RhF	rheumatoid factor
RIA	radioimmunoassay
RiCoF	ristocetin cofactor

Symbols & abbreviations

RIF	right iliac fossa
RIPA	ristocetin-induced platelet aggregation
RNP	ribonucleoprotein
RPGN	rapidly progressive glomerulonephritis
RT-PCR	reverse transcriptase polymerase chain reaction
RUQ	right upper quadrant
s	seconds
SAECG	signal-averaged ECG
SAH	subarachnoid haemorrhage
SC	subcutaneous
SCA	sickle cell anaemia
SCD	sickle cell disease
SDH	subdural haemorrhage
SHBG	sex-hormone-binding globulin
SLE	systemic lupus erythematosus
SmIg	surface membrane immunoglobulin
SOB	short of breath
SOL	space-occupying lesion
SM	smooth muscle
SPECT	single photon emission computed tomography
stat	*statim* (immediate; as initial dose)
STEMI	ST-elevation myocardial infarction
sTfR	soluble transferrin receptor assay
SVC	superior vena cava
SVCO	superior vena caval obstruction
SXR	skull x-ray
T°	temperature
$t^1/_2$	half-life
T4	thyroxine
TA	temporal arteritis
TB	tuberculosis
tds	*ter die sumendum* (to be taken 3 times a day)
TdT	terminal deoxynucleotidyl transferase
TENS	transcutaneous nerve stimulation
TFT	thyroid function test(s)
TIAs	transient ischaemic attacks
TIBC	total iron binding capacity
TN	trigeminal neuralgia
TNF	tumour necrosis factor

TOE	transoesophageal echocardiogram
TPA	tissue plasminogen activator
TPO	thyroid peroxidase
TRAB	thyrotropin receptor antibodies
TRALI	transfusion-associated lung injury
TRAP	tartrate-resistant acid phosphatase
TSH	thyroid-stimulating hormone
TT	thrombin time
TTE	transthoracic echocardiography
TTP	thrombotic thrombocytopenic purpura
TXA	tranexamic acid
u/U	units
UC	ulcerative colitis
U&E	urea and electrolytes
UKPDS	United Kingdom Prospective Diabetes Study
URTI	upper respiratory tract infection
UTI	urinary tract infection
USS	ultrasound scan
VIII:C	factor VIII clotting activity
VIP	vasoactive intestinal peptide
Vit K	vitamin K
VSD	ventricular septal defect
VTE	venous thromboembolism
vWD	von Willebrand's disease
vWF	von Willebrand factor
vWFAg	von Willebrand factor antigen
WBC	white blood count *or* white blood cells
WHO	World Health Organisation
WM	Waldenström's macroglobulinaemia
XDPs	cross-linked fibrin degradation products

Approach to investigation

Why do tests?

Patients seldom present to their doctors with *diagnoses*—rather, they have symptoms or signs. The major challenge of medicine is being able to talk to the patient and obtain a history and then carry out a physical examination looking for pointers to their likely underlying problem. Our elders and, some would argue, betters in medicine had less tests available to them then we have today, and their diagnoses were often made solely from the history and examination. Of course, they would claim that their clinical acumen and skills were greater than ours and that we rely too heavily on the huge armoury of laboratory and other investigations available today. This, in part, is probably true, but we cannot ignore the fact that advances in science and technology have spawned a bewildering array of very useful and sophisticated tests that help us to confirm our diagnostic suspicions.

By 'test' we mean the measurement of a component of blood, marrow or other body fluid or physiological parameter to determine whether the patient's value falls within or outside the normal range, either suggesting the diagnosis or, in some cases, actually making the diagnosis for us.

Factors affecting variable parameters in health

Many measurable body constituents vary throughout life. For example, a newborn baby has an extremely high haemoglobin concentration which falls after delivery; this is completely normal and is *physiological* rather than pathological. A haemoglobin level this high in an adult would be pathological since it is far outside the normal range for the adult population.

Factors affecting measurable variables

- Age.
- Sex.
- Ethnicity.
- Altitude.
- Build.
- Physiological conditions (e.g. at rest, after exercise, standing, lying).
- Sampling methods (e.g. with or without using tourniquet).
- Storage and age of sample.
- Container used, e.g. for blood sample, as well as anticoagulant.
- Method of analysis.

Reference ranges (normal values)

These are published for most measurable components of blood and other tissue and we have included the normal ranges for most blood and CSF analytes at the end of the book.

What makes a test useful?

A really good test, and one which would make us appear to be out-standing doctors, would be one which would *always* be positive in the presence of a disease and would be *totally* specific for that disease alone; such a test would never be positive in patients who did not have the dis-order. What we mean is that what we are looking for are *sensitive* tests that are *specific* for a given disease. Sadly, most tests are neither 100% sen-sitive nor 100% specific but some do come very close.

How to use tests and the laboratory

Rather than request tests in a shotgun or knee-jerk fashion, where every box on a request form is ticked, it is far better to use the laboratory selec-tively. Even with the major advances in automation where tests are batched and are cheaper, the hospital budget is finite and sloppy requesting should be discouraged.

Outline your differential diagnoses: what are the likeliest diseases given the patient's history, examination findings and population the patient comes from?

Decide which test(s) will help you make the diagnosis: request these and review the diagnosis in the light of the test results. Review the patient and arrange further investigations as necessary.

The downside of tests

It is important to remember that tests may often give 'normal' results even in the presence of disease. For example, a normal ECG in the presence of chest pain does *not* exclude the occurrence of myocardial infarction with 100% certainty. Conversely, the presence of an abnormality does not nec-essarily imply that a disease is present. This, of course, is where clinical experience comes into its own—the more experienced clinician will be able to balance the likelihood of disease with the results available even if some of the test results give unexpected answers.

Sensitivity & specificity	
Sensitivity	% of patients with the disease and in whom the test is positive
Specificity	% of people without the disease in whom the test is negative

Quick-fix clinical experience

This simply does not exist. Talking to patients and examining them for physical signs and assimilating knowledge gained in medical school are absolute requirements for attainment of sound clinical judgement. Those students and doctors who work from books alone do not survive effec-tively at the coal face! It is a constant source of irritation to medical stu-dents and junior doctors, when a senior doctor asks for the results of an investigation on the ward round and you find this test is the one that clinches the diagnosis. How *do* they do it? Like appreciating good wine—they develop a nose for it. You can learn a great deal by watching your registrar or consultant make decisions. This forms the basis of your *own* clinical experience.

Laboratory errors and how to avoid them

It is a fact of life that the sophisticated automated analysers in current use are not 100% accurate 100% of the time—but they come pretty close. In order to keep errors to a minimum, precautions need to be taken when sampling biological material, e.g. blood.

Minimising spurious results using blood samples
- Use correct bottle.
- Fill to line (if anticoagulant used). This is less of a worry when vacuum sample bottles are used since these should take in exactly the correct amount of blood, ensuring the correct blood : anticoagulant ratio. This is critical for coagulation tests.
- Try to get the sample to the lab as quickly as possible. Blood samples left lying around on warm windowsills, or even overnight at room temperature, will produce bizarre results, e.g. crenated RBCs and abnormal-looking WBCs in old EDTA samples.
- Try to avoid rupturing red cells when taking the sample (e.g. using narrow gauge needle, prolonged time to collect whole sample) otherwise a 'haemolysed' sample will be received by the lab. This may cause spurious results for some parameters (e.g. $[K^+]$).
- Remember to mix (not shake) samples containing anticoagulant.

Variations in normal ranges in health
As discussed earlier, most of the normal ranges for blood parameters discussed in this book are for non-pregnant adults. The reason for this is that blood values, e.g. Hb, RCC are high in the newborn and many FBC, coagulation and other parameters undergo changes in pregnancy.

Part 1
The patient

3

Abdominal distension

Patients may describe generalised abdominal swelling or localised fullness in a specific area of the abdomen. In the history enquire specifically about
• change in bowel habit • weight loss • associated pain.

Generalised swelling

Consider
- Fat.
- Fluid.
- Faeces.
- Flatus.
- Fetus.
- Full bladder.

Ascites: fluid in the peritoneal cavity. Look for shifting dullness and fluid thrill on percussion, stigmata of chronic liver disease, lymphadenopathy, oedema and assess JVP.

Causes
- Malignancy.
- Cirrhosis/portal hypertension.
- Hypoproteinaemia.
- Right heart failure.

Investigations
- U&E.
- LFTs.
- Serum albumin.
- Ascitic tap for protein (transudate *vs.* exudate), cytology, MC&S.
- USS abdomen.

Flatus
Gaseous distension. Need to exclude bowel obstruction. Assess for colicky abdominal pain, bowel habit, flatus and vomiting. Look for resonant distension on percussion, altered or absent bowel sounds, focal tenderness with rebound and guarding. Always check for herniae and perform PR examination in suspected obstruction.

Causes
- *Intraluminal*: faecal impaction, gallstone ileus.
- *Luminal*: inflammatory stricture (e.g. Crohn's), tumour, abscess.
- *Extraluminal*: herniae, adhesions, pelvic mass, lymphadenopathy, volvulus, intussusception.
- Paralytic ileus: drug induced, electrolyte disturbances.
- Age-related causes of obstruction.
- *Neonatal*: congenital atresia, imperforate anus, volvulus, Hirschsprung's, meconium ileus.
- *Infants*: intussusception, Hirschsprung's, herniae, Meckel's diverticulum.
- *Young/middle age adults*: herniae, adhesions, Crohn's.
- *Elderly*: herniae, carcinoma, diverticulitis, faecal impaction.

Investigations
- FBC.
- U&E.

- AXR (erect and supine).
- Consider barium enema, barium follow-through, sigmoidoscopy, surgical intervention for complete acute obstruction.

Localised swelling/masses: common causes according to site

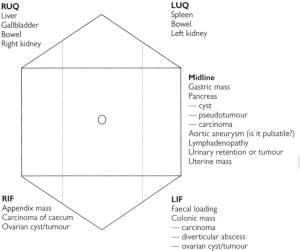

RUQ
Liver
Gallbladder
Bowel
Right kidney

LUQ
Spleen
Bowel
Left kidney

Midline
Gastric mass
Pancreas
— cyst
— pseudotumour
— carcinoma
Aortic aneurysm (is it pulsatile?)
Lymphadenopathy
Urinary retention or tumour
Uterine mass

RIF
Appendix mass
Carcinoma of caecum
Ovarian cyst/tumour

LIF
Faecal loading
Colonic mass
— carcinoma
— diverticular abscess
— ovarian cyst/tumour

Fig. 1.1

Investigate according to site
- Consider USS abdomen and pelvis.
- CT scanning.
- Barium studies.
- IVU.

📖OHCM pp50, 502.

Abdominal pain

Abdominal pain may be *acute* or *chronic*. Severe, acute pain may indicate a surgical emergency including perforation, peritonitis or obstruction. Assess nature and radiation of pain, clinical status of patient including fever, tachycardia and hypotension.

Common causes of abdominal pain according to site

Epigastric pain
Peptic ulcer disease, gastritis or duodenal erosions, cholecystitis, pancreatitis.

Periumbilical
Pancreatitis, mesenteric artery ischaemia (older patient with vascular disease).

RUQ pain
Biliary colic, cholecystitis, hepatitis, peptic ulcer.

LUQ pain
Splenic, peptic ulcer.

Loin pain
Renal colic (colicky radiating loin→groin), pyelonephritis, renal pathology.

LIF pain
Constipation, diverticular disease, irritable bowel syndrome, pelvic referred pain, inflammatory bowel disease.

RIF pain
Appendicitis, pelvic referred pain, inflammatory bowel disease (e.g. Crohn's of terminal ileum).

Suprapubic
UTI, cystitis, salpingitis.

Generalised
Gastroenteritis, irritable bowel, constipation, generalised peritonitis.

6 Pitfalls
Metabolic causes—e.g. diabetic ketoacidosis, hypercalcaemia, Addison's disease, porphyria, lead poisoning.
Atypical referred pain—e.g. myocardial infarction, pneumonia.

Investigations
- FBC.
- U&E, e.g. deranged electrolytes following vomiting, diarrhoea or bowel obstruction.
- Plasma glucose.
- Serum amylase (↑ in pancreatitis and bowel obstruction).
- Urinanalysis and MSU, e.g. haematuria, proteinuria, glucose.
- LFTs (consider obstructive vs. hepatitic picture).
- Plain AXR (erect and supine to assess for perforation and bowel obstruction).
- KUB for renal tract calculi.
- USS abdomen, particularly for biliary tract, gallbladder and renal tract.
- IVU to assess for renal tract calculi/pathology.

📖OHCM pp50, 462.

Alteration of behaviour

This is usually reported by a relative or friend rather than by the patient. Often the patient will have little or no insight into the disease and taking a history can be difficult. In addition to a full general and neurological physical examination a mental state examination is required.

Find out if this is the first episode of altered behaviour or if the episodes are recurrent. Is there a gradual change in behaviour (and personality) over time?

Acute delirium

Causes
- Sepsis (common).
- Acute intracranial event, e.g. haemorrhage.
- Metabolic disturbance, e.g. uraemia, hypercalcaemia (common).
- Intracerebral tumour (including meningioma).
- Drugs—especially interactions in elderly.
- Alcohol (and withdrawal syndrome).
- Hypoxia (common).
- Hypoglycaemia (iatrogenic in diabetic patients receiving insulin treatment or oral insulin secretagogues or insulinoma and other causes, 📖pxx).

Dementia
- Alzheimer's (common), Pick's (rare).
- Vascular, e.g. multi-infarct.
- Huntingdon's chorea.
- Vitamin B_{12} deficiency (severe).
- Hypothyroidism (severe).
- Wilson's disease.
- Alcoholism.
- Normal pressure hydrocephalus.

7

Note: 'Frontal lobe syndrome' from SOL, e.g. meningioma. Presents with disinhibition, impaired social functioning, primitive reflexes, e.g. grasp reflex.

Anxiety states

Usually psychogenic but consider organic possibilities such as
- Phaeochromocytoma (rare).
- Hyperthyroidism (common).
- Paroxysmal atrial tachycardia (fairly common).
- Alcohol withdrawal (usually history of excessive alcohol intake).

Psychosis
- Schizophrenia.
- Bipolar disorder or pseudo-dementia in
  - SLE.
  - Cushing's syndrome.
  - Multiple sclerosis.
  - Thyrotoxicosis ('apathetic' thyrotoxicosis in the elderly).

Temporal lobe epilepsy
- Temporary disturbance of content of consciousness.

Investigations: guided by history and examination
- U&E.

- Glucose (in non-diabetics take fasting venous plasma in fluoride oxalate tube with simultaneous serum or plasma for insulin concentration—📖pxx for details of investigating suspected insulinomas and other causes of spontaneous hypoglycaemia).
- CXR.
- LFTS.
- TFTS.
- FBC.
- ESR.
- Urinalysis (protein, nitrites, glucose).
- Cranial CT scan.
- Serum vitamin B_{12}.
- Arterial blood gases (ABGS) ± carboxyhaemoglobin.
- Blood cultures.

Consider
- Syphilis serology.
- HIV test.
- Urine drug screen (📖Chapter 11).
- Blood ethanol level (may be low in withdrawal state).
- EEG.
- 24h ECG.
- Sleep study.

Alteration in bowel habit

A change in bowel habit in an adult should always alert you to the possibility of bowel cancer. Ask about associated features—PR bleeding, tenesmus, weight loss, mucus, abdominal pain or bloating.

Has the patient started any new medications, including 'over the counter'? Look for signs of systemic disease.

Consider
- Carcinoma of the colon.
- Diverticular disease.
- Irritable bowel syndrome (IBS).
- Constipation with overflow diarrhoea.
- All of the above may present with alternating diarrhoea and constipation.

Investigations
- Digital rectal examination.
- Proctoscopy.
- Sigmoidoscopy (rigid/flexible).
- Colonoscopy.
- Barium enema.

📖 *Diarrhoea* (p28), *Constipation* (p26), *Incontinence: faecal* (p49).

Anaemia

Reduced Hb, no specific cause implied (and not a diagnosis, so don't be complacent): ♂ <13.5g/dL, ♀ <11.5g/dL. Often associated with non-specific symptoms such as fatigue, poor concentration, shortness of breath and dizziness. Older patients may experience palpitations and exacerbation of angina, congestive cardiac failure or claudication.

Signs

Pallor of conjunctivae and skin creases, nail pallor and koilonychia (spoon-shaped nails, rare finding in severe chronic iron deficiency), angular cheilitis and glossitis. Difficult to gauge anaemia from skin signs *alone*.

Causes

Two common approaches to assess anaemia.

1. Red cell dynamics
- ↑ RBC loss/breakdown, e.g. haemolysis (congenital or acquired) or bleeding.
- ↓ red cell production, e.g. vitamin/mineral deficiency, marrow suppression/infiltration, myelodysplasia, haemoglobin disorders (e.g. thalassaemia), chronic disease, renal failure.

2. Red cell indices

Microcytic/hypochromic	↓ MCV, ↓ MCHC E.g. Fe deficiency, thalassaemia, anaemia of chronic disease
Macrocytic	↑ MCV Reticulocytosis (polychromasia on blood film), B_{12}/folate deficiency, chronic liver disease, hypothyroidism, alcohol, myelodysplasia
Normocytic, normochromic	↔ MCV & MCHC Anaemia of chronic disease (e.g. chronic infection, inflammatory disease or malignancy), acute blood loss, renal failure, myeloma

Investigations

FBC and film
Assessment of RBC indices helps direct investigation as above.

Microcytic
- Check iron stores (ferritin or soluble transferrin receptor assay). *Note*: ferritin is ↑ in acute inflammation and may be misleading. Iron/TIBC no longer used for assessment of iron deficiency (📖p176).
- Consider thalassaemia screening if not iron deficient.

9

- If iron deficient assess dietary history (vegetarians) and look for risk factors for blood loss and increased demands.
- Premenopausal women—assess menstrual losses.
- Pregnancy/infants/adolescence consider physiological (↑ requirements).
- All others: look for source of blood loss. GI tract is most common source. Consider OGD and/or colonoscopy guided by symptoms and barium studies.

Macrocytic
- Reticulocyte count.
- Serum B_{12} and red cell folate levels.
- If folate deficient: assess dietary history and physiological requirements.
- If B_{12} deficient: rarely dietary cause alone, usually an associated pathology. Pernicious anaemia is the most common cause: check *parietal cell antibodies* (90% patients with PAare +ve, but seen in other causes of gastric atrophy, especially in older individuals) and/or *intrinsic factor antibodies* (+ve in only 50% with PA but specific). Consider ileal disease and malabsorption.
- LFTs.
- Thyroid function.

Normocytic
- Blood film.
- ESR.
- Renal function.
- Consider myeloma screen in older adults (Igs, protein electrophoresis, urine BJP. Skeletal survey of value if paraprotein or BJP).
- Autoimmune screen to exclude connective tissue disease.

Haemolysis screen
- FBC, MCV (↑ due to reticulocytosis).
- Blood film (spherocytes, polychromasia, bite cells and red cell fragmentation).
- Reticulocyte count.
- Bilirubin and serum LDH.
- Haptoglobins (absent in haemolysis).
- DAT (old term is direct Coombs' test).

Consider
- Congenital haemolytic anaemias: membrane defects, enzyme deficiencies (e.g. G6PD, pyruvate kinase).
- DIC/microangiopathic haemolysis—DIC screen.

Ankle oedema

Swollen ankles are a very common complaint. Is the swelling unilateral or bilateral? Does it pit with digital pressure? Is there associated breathlessness? Is there ascites?

Causes of unilateral ankle oedema
- Chronic venous insufficiency (especially post-DVT).

- DVT.
- Cellulitis.
- Compression of large vein by tumour or lymph nodes.
- Lymphatic obstruction:
  - Congenital.
  - Infection (e.g. filariasis).
  - Malignant infiltration.
- Milroy's disease (📖OHCM section 19).

Causes of bilateral ankle oedema
- Right ventricular failure—2° to chronic lung disease.
- Congestive cardiac failure (CCF)—cardiomyopathy, constrictive pericarditis, etc.
- Hypoalbuminaemia—nephrotic syndrome, hepatic cirrhosis, protein-losing enteropathy, malnutrition (starvation or malabsorption), (gravity).
- Dependent oedema (immobility).
- Drugs—Ca^{2+} channel blockers, NSAIDS.
- Idiopathic/cyclical oedema syndrome.
- Pregnancy.
- Wet beriberi (rare in Western societies but commoner in Africa).

Essential investigations
- U&E.
- LFTS.
- Urine dipstick for proteinuria.
- Urine protein/creatinine ratio or 24h urine protein excretion.
- CXR.
- 12-lead ECG.
- Echocardiogram.

Consider
- Liver USS.
- Doppler studies of leg veins.
- Contrast venography.
- Filariasis serology/blood film.
- Xylose breath test.
- OGD with small bowel biopsy.

▶All the causes of unilateral ankle oedema may also cause bilateral oedema.

Anorexia

This describes a loss of appetite for food, and is associated with a wide range of disorders. In fact, anorexia is a fairly common consequence of underlying disease, and represents a general undernourishment. Anorexia *per se* is associated with increased morbidity especially when present in patients undergoing surgery; post-operative infection is commoner, as is prolongation of the hospital stay.

The extent to which it will be investigated depends on the general status of the patient, presence and duration of any symptoms or signs. Clinical judgement will help!

Causes
- Anorexia nervosa.
- Depressive illness.
- Stress.
- Cancers: any, including carcinoma of stomach, oesophagus, metastatic, leukaemia or lymphoma.
- Drugs, including chemotherapy.
- Radiotherapy.
- Renal failure.
- Hypercalcaemia.
- Infections.
- Cigarette smoking.

Investigations
- Full history and examination.
- FBC—looking for anaemia or non-specific changes seen in underlying disease.
- ESR—may be elevated in inflammatory disorders.
- U&E.
- LFTs.
- Serum Ca^{2+}.
- CXR (e.g. lung cancer, TB, etc.).
- Cultures of blood, sputum, urine, stool if pyrexial and/or localising symptoms or signs.

Anuria

Anuria denotes absent urine production. Oliguria (<400mL urine/24h) is more common than anuria. A catheter must be passed to confirm an empty bladder.

Causes
- Urinary retention—prostatic hypertrophy, pelvic mass, drugs, e.g. tricyclic antidepressants, spinal cord lesions.
- Blocked indwelling urinary catheter.
- Obstruction of the ureters—tumour, stone, sloughed papillae (bilateral).
- Intrinsic renal failure—acute glomerulonephritis, acute interstitial nephritis, acute tubular necrosis, rhabdomyolysis.
- Pre-renal failure—dehydration, septic shock, cardiogenic shock.

An urgent ultrasound of the renal tract must be performed and any physical obstruction relieved as quickly as possible, directly (urethral catheter) or indirectly (nephrostomy). ▶▶*Renal function and serum electrolytes must be measured without delay.*

Further tests as clinically indicated
- FBC.
- Blood cultures.
- Arterial blood gases (ABGS).
- Uric acid.
- Autoimmune profile.
- ESR.
- CK.
- PSA (prostatic carcinoma).
- Serum Ca^{2+} & PO_4^{3-}.
- 12-lead ECG.
- CXR.
- CVP measurement via central line (to guide IV fluids).
- MSU (UTI).
- Urine microscopy (for casts).
- Urine osmolality, sodium, creatinine, urea concentrations.
- IVU (p516).
- Urinary stone analysis, if available.
- CT pelvis.
- Renal biopsy (if intrinsic renal disease suspected, normal-sized kidneys).

13

OHCM p260.

Ataxia

Ataxia is an impaired ability to coordinate limb movements. There must be no motor paresis (e.g. monoparesis) or involuntary movements (e.g. the characteristic cog-wheel tremor in Parkinson's disease is *not* ataxia).

Ataxia may be
- Cerebellar.
- Vestibular.
- Sensory.

Note: Many forms of ataxia are hereditary (but are uncommon).

Hereditary causes
- Friedreich's ataxia.
- Ataxia telangiectasia.
- Spinocerebellar ataxia.
- Corticocerebellar atrophy.
- Olivopontocerebellar atrophy.
- Hereditary spastic paraplegia.
- Xeroderma pigmentosa.

Investigations
- Family studies.

- Genetic analysis (discuss with regional genetics laboratory—counselling may be required).

Vestibular ataxia
- Acute alcohol intoxication.
- Labyrinthitis.

Sensory ataxia
- Loss of proprioception—peripheral neuropathy, dorsal column disease.
- Visual disturbance.

Investigations
- Venous plasma glucose (diabetic neuropathy).
- Serum vitamin B_{12} (subacute combined degeneration of the cord—rare, but serious).
- LFTs.
- Cryoglobulins.

Cerebellar ataxia
- Demyelinating diseases, e.g. multiple sclerosis (MS).
- Cerebellar infarct or haemorrhage.
- Alcoholic cerebellar degeneration.
- Cerebellar tumour—primary in children, metastases in adults. *Note:* Von Hippel Lindau disease (📖OHCM section 19).
- Nutritional deficiency:
  - Vitamin B_{12}.
  - Thiamine.
- Cerebellar abscess.
- Drugs (supratherapeutic blood levels):
  - Carbamazepine.
  - Phenytoin.
- Tuberculoma.
- Paraneoplastic syndrome.
- Developmental.
- Arnold Chiari malformation.
- Dandy Walker syndrome.
- Paget's disease of skull.
- Wilson's disease (hepatolenticular degeneration).
- Hypothyroidism.
- Creutzfeldt-Jacob disease and other chronic infections.
- Miller Fisher syndrome.
- Normal pressure hydrocephalus.

Ataxia should be distinguished from movement disorders, e.g.
Chorea
- Huntingdon's, Sydenham's, thyrotoxicosis (very rare).

Athetosis

Hemiballismus
- Characteristic movement disorder; rare.

Tardive dyskinesia
- Chronic phenothiazine therapy.

Investigations
- Cranial CT.

- MRI brain (if demyelination suspected).
- CXR (cerebellar metastases from bronchogenic carcinoma; paraneoplastic syndrome).
- TFTs.
- Triple evoked potentials (demyelination).
- Lumbar puncture (📖p384).
- LFTs.
- Serum drug concentrations esp. anticonvulsants.
- Serum vitamin B_{12}.
- Erythrocyte transketolase (↓ in thiamine deficiency, e.g. alcoholism).
- Isotope bone scan (Paget's, metastases).
- Serum alkaline phosphatase (ALP)—bone isoenzyme (Paget's, metastases).
- Urine hydroxyproline (Paget's disease—reflects bone turnover).
- Caeruloplasmin (Wilson's disease).
- Serum and urine copper (Wilson's disease).

Consider whether the movement disorder is psychogenic (uncommon) rather than due to neuropathology. Uncommon and should not be confidently assumed.

15

📖OHCM p373.

Bradycardia

If the heart rate is <60 beats/min, the patient, by definition, has a bradycardia (an arbitrary definition). Bradycardia may be transient, chronic or intermittent. A slow pulse can be physiological (in trained athletes) but may also be indicative of potentially serious cardiac disease.

Bradycardia may result from
- Increased vagal tone.
- Decreased sympathetic drive.
- Cardiac drug therapy is a prominent cause, e.g.
  - β-adrenergic blockers (Note: β-blocker eye drops (used in treatment of glaucoma) may be systemically absorbed causing bradycardia).
  - Digoxin (AV block).
  - Diltiazem.
  - Verapamil.
  - Amiodarone (Note: may also cause iatrogenic hypothyroidism).

▶Injudicous combinations of these drugs may lead to serious bradycardia or heart block. Consider self-accidental or deliberate self-poisoning (includes opiates).

Other causes
- During normal phases of sleep.
- After fever (typhoid).

- As a reflex response in hypertension (nephritis/phaeochromocytoma).
- Complicating acute inferior myocardial infarction (usually transient).
- Transient—vasovagal, sick sinus syndrome.
- Hypothyroidism (sinus bradycardia).
- Increased intracranial pressure, e.g. cerebral tumour.
- Hypothermia (Note: myxoedema coma).
- Obstructive jaundice.
- Hyperkalaemia (severe).
- Phaeochromocytoma—with hypertension (α-adrenergic effect; rare—tachycardia more common).
- Anorexia nervosa.

A thorough history and examination is mandatory (e.g. dizzy spells, black-outs; preceding or intercurrent chest pain; headache and other causes include ↑ intracranial pressure ↑ ICP); cardiac amyloid, myocarditis, diphtheria, Chagas' disease (⊞OHCM section 15).

Investigations
- 12-lead ECG—look for junctional rhythm or heart block (1st degree, 2nd degree or complete); atrial fibrillation with slow ventricular response (may be difficult to distinguish clinically from sinus bradycardia).

If there is a history of chest pain check cardiac enzymes
- Serum creatine kinase (if >6h of onset of MI).
- Serum troponin I (if >8h of onset of symptoms).
- Continuous monitoring of cardiac rhythm on CCU.

Further investigations will be determined by ECG and clinical features
- Check core temperature with low-reading thermometer (?hypothermia).
- J waves on ECG.
- U&E.
- TFTs (?hypothyroid).
- LFTs (if cholestatic jaundice).
- 24h ECG, e.g. in suspected sick sinus syndrome.
- Cranial CT if ↑ ICP strongly suspected, e.g. if papilloedema.

⊞OHCM pp88, 118.

Breathlessness

Dyspnoea is the perception of breathlessness and may be *exertional* or, when more advanced, occur *at rest*. It may only occur when lying down (orthopnoea). Is the breathlessness a recent development? Is it episodic?

Ask how far the patient can walk without stopping (often an unreliable history) and how many pillows he/she uses in bed at night (in orthopnoea). Look for digital clubbing, central cyanosis and chest wall deformities.

Pulmonary causes
- Pneumonia, e.g. bacterial, viral.

- Bronchitis—acute or chronic.
- COPD.
- Acute asthma.
- Pneumothorax—even a small pneumothorax may acutely exacerbate dyspnoea in patients with pre-existing chronic pulmonary disease.
- Interstitial lung disease—e.g. sarcoidosis, fibrosing alveolitis, extrinsic allergic alveolitis, pneumoconiosis.
- Bronchogenic carcinoma.
- Foreign body obstructing bronchus (esp. children—peanut in right main bronchus).
- Pleural effusion—unilateral or bilateral.
- Ascites (diaphragmatic 'splinting').
- Lymphatic carcinomatosis (Note: CXR may appear normal in early stages).
- Pulmonary embolism ± infarction—single, multiple, recurrent.
- Pulmonary hypertension—1° or 2°.
- Pulmonary oedema—acute or chronic.
- Adult respiratory distress syndrome (ARDS).

Note: Remember metabolic acidosis—diabetic and alcoholic ketoacidosis, lactic acidosis (in metformin-treated patients, especially if renal impairment).

Also
- Salicylate poisoning.
- Methanol (metabolised to formic acid).
- Ethylene glycol (metabolised to oxalic acid).

Other causes
- Associated with angina pectoris/acute coronary syndromes.
- Acute myocardial infarction (MI).
- Valvular heart disease, VSD.
- Anxiety.
- Hyperventilation syndrome.
- Obesity.
- Kyphoscoliosis.
- Metabolic acidosis—e.g. severe salicylate poisoning, DKA, lactic acidosis, hepatic or renal failure (acute or chronic).
- Anaemia (📖pp9, 167).
- Diaphragmatic/respiratory muscle paralysis, e.g. Guillain-Barré syndrome.
- Generalised neuromuscular disease, e.g. motor neurone disease (MND).
- Acute laryngeal oedema, e.g. angio-oedema, diphtheria.
- Laryngeal obstruction, e.g. laryngeal carcinoma.
- External compression of larynx, e.g. retrosternal goitre.
- Laryngeal spasm, e.g. ↓ serum Ca^{2+}.

Note: Occasionally, diabetic ketoacidosis may present in the absence of marked hyperglycaemia. However, true 'euglycaemic' ketoacidosis is rare

(<1% of all cases. In alcoholic ketoacidosis, plasma glucose may not be elevated and Ketostix® reaction may be misleading (📖p151).

Preliminary investigations should include
- CXR.
- ABGs (± blood lactate).
- 12-lead ECG.
- FBC.
- Venous plasma glucose.
- Ca^{2+}.

Other tests may be indicated
- CT chest.
- V/Q scan.
- Spiral CT (if acute PE suspected).
- Bronchoscopy.
- Lung biopsy.
- Peak flow rate.
- Respiratory function tests.
- Echocardiogram.
- Serum salicylate levels.
- U&E.
- LFTs.
- ESR.

📖OHCM pp5, 56, 768.

Bruising

Easy bruising is a common complaint and warrants careful assessment of onset and nature. Recent onset of spontaneous and unusual bruising or bleeding may suggest a serious acquired defect. A lifelong history of bruising and bleeding (e.g. post-tonsillectomy, dental extraction or surgery) may imply a congenital defect. Family history may be informative.

Examine: skin, mouth, dependent areas and fundi for mucocutaneous bleeding and purpura (non-blanching haemorrhages into the skin).

Platelet causes
- Thrombocytopenia or platelet dysfunction (e.g. aspirin).
- Marrow failure, infiltration, ITP, DIC, hypersplenism, drugs or alcohol.

Vascular causes
- Congenital, e.g. Osler-Weber-Rendu syndrome.
- Acquired, e.g. senile purpura, vasculitis (Henoch Schönlein purpura, infection), diabetes, corticosteroid therapy, scurvy, connective tissue diseases.

Coagulopathy
- Congenital—mucocutaneous bruising is suggestive of a platelet-mediated defect (e.g. von Willebrand's disease, Glanzmann's thrombasthenia) rather than clotting factor deficiency (e.g. haemophilia A and B).
- Acquired, e.g. DIC, vitamin K deficiency.

Hyperviscosity
- Myeloma, Waldenström's macroglobulinaemia (low grade lymphoma that produces ↑ IgM), ↑↑WBC in leukaemia.

Investigations
- FBC and film.
- Coagulation—INR and APTR.
- Bleeding time, measures platelet and vascular phase.
- DIC screen including fibrinogen, thrombin time, D-dimers or FDPs.

Consider further tests and referral to haematology for
- Factor assays.
- Platelet aggregation studies to assess platelet function.

📖 OHCM p646.

Calf swelling

Assess whether swelling is bilateral or unilateral, precipitating factors and duration of onset. Careful examination of the affected leg should be extended to a full examination, particularly of abdominal and cardiovascular systems.

Causes

Venous and lymphatic
- Deep vein thrombosis (DVT).
- Superficial thrombophlebitis.
- Varicose veins.
- Post-phlebitic limb (post-DVT).

Soft tissue/musculoskeletal
- Calf haematoma or trauma.
- Ruptured Baker's cyst (synovial effusion in the popliteal fossa associated with RA).
- Cellulitis (associated fever, sepsis, tachycardia).

Systemic
- Congestive cardiac failure (bilateral limb oedema, ↑ JVP and signs of LVF).
- Hepatic failure.
- Hypoalbuminaemia.
- Nephrotic syndrome.
- Pregnancy: increased dependent oedema but note also an ↑ thrombotic risk and DVT should be excluded.

Deep vein thrombosis (DVT)
Usually affects lower limb and can extend proximally into iliofemoral veins and IVC with higher risk of associated PE and higher incidence of post-phlebitic limb. Occasionally seen affecting upper limb but this is atypical.

Risk factors for DVT
- Age >60 years.
- Previous DVT or PE.
- Recent major surgery, especially orthopaedic lower limb, abdo and pelvic.
- Marked immobility.
- Malignancy.
- Pregnancy and post-partum.
- High dose oestrogen oral contraceptive pill.
- Family history of VTE.

Investigation

USS doppler studies, impedance plethysmography, venography, exclude PE. If any associated symptoms arrange V/Q scan, spiral CT, pulmonary angiography. Thrombophilia screening for younger patients (age <55), atypical site and extensive clots, spontaneous onset, family history.

Chest pain

Chest pain, particularly acute pain, is common. A detailed history coupled with careful clinical examination can often clarify the diagnosis with a high degree of probability. Most commonly, symptoms are attributable to musculoskeletal causes, cardiac ischaemia or pleuritic disease.

Be sure to ask about
- Onset.
- Duration.
- Character.
- Site.
- Radiation.
- Associated features.
- Previous episode.
- Response to analgesia, antacids or GTN.

Cardiac causes
- Acute myocardial infarction.
- Angina pectoris.
- Syphilitic aortitis/angina (very rare).
- Acute pericarditis.
- Thoracic aortic dissection (severe interscapular pain).
- Mitral valve prolapse (rare cause of chest pain).
- Aortic stenosis (via coronary ischaemia).
- Hypertrophic obstructive cardiomyopathy (cardiac ischaemia).

Pulmonary causes
- Pulmonary embolism (associated infarction causes pleuritic pain).
- Pleurisy.
- Pneumonia.
- Pulmonary metastases (in bone).
- Bronchial carcinoma (*Note*: Pancoast's syndrome—📖OHCM section 19).
- Pleural tumour, e.g. mesothelioma.
- Tracheitis.
- Acute bronchitis.

- Mediastinal malignancy.
- Pulmonary tuberculosis (TB).
- Mediastinal surgical emphysema.

Gastrointestinal causes
- Oesophageal spasm, oesophagitis, infection (e.g. *Candida*) or reflux.
- Mallory-Weiss tear of oesophagus.
- Perforated duodenal ulcer.
- Acute pancreatitis.
- Cholecystitis.
- Biliary colic.

Other causes
- Muscular pain, costochondritis or rib fracture.
- Bornholm disease.
- Acute shingles.
- Post-herpetic neuralgia.
- Cervical disc disease, osteoarthritis.
- Ankylosing spondylitis.
- Vertebral collapse.
- Thoracic outlet syndrome.
- Shoulder pain (▶Pancoast's syndrome).
- Breast pain—intrinsic tumour, mastitis.
- Chest wall malignancy.
- Anxiety state (a diagnosis that should follow exclusion of other causes).

Investigations
- 12-lead ECG.
- CXR.
- Cardiac enzymes.
- Troponin T or I.
- Exercise tolerance test.
- Coronary angiogram.
- Myoview scan.
- D-dimers.
- V/Q scan.
- Leg doppler scan.
- ABGs.
- CT thorax.
- Pulmonary angiogram.
- Sputum culture (▶acid and alcohol fast bacilli, AAFB).
- Sputum cytology.
- Bronchoscopy.
- FBC (anaemia may precipitate or aggravate angina).
- Thoracoscopy.
- Pleural tap.
- Pleural biopsy.
- Cervical spine x-ray.
- Upper GI endoscopy.

- Serum or urine amylase.
- LFTs.
- Abdominal USS.

Note: A typical presentations of cardiac ischaemia are well recognised; the 12-lead ECG may be normal at presentation of acute cardiac ischaemia. Sometimes a period of observation in hospital is required to exclude serious pathology. Increased availability of specific cardiac muscle protein (troponin I or T) helps to stratify risk in patients with acute coronary syndromes.

Care should be taken to ensure that blood for estimation of cardiac enzymes (total CK or the specific myocardial isoenzyme, CK-MB) is not taken too early, i.e. before a significant elevation can occur (serum CK rises at 3–6h and peaks at ~24h after the onset of acute MI). Repeated testing after an appropriate interval may be required.

The severity of pain is not always a reliable indicator of the seriousness of the disease. For example, acute MI in patients with diabetes of long duration may present with minimal pain (attributed to autonomic neuropathy). Conversely, severe chest pain may result from oesophageal acid reflux.

📖 OHCM pp76, 770.

Clubbing

Digital clubbing can affect fingers or toes. There is an increase in the soft tissue so that the distal phalanx becomes larger in all directions. The angle between the nail and the nail bed is lost, the nail becomes curved, both longitudinally and laterally, and there is increased sponginess of the nail bed.

Thoracic causes
- Bronchogenic carcinoma, especially squamous cell.
- Asbestosis ± mesothelioma.
- Pleural or mediastinal tumour.
- Thoracic lymphoma.
- Bronchiectasis.
- Cystic fibrosis (CF).
- Lung abscess.
- Empyema.
- Pulmonary TB.
- Pulmonary fibrosis.
- Pulmonary sarcoidosis.

Cardiac & vascular causes
- Bacterial endocarditis.
- Thoracic vascular malformation—axillary AV malformation may cause unilateral clubbing.
- Congenital cyanotic heart disease.

Gastrointestinal causes
- 1° biliary cirrhosis.
- Chronic active hepatitis.
- Oesophageal, gastric, colonic carcinoma.
- Colonic amoebiasis.
- Coeliac disease.
- Familial polyposis coli, Gardner's syndrome.

Miscellaneous causes
- Thyrotoxicosis (thyroid acropachy—rare).
- Polycythaemia rubra vera.
- Hypervitaminosis A.
- Syringomyelia.
- SLE.
- Familial.

Investigations should include
- CXR.
- ABGs.

On clinical suspicion
- Bronchoscopy.
- CT chest.
- Echocardiogram.
- Abdominal USS.
- Liver biopsy.
- FBC.
- ESR.
- LFTs.
- TFTs.
- Serum ACE.
- Blood cultures (multiple if bacterial endocarditis suspected).
- Colonoscopy.
- OGD.

The combination of digital clubbing with bone pain in the wrists or ankles and x-ray appearances of a proliferative periostitis is termed hypertrophic pulmonary osteoarthropathy (HPOA).

📖 OHCM pp37, 54.

Coma

The Glasgow Coma Scale (GCS) is used to assess level of consciousness. Minimum score is 3, maximum 15.

Assess level of consciousness and determine whether this is stable, fluctuating, improving or deteriorating on serial assessments.

Cerebral causes
- Intracranial haemorrhage (SAG, SDH, EDH, intracerebral bleed).
- Large cerebral infarct.
- Pontine haemorrhage (pinpoint pupils).
- Cerebral venous sinus thrombosis.
- Hypertensive encephalopathy.

Glasgow Coma Scale		
Eye opening	1	Nil
	2	To pain
	3	To voice
	4	Spontaneously
Motor response	1	Nil
	2	Extension
	3	Flexion
	4	Withdrawal from pain
	5	Localising to pain
	6	Voluntary
Vocal response	1	Nil
	2	Groans
	3	Inappropriate words
	4	Disorientated speech
	5	Orientated speech

- Cerebral tumour (associated local cerebral oedema may respond to dexamethasone).
- Head injury.
- Cerebral infection—encephalitis, meningitis, cerebral malaria, brain abscess.
- Post-ictal state.
- Sub-clinical status epilepticus (*Note*: an EEG diagnosis).
- Cerebral vasculitis, e.g. SLE.
- End-stage multiple sclerosis.
- Leucodystrophy.
- Creutzfeldt-Jakob disease (including variant CJD).

Metabolic causes

- Drugs (usually in deliberate overdose, 📖Ch11).
- Alcohol excess (*Note*: remember hypoglycaemia as a cause of coma in alcoholics, as well as extradural haematoma).
- Hypoglycaemia (iatrogenic, overdose of insulin or sulphonylureas, insulinoma, IGF 2-associated hypoglycaemia in certain tumours).
- Diabetic ketoacidosis (coma in ~10% of cases—adverse prognostic sign).
- Hyperosmolar non-ketotic coma (may present as severe dehydration ± coma).
- Uraemia.
- Late stages of hepatic encephalopathy.
- Severe hyponatraemia (relatively common—esp. inappropriate ADH syndrome).
- Hypothyroidism (*myxoedema coma*—rare).
- Hypercalcaemia.
- Inborn error of metabolism, e.g. porphyria, urea cycle disorders.
- Type 2 respiratory failure (CO_2 narcosis).
- Hypothermia (severe).
- Hyperpyrexia (neuroleptic malignant syndrome, NMS after anaesthesia).
- Severe nutritional deficiency—thiamine, pyridoxine, vitamin B_{12}.

Investigations
- Venous plasma glucose (exclude hypoglycaemia with fingerstick + reflectance meter, confirm with venous plasma fluoride-oxalate sample).
- U&E.
- LFTs.
- Serum Ca^{2+}.
- Serum osmolality.
- Urine Na^+.
- Blood cultures.
- Clotting screen (📖pp205–207).
- ABGs.
- Drug screen (serum, urine).
- Cranial CT scan.
- Lumbar puncture (LP).
- CXR (bronchogenic carcinoma with cerebral metastases).
- 12-lead ECG.
- EEG.
- Erythrocyte transketolase ($\downarrow$ in thiamine deficiency).
- Serum NH_3 ($\uparrow$ in urea cycle disorders).
- Brain biopsy.

Always assess **A**irway, **B**reathing, **C**irculation before assessment of the cause of $\downarrow$ consciousness. Consider psychogenic unresponsiveness.

📖OHCM pp772, 774, 812.

Confusion

A reliable witness, family member or carer may be vital in assessing a patient with confusion, and care must be taken to discriminate between acute and chronic symptoms. Acute confusional states carry a very broad differential diagnosis and require careful initial evaluation. Any systemic illness can precipitate a confusional state.

Causes

Hypoxaemia	Acute infection, asthma, COPD, etc.
Head injury	Cerebral trauma
Vascular	CVA, TIA, intracerebral, subdural haemorrhage
Infection	– systemic
	– meningitis or encephalitis
Endocrine/metabolic	Diabetic ketoacidosis, hypoglycaemia, thyrotoxicosis or myxoedema, uraemia, hypercalcaemia, hyponatraemia
etOH and drug abuse	Acute intoxification and withdrawal. Also, consider overdose
Iatrogenic	Full and recent medication history (especially opiates, analgesia and sedatives)

Post-ictal state
Cerebral tumour
Psychiatric
Wernicke's encephalopathy

Investigations
- FBC, U&E, LFTs, serum Ca^{2+}, BM stix and blood glucose.
- ABGs.
- MSU, blood cultures, sputum culture.
- CXR.
- ECG.
- Thyroid function.
- Drug/toxicology screen—blood and urine.
- CT scan.
- Lumbar puncture.

▶▶Always look for *MedicAlert*™ bracelet, necklace or card.

📖OHCM pp362, 440.

Constipation

Patients may use the term constipation to mean infrequent, hard, small volume or difficult to pass faeces. Patients vary enormously in their threshold to seek medical advice about bowel habit.

Ask about • associated pain • PR bleeding • tenesmus • weight loss.

Causes
- Carcinoma of the colon.
- Diverticular disease.
- Anorectal disease—fissure or haemorrhoid.
- Benign stricture.
- Rectocoele.
- Sigmoid volvulus.
- Hernia.
- Drugs, especially analgesics.
- Poor fluid intake.
- Low fibre diet.
- Change in diet.
- Immobility.
- Irritable bowel syndrome.
- Megarectum.
- Hirshsprung's disease.
- Spinal cord lesion.
- Stroke.
- Jejunal diverticulosis.
- Hypothyroidism.
- Diabetic neuropathy.
- Hypercalcaemia, hyperparathyroidism, hypokalaemia.
- Uraemia.
- Porphyria.

- Pregnancy.
- Multiple sclerosis.
- Parkinson's disease.
- Dermatomyositis.
- Myotonic dystrophy.
- Scleroderma.
- Psychological.

Investigations
- Digital rectal examination.
- Proctoscopy.
- Sigmoidoscopy.
- Colonoscopy.
- Barium enema.
- U&E.
- Ca^{2+}.
- TFTs.
- FBC.
- Bowel transit time studies.
- Anorectal manometry.
- Electrophysiological studies.
- Defaecating proctography.

▶▶Elderly patients are more prone to constipation.

📖OHCM p204.

Cyanosis

Cyanosis refers to blue/purplish discoloration of tissues due to ↑ in deoxygenated Hb content in blood (usually when >5g/dL). Central cyanosis refers to discoloration of mouth and tongue as well as peripheries. Cyanosis is easier to detect in individuals with polycythaemia and normal Hb, and may be missed if the patient has significant anaemia.

Causes of central cyanosis
- Pulmonary disease causing impaired O_2 transfer.
  - e.g. severe pneumonia, asthma, COPD, pulmonary oedema, PE.
- R→L shunting of deoxygenated blood, e.g. VSD, PDA.

Investigate and treat according to likely cause
- ABGs.
- FBC.
- CXR.
- ECG.

Note: Rare cause—methaemoglobinaemia. Cyanosis with normal PaO_2. Methaemoglobin (ferric iron, Fe^{3+}) holds tightly onto O_2 causing tissue hypoxia but with apparent normal PaO_2. This condition may be congenital (usually well and asymptomatic) or acquired due to ingestion of oxidising agents, e.g. phenacetin, inorganic nitrates and local anaesthetics. Treatment is to remove the cause and give methylene blue.

Causes of peripheral cyanosis
As above but can also be related to peripheral circulation and vasculature, reflecting poor perfusion.

Peripheral cyanosis is seen in
- Cold conditions.
- Shock.
- Mitral stenosis.
- Raynaud's.
- Hypovolaemia.
- Peripheral arterial disease.

📖OHCM pp54, 178.

Diarrhoea

Patients may use the term diarrhoea to describe loose stools, increased frequency of defaecation, increased volume of stool, steatorrhoea, melaena or faecal incontinence (📖p49).

Ask about
- Duration.
- Associated features (abdominal pain, vomiting, mucus or blood per rectum).
- Systemic symptoms.
- Recent foreign travel.
- Suspect food.
- Is anyone else in the household affected?

Causes
- Infection (including 'traveller's diarrhoea').
- Inflammatory bowel disease.
- Diverticular disease.
- Colonic carcinoma.
- Other tumour, especially villous adenoma.
- Coeliac disease.
- Tropical sprue.
- Irritable bowel syndrome (IIBS).
- Ischaemic colitis/bowel infarction.
- Laxative use!
- Other drugs, e.g. metformin, orlistat.
- Over indulgence in fruit or vegetables.
- Overflow secondary to constipation.
- Carcinoid syndrome (uncommon).
- Gastrinoma (rare).
- VIPoma (rare).
- Glucagonoma (very rare).
- Hyperthyroidism (common).
- Medullary carcinoma of the thyroid (uncommon).
- Bile salt diarrhoea (previous ileal disease or surgery).

- Dumping syndrome (previous gastric surgery).
- Gut motility disorders.
- Malabsorption (CF, pancreatitis, lymphangiectasia, coeliac).
- Lactose intolerance.
- Scleroderma.
- Amyloidosis.
- Whipple's disease.

Investigations
- Stool culture, hot stool for parasites.
- *Clostridium difficile* toxin in stool.
- High rectal swab for parasites (Note: giardiasis is diagnosed on duodenal biopsy.
- Rectal examination, proctoscopy, sigmoidoscopy ± biopsy.
- Colonoscopy.
- AXR.
- Barium enema.
- Small bowel follow-through contrast studies.
- Upper GI endoscopy.
- Small bowel biopsy.
- FBC and blood film.
- ESR.
- CRP.
- Serum ferritin and folate.
- U&E (exclude haemolytic-uraemic syndrome especially in children).
- Urine screen for laxatives.
- Antigliadin and antiendomysial antibodies (coeliac disease).
- TFTs.
- Serum gut hormone profile (gastrin, VIP, glucagon—seek expert advice).
- 24h urine for 5HIAA (5-hydroxindole acetic acid).
- Serum calcitonin (medullary carcinoma of thyroid).
- Lactose hydrogen breath test (for lactose intolerance).
- ^{14}C- xylose breath test (bacterial overgrowth in small bowel).
- CT abdomen.
- Mesenteric angiography (ischaemia).

29

Investigation must be guided by history and examination findings. If the patient is an inpatient they should be isolated until infection is excluded. Consider HIV and other immune disorders if an unusual bowel organism is found.

Dizziness & blackouts

Patients may use the term 'dizziness' loosely to convey many different feelings. Try to elicit whether they mean vertigo ('the room was spinning around'), near syncope ('I felt faint', 'light headed'), or something quite different!

If the patient complains of blacking out it is important to determine whether they lost consciousness, if so for how long, or if they felt faint prior to collapsing.

If there has been loss of consciousness consider
- Subarachnoid haemorrhage (📖OHCM section 10).
- Syncope—cardiac, neurological or simple faint (📖p33).
- Hypoglycaemia (especially in diabetic patients).
- Epileptic fit.
- Head injury.
- Alcohol or illicit drugs (*Note*: self-poisoning).

Investigations
- ECG.
- Venous plasma glucose.
- ESR.
- CT head.
- LP.
- 24h cardiac tape.
- Tilt table test.

If the complaint is of dizziness establish if it is *vestibular*—vertigo, episodic, precipitated by change in position, associated nausea, vomiting, deafness or tinnitus—or *non-vestibular*—'light headed', constant, associated with hyperventilation, palpitations, syncope, sweating, pallor, headache.

Examine the nervous and cardiovascular systems carefully. Look at the tympanic membranes. Check for orthostatic hypotension.

Vestibular causes
- Labyrinthitis.
- Meniere's disease.
- Acoustic neuroma or other cerebello-pontine angle tumour.

Investigations
- Hallpike manoeuvre (📖OHCM section 10).
- Audiometry.
- MRI or CT of cerebello-pontine angle.

Non-vestibular causes
- Drugs, e.g. phenytoin in excessive doses.
- Cerebellar disease (infarct, degenerative, demyelinating, etc).
- Transient cardiac arrhythmia.
- MS.
- Temporal lobe epilepsy.
- Anxiety or depression.
- Panic attacks or hyperventilation syndrome.

Investigations
- Blood anticonvulsant concentrations.
- Cranial CT or MRI.
- 12-lead ECG.
- 24h cardiac tape.
- EEG (📖pp401–407).

The cause of dizziness is often not found.

▶In the UK, driving regulations prohibit driving for 4 weeks after a simple faint. If a cardiac or neurological cause is suspected driving must cease until investigated and treated.

Dysarthria & dysphasia

Dysarthria is difficulty in articulating words. The patient may complain of 'slurred speech'. Dysphasia is a difficulty in the formation of speech due to interference with higher mental function. These disturbances often occur together, most commonly in the context of a stroke.

Damage to Wernicke's area causes a *receptive dysphasia*. Speech may be fluent but meaning is lost. Damage to Broca's area causes an *expressive dysphasia*. Speech is non-fluent and the patient is aware they are not using the right words.

Causes of dysphasia include stroke (usually with right hemiparesis, arm more affected than leg) or space-occupying lesion. Psychosis, especially schizophrenia, may cause a similar picture—so-called 'word salad'.

Causes of dysarthria
- Stroke (internal capsule or extensive lesion of motor cortex—acute).
- MND.
- Mid-brain or brainstem tumour.
- Parkinson's disease.
- Cerebellar disease (haemorrhage, infarct, multiple sclerosis, hereditary ataxia, alcoholic or paraneoplastic degeneration).
- Syringobulbia (chronic, progressive).
- Neuromuscular (myasthenia gravis, dermatomyositis, myotonic dystrophy).
- Acute alcohol or drug intoxication.

Dysarthria may be more obvious when the (English-speaking!) patient is invited to say 'Baby hippopotamus', 'British constitution', etc.

Investigations
- Cranial CT scan.
- Venous plasma glucose.
- ESR.
- Serum lipids.
- 12-lead ECG.
- Echocardiogram.
- Carotid doppler studies (especially if bruit).
- CXR.
- LFTs.

Less commonly
- Serum muscle enzymes (polymyositis).
- Autoimmune profile.

- EMG.
- Skeletal muscle biopsy.

📖OHCM p344.

Dysphagia

Dysphagia is difficulty in swallowing. The patient may have associated odynophagia (painful swallowing) or regurgitation of food (immediate or delayed?). Elicit whether the dysphagia is for liquid, solids or both. Is it intermittent or progressive? Are there associated symptoms?

A careful physical examination is mandatory. Pay special attention to the lower cranial nerves; search for lymph nodes in the supraclavicular fossae. Palpate the thyroid and percuss for retrosternal enlargement.

Causes
- Oesophageal carcinoma.
- Benign oesophageal stricture secondary to chronic acid reflux.
- Barrett's oesophagus.
- Achalasia or diffuse spasm.
- Stroke (bilateral internal capsule CVAs—pseudo-bulbar palsy).
- Oesophageal web (+ iron deficiency anaemia = Plummer Vinson (Patterson Kelly Brown) syndrome).
- Pharyngeal pouch.
- Muscular problem (myasthenia gravis, dermatomyositis, myotonic dystrophy).
- Bulbar palsy (MS, MND, poliomyelitis).
- Scleroderma (including CREST syndrome—📖OHCM section 11).
- Infection (usually acute pain on swallowing).
- Mediastinal mass (goitre, carcinoma of the bronchus, enlarged left atrium, aortic aneurysm).

Investigations
- FBC.
- ESR.
- Upper GI endoscopy.
- Barium swallow.
- CXR.
- Oesophageal manometry studies (📖p353).
- Cranial CT or MRI (if neurological signs).
- Acetylcholine (ACh) receptor antibodies and Tensilon (edrophonium). test if myasthenia gravis suspected (📖p413).

Note: Consider HIV testing if there is oesophageal candida, herpes simplex or cytomegalovirus infection in the oesophagus.

📖OHCM pp196, 382.

Facial pain

Is the pain unilateral or bilateral? Is it constant or intermittent? Are there precipitating factors or trigger points?

A full examination of the head and neck is required in addition to a detailed neurological and systemic examination.

Causes
- Trigeminal neuralgia (TN).
- Temporal arteritis (TA). ▶▶Risk of visual loss (📖OHCM section 11).
- Herpes zoster (shingles or post-herpetic neuralgia).
- Dental caries, sepsis.
- Sinusitis.
- Temporomandibular joint dysfunction.
- Cluster headache.
- Glaucoma.
- Angina pectoris.
- Tonsillitis.
- Syringobulbia.
- Atypical facial neuralgia.
- Migraine.

Investigations
- ESR—urgent in suspected TA.
- Temporal artery biopsy if TA strongly suspected. (▶▶Must be performed rapidly—*within days*—if steroid treatment is commenced. However, do not withhold corticosteroid therapy for this reason!) Because of 'skip' lesions, false negative biopsies may be encountered. Be guided by the full clinical picture rather than reliance on a single test.
- Plain radiographs or CT imaging of frontal or maxillary sinuses.
- MRI to exclude MS, basilar aneurysm, trigeminal schwannoma, neurofibroma as causes of TN.
- MRI of cervical spinal cord to exclude syringobulbia if pain is accompanied by brainstem signs.

📖*Headache* (p43).
📖OHCM pp58–59.

33

Faints

The circumstances surrounding the 'faint', 'collapse' or 'blackout' are often good clues to the cause. The history of an eyewitness can be particularly valuable.

Simple (vasovagal) faint
- Hot room, crowded, emotional, painful circumstances.
- Occurs whilst standing (or sitting).
- Brief loss of consciousness.
- Classic stigmata of generalised tonic-clonic epilepsy are usually absent.

Cardiac cause
- Chest pain, palpitations, breathlessness may precede collapse.
- Brief, rapid loss of consciousness; prompt recovery in transient arrhythmia.
- Classic sequential pallor, cyanosis and flushing in Stokes-Adams attacks.

Neurological cause
- Limb or facial weakness, dysphasia, etc.
- Central cyanosis, tonic-clonic convulsions.
- Gradual return to normal level of consciousness, e.g. post-ictally.

▶Remember hypoglycaemia (neuroglycopenia).

A detailed physical examination, paying particular attention to cardiovascular and neurological systems, should be performed.

Postural blood pressure response should be carefully recorded (i.e. after lying supine for at least 5min and again on standing—care to avoid collapse in patients with marked postural hypotension).

- A 12-lead ECG should be performed in all adults.

Other investigations as clinically indicated
- 24h ambulatory ECG.
- Echocardiogram (to exclude aortic stenosis if murmur audible).
- Tilt table test (p322).
- Carotid doppler studies.
- V/Q scan (if any suspicion of pulmonary embolism).
- Cranial CT.
- EEG.

Consider cough- or micturition-, effort- or carotid sinus syncope syndromes. In the UK, regulations prohibit driving for 4 weeks after a simple faint. If a cardiac or neurological cause is suspected driving must cease until appropriately investigated and treated.

OHCM p334.

Fever of unknown origin (FUO or PUO)

Defined as T° >38.3°C on several occasions lasting 3 weeks or more. It is very important to take a full history and consider infectious contacts, recent travel abroad, recent surgery and dental treatment, sexual history and risk factors for HIV.

Signs
Examine for heart murmurs, splinter haemorrhages, splenomegaly, lymphadenopathy and rashes/pruritus.

Causes

Infection	Abscesses (e.g. subphrenic, pelvic, lung), osteomyelitis, TB, endocarditis, parasites, rheumatic fever, brucellosis, toxoplasmosis, Lyme disease, histoplasmosis, viral (esp. EBV, CMV, hepatitis and HIV).
Malignancy	Lymphoma, leukaemia, hypernephroma, ovary, lung, hepatoma.
Connective tissue	PAN, SLE, RA, Still's disease, temporal arteritis.
Other	Sarcoidosis, atrial myxoma, drug fever, inflammatory bowel disease, factitious.

Investigations
- Re-take the history and re-examine the patient (something might have been missed or new symptoms/signs may have developed).
- FBC, ESR.
- U&E, LFTs, Ca^{2+}.
- CXR.
- MSU, urinanalysis.
- Serology for *Brucella* and *Toxoplasma*.
- All biopsy material should be sent for culture, including TB.
- Blood cultures (serial may be necessary).
- Monospot/Paul Bunnell.
- Autoimmune profile (ANA, RF, ANCA, etc.).
- Bone marrow aspirate/trephine/culture for TB with ZN stain.
- Abdominal USS (?masses).

Extend investigations as below according to symptoms and signs
- Consult microbiology or infectious disease consultant for advice.
- Stool cultures and fresh stool for ova, cysts and parasites.
- Repeat serological investigation for changing titres (2–3 weeks).
- Thick and thin blood film for malaria and parasites.
- Mantoux.
- Transthoracic or TOE to exclude endocarditic vegetations.
- CT chest, abdomen and pelvis.

▶▶Always re-examine the patient for evolving new signs if cause remains unknown.

📖OHCM p554.

35

First fit

▶▶A first fit in an adult requires careful evaluation since the probability of an underlying structural lesion increases with age.

Take a careful history, preferably from a witness as well as the patient. Most lay persons will recognise a generalised tonic-clonic fit. However, the occurrence of a few 'epileptiform' movements in patients with syncopal episodes (Faints p33) may cause diagnostic uncertainty.

Be sure to ask about
- Aura preceding episode. ►Temporal lobe epilepsy—olfactory or gustatory auras (not necessarily followed by convulsions).
- Loss of consciousness—how long? Often overestimated by witnesses!
- Tongue biting.
- Focal or generalised convulsive movements. Note: A clear history of a tonic-clonic fit commencing in a limb and progressing to a more generalised convulsion is highly suggestive of a structural intracerebral lesion; cranial imaging is mandatory.
- Central cyanosis (tonic phase).
- Urinary incontinence.
- Injuries.
- Post-ictal confusion.
- History of trauma.
- Alcohol intake. Remember: alcohol withdrawal fits as well as acute intoxication.
- Drug history—prescribed and recreational.
- History of insulin-treated diabetes or type 2 diabetes treated with oral secretagogues, i.e. sulphonylureas, repaglinide, nateglinide. Note that metformin and thiazolidinediones as monotherapy do not cause significant hypoglycaemia.

A full general and neurological examination is needed, specifically including
- Fever.
- Meningism, i.e. nuchal rigidity, +ve Kernig's sign (meningoencephalitis).
- Cutaneous rash or ecchymoses (?bleeding diathesis).
- Evidence of head trauma (preceding fit or as a consequence).
- Signs of chronic liver disease.
- Focal neurological deficit. ►Third nerve palsy in intracranial space- occupying lesion (SOL), including aneurysm of the posterior communicating artery. Sixth nerve lesion may act as a 'false localising sign' in ↑ ICP.
- *MedicAlert*™ bracelet (history of epilepsy or diabetes—search personal belongings).

Bilateral extensor plantar reflexes can occur after a generalised fit without a structural brain lesion and there may be a transient hemiparesis (Todd's paresis).

Causes
- Epilepsy (OHCM section 10).
- Hypoglycaemia (acute, severe, history of diabetes?).
- Hyponatraemia (usually <110mmol/L or rapid development).
- Hypocalcaemia (OHCM section 17).
- Hypomagnesaemia (may accompany hypocalcaemia).
- Hypophosphataemia (rare).
- Alcohol withdrawal. ►►Risk of associated hypoglycaemia.
- Discontinuation of anticonvulsant medication.
- Infection—viral encephalitis or bacterial meningitis. ►►Consider intracerebral abscess, tuberculoma in predisposed patients.

- Encephalopathy—hepatic, uraemic, hypertensive, thyrotoxic (rare—'thyroid storm').
- Eclampsia.
- Porphyria.
- Cerebral SLE.
- Head injury.
- Hypoxia.
- Cerebral tumour.
- Stroke—cerebral infarct, haemorrhage.

Investigations
- Venous plasma glucose (fingerprick test at bedside useful as 'screen'—but can be unreliable).
- U&E.
- Serum Ca^{2+}, Mg^{2+}, PO_4^{3-}.
- Cranial CT or MRI scan.
- EEG.
- LP (📖p384).
- CXR.
- Serum PRL (may be ↑ after generalised convulsions, but not pseudo-seizures).
- ABGs—REMEMBER transient lactic acidosis following generalised tonic-clonic convulsion.
- Blood ethanol (may be undetectable in withdrawal state).
- Serum or urine drug screen.

'Pseudo-seizures' may be encountered in patients with atypical recurrent fits (usually long history of epilepsy) and this is unlikely in an adult presenting with a first fit. In UK, the national driving license authority prohibits driving for 12 months following a first fit.

📖OHCM p364.

Galactorrhoea

Denotes inappropriate breast milk production, i.e. in the absence of pregnancy. The most common cause is hyperprolactinaemia (↑ PRL) due to a pituitary microprolactinoma of <10mm diameter (📖p132). Prolactinomas (usually macroadenomas) may cause galactorrhoea in men.

Note: Other disease in the pituitary region, certain drugs and several systemic disorders may be associated with ↑ PRL (📖OHCM section 9).

Causes
Normoprolactinaemic galactorrhoea
- This has been described in pre-menopausal women occurring after the conclusion of:
  — Treatment with the combined contraceptive pill.

— Breastfeeding (for >6 months afterwards).
- Increased sensitivity of lactogenic tissue prolactin (PRL) is postulated but the mechanism remains uncertain. In part, this may reflect difficulties that can arise in determining whether PRL is persistently elevated. Menstrual disturbances have been described.

Hyperprolactinaemia
- The differential diagnosis and investigation of hyperprolactinaemia is considered on p132.

Investigations
- Serum PRL (*Endocrinology & Metabolism* 📖p132).
- Repeated measurements under controlled conditions may be required since PRL is a 'stress' hormone and may be increased by venepuncture.

Note: If ↑ PRL is confirmed, further investigations to exclude causes other than prolactinoma are required.

- Pituitary imaging (CT, or preferably, MRI) and visual field testing (Goldmann) may also be indicated if a macroprolactinoma is suspected (PRL concentrations usually very high).

Note: If there is doubt about the nature of the nipple discharge further specialised investigations may be required on the fluid, including:
- Casein.
- Lactose.
- Microscopy.

Clear fluid may result from benign breast disease.

Note: Bloody discharge should prompt urgent specialist investigations to exclude carcinoma of the breast:
- Mammography.
- Biopsy.
📖OHCM p312.

Kleinberg DL *et al.* (1977) Galactorrhoea: a study of 235 cases, including 48 with pituitary tumors. *NEJM* **296**, 589–600.

Gout

Gout is a disease of deposition of monosodium urate monohydrate crystals in tissues and relates to hyperuricaemia. Hyperuricaemia is due to an imbalance between purine synthesis and uric acid excretion. Episodes of acute gout may be precipitated by alcohol, trauma, dietary changes, infection, chemotherapy or surgery. More common in men and very rare in pre-menopausal women.

Clinical features
- Inflammatory arthritis, classically a monoarthritis or oligoarthritis affecting 1st MTP joint of foot but can affect any joint including the spine.

- Tenosynovitis.
- Bursitis or cellulitis.
- Tophi—urate deposits in tendons, ear pinna and joints.
- Urolithiasis and renal disease.

Investigation
- ESR (may be ↑).
- Urate crystals demonstrated in synovial fluid or tissues—negatively birefringent on polarised light microscopy.
- Serum urate (not always ↑ in acute episode, and normal urate level does not exclude the diagnosis).
- XR—soft tissue swelling and punched out bony erosions.
- AIP (to exclude rheumatoid).
- Microscopy of synovial fluid (Gram stain and culture).

Treatment

Acute episode
- NSAIDs, colchicine, intra-articular steroids or oral steroids.
- Avoid precipitating factors and purine-rich foods.
- Urate lowering therapy indicated for tophi, recurrent attacks and urine/renal disease, e.g.
  - Allopurinol (xanthine oxidase inhibitor).
  - Probenecid (uricosuric).

Note: Asymptomatic hyperuricaemia is more common than gout and a high serum urate with coexistent arthritis is not necessarily due to crystal deposition. Consider important other causes especially infective arthritis and pseudo-gout.

Pseudo-gout
Calcium pyrophosphate crystal deposition causing acute arthritis or chondrocalcinosis. Crystals are weakly +ve birefringent on polarised light microscopy. Associations include old age, dehydration, hyperparathyroidism, hypothyroidism, haemochromatosis, acromegaly, rheumatoid arthritis and osteoarthritis.

📖OHCM p404.

Gynaecomastia

Gynaecomastia is benign bilateral hyperplasia of glandular and fatty breast tissue in the male. The balance between androgens and oestrogens is thought to be of importance in the pathogenesis; many conditions may influence this ratio. Most commonly, it appears transiently during normal puberty (detectable at some stage in ~50% cases). Gynaecomastia may also be caused by specific endocrine disease or be associated with certain chronic diseases. Treatment with certain drugs is a common cause (~30% of cases) and arises via several mechanisms. Investigations will be guided by the individual circumstances. A careful drug history and thorough physical examination are required, particularly in the post-adolescent period.

When indicated, and after excluding causes such as congenital syndrome and drug therapy, investigations are principally directed at:
- Excluding endocrine carcinoma (rare).
- Identifying associated chronic diseases.

Note:
- Simple obesity is not usually a cause of true gynaecomastia, i.e. the glandular element is not increased.
- ↑ Serum prolactin (PRL) in isolation does not cause gynaecomastia.
- Unilateral, eccentric breast enlargement should prompt exclusion of breast carcinoma (rare).

Causes include
- Physiological states (transient):
    - Newborn.
    - Puberty.
    - Advanced age.
- Klinefelter's syndrome (47, XXY; mosaics).
- Secondary hypogonadism, e.g mumps orchitis.
- Androgen resistance syndromes, e.g. testicular feminisation.
- ↑ Tissue aromatase activity (converts androgens to oestrogens).
- Oestrogen-producing tumours:
    - Leydig cell tumour.
    - Sertoli cell tumour.
    - Adrenal carcinoma.
- Chronic liver disease.
- Chronic renal failure.
- Panhypopituitarism.
- Tumours producing human chorionic gonadotrophin (hCG).
- Drugs: oestrogens (prostatic carcinoma, transsexuals), spironolactone, cimetidine, digoxin, cytotoxic agents, marijuana.
- Hyperthyroidism (↑ serum sex-hormone-binding globulin, SHBG).
- Primary hypothyroidism.
- Cushing's syndrome.
- Carcinoma of bronchus.
- Idiopathic.

Investigations
- Testosterone.
- FSH.
- LH.
- LFTs.
- TFTs.
- Oestradiol.
- β-hCG.
- PRL.
- SHBG (affinity of SHBG is higher for testosterone than for oestrogens, therefore ↑ SHBG causes disproportionate ↓ in free testosterone levels).
- Dehydroepiandrosterone sulphate (DHEAS).

- Androstenedione.
- Testicular USS.
- CXR.
- Abdominal CT or MRI imaging (for suspected adrenal tumours).
- Pituitary imaging.
- Karyotype.
- Urinary 17-oxo-steroids.

If carcinoma of breast is suspected
- Mammogram.
- Fine needle aspiration.

📖OHCM p306.

Braunstein GD. (1994) Gynecomastia. *NEJM* **328**, 490–495.

Haematemesis

This literally means *vomiting blood*, and is often associated with melaena (passage of black tarry stools). **41**

Causes
- Chronic peptic ulceration (e.g. DU or GU) accounts for 50% of cases of bleeding from the upper GI tract.
- Acute gastric ulcers or erosions.
- Drugs (e.g. NSAIDs) or alcohol.
- Reflux oesophagitis.
- Mallory Weiss tear.
- Oesophageal varices.
- Gastric carcinoma (uncommon).

Investigations after admission and stabilisation of the patient
- Full history, including drugs, alcohol, past history, indigestion, etc.
- FBC.
- U&E.
- Cross-match blood.
- Urgent upper GI tract endoscopy.
- Check *Helicobacter pylori* serology ± urea breath test.

📖OHCM pp208, 210, 802.

Haematuria

In health adults pass between 500,000 and 2,000,000 red cells over a 24h period. Haematuria implies the passage of excess blood that may be detectable using dipsticks (microscopic haematuria) or may be obvious to the naked eye (macroscopic haematuria).

Causes

- Many.
- Glomerular disease, e.g. 1° glomerulonephritis, 2° glomerulonephritis (SLE, vasculitis, infection).
- Vascular or interstitial disease due to hypersensitivity reactions, renal infarction, papillary necrosis or pyelonephritis.
- Trauma.
- Renal epithelial or vascular tumours.
- Lower renal tract disease, e.g. tumours, stones, infection, drug toxicity (e.g. cyclophosphamide), foreign bodies or parasites.
- Systemic coagulation abnormalities, e.g. platelet or coagulation factor abnormalities such as profound thrombocytopenia or DIC.

Investigations

- Urinalysis—dipstick, microscopic examination, culture.
- Radiology* e.g. KUB or IVU.
- Specialist investigation* e.g. angiography, CT or MRI scanning.
- Cystoscopy*.

*Ideally these tests should be arranged after discussion with either a nephrologist or urologist.

📖OHCM p246.

Haemoptysis

This describes *coughing up blood* or blood-stained sputum, and can vary from faint traces of blood to frank bleeding. Before embarking on investigations it is essential to ensure that the blood is coughed up from the respiratory tract and is not that of epistaxis or haematemesis (easily confused).

Causes

- Infective, e.g. acute respiratory infection, exacerbation of COPD.
- Pulmonary infarction, e.g. PE.
- Lung cancer.
- Tuberculosis.
- Pulmonary oedema.
- Bronchiectasis.
- Uncommon causes, e.g. idiopathic pulmonary haemosiderosis, Goodpasture's syndrome, microscopic vasculitis, trauma, haematological disease (e.g. ITP or DIC).

Investigations

- Colour of blood provides clues (pink frothy in pulmonary oedema, rust-coloured in pneumonia).
- Check O_2 saturation.
- FBC (? ↓ platelets).
- ESR.
- Coagulation screen.
- Sputum culture.

- CXR.
- Arrange bronchoscopy after discussion with respiratory team.

📖OHCM pp60–61.

Headache

📖 *Facial pain* (p33).

Headache is an extremely common complaint. Most patients self-medicate and only a small proportion will seek medical advice. Headache may be acute or chronic, constant, recurrent or gradually progressive. It may arise from structures within the cranial vault or from external causes (📖OHCM section 7).

Causes differ according to age; temporal arteritis is very uncommon in patients under ~55 years, for example. Migraine may be associated with classic features (📖OHCM section 7). Remember to enquire about the combined oral contraceptive pill—may exacerbate migraine. 'Tension' headaches predominate.

Causes in adults include
- 'Tension' headache (very common; usually recurrent and stereotyped).
- Migraine. Although common, many patients who believe they have 'migraine' probably have 'tension' headaches. Classic migraine predominantly affects adolescents and young adults.
- Cluster headaches.
- As part of a generalised viral illness, e.g. 'flu.
- Causes of ↑ ICP (📖OHCM section 7).
- Acute infective meningitis (bacterial, viral most commonly).
- Encephalitis (most commonly viral, e.g. herpes simplex).
- Intracerebral haemorrhage.
- Post-traumatic (common).
- Intracerebral tumour (primary or secondary, benign or malignant).
- Acute subarachnoid haemorrhage.
- Subdural haematoma.
- Acute glaucoma.
- Acute sinusitis.
- Rubeosis iridis (secondary glaucoma in patients with advanced diabetic eye disease).
- Trigeminal neuralgia.
- Referred pain, e.g. from dental caries or sepsis.
- Arterial hypertension; malignant or accelerated phase; essential hypertension is rarely the cause of headache.
- Temporal arteritis (TA). ▶▶Visual loss preventable with prompt corticosteroid therapy (📖OHCM section 7).
- Venous sinus thrombosis.
- Benign intracranial hypertension (mimics intracerebral tumour).

- Pneumonia caused by *Mycoplasma. pneumoniae* may be associated with headache (meningoencephalitis).
- Nocturnal hypoglycaemia (often unrecognised) may cause morning headaches in patients with insulin-treated DM.
- Analgesia-withdrawal headache (📖OHCM section 7).
- Hangover following alcohol excess.
- Otitis media.
- Chronic hypercalcaemia (rare).

Investigations
- ESR (▶▶temporal arteritis—exclude with urgency).
- CRP.
- FBC.
- U&E.
- Throat swabs.
- Blood cultures (if febrile).
- Lumbar puncture (📖p384).
- SXR ± cervical spine XR.
- Sinus x-rays (may be local tenderness in sinusitis).
- Cranial CT (📖p394).
- CXR (cerebral metastases from bronchogenic carcinoma).
- Urinalysis.
- Intra-ocular pressure measurement and refraction.
- Cerebral angiography (if aneurysm or AV malformation).
- Serum Ca^{2+}.

📖OHCM pp330, 354, 766.

Heart failure

Heart failure may be acute or chronic. The prevalence of heart failure in the elderly is ~10% in industrialised nations.

The term 'heart failure' includes the clinicopathological syndromes of
- Congestive cardiac failure.
- Left ventricular failure/pulmonary oedema (these terms are not synonymous!).
- Right heart failure (including cor pulmonale).

The concepts of 'pre-load' and 'after-load' are helpful in considering the pathophysiology of heart failure.

Note
- Fluid overload in CRF is sometimes misinterpreted as evidence of cardiac failure.
- The development of arrhythmias, e.g. AF (📖OHCM section 5) may precipitate heart failure in predisposed patients.
- Anaemia and thyrotoxicosis (▶amiodarone!) may exacerbate cardiac syndromes including heart failure.
- Commonly used drugs such as β-adrenergic blockers, NSAIDs, some Ca^{2+} antagonists may precipitate or exacerbate heart failure.

- RAS can present as 'flash' pulmonary oedema.
- Exclude hypoalbuminaemia as a cause of generalised oedema.
- Not all cases of pulmonary oedema have a cardiac cause.
- Ankle oedema in the elderly does not necessarily denote cardiac failure.
- Cocaine use may cause acute pulmonary oedema (and acute coronary syndromes).
- Diabetes is a potent risk factor for heart failure.

Causes
- CHD (most common cause in Western societies; acute or chronic).
- Hypertensive heart disease.
- Valvular heart disease, e.g. aortic stenosis.
- Congenital heart disease.
- Cardiomyopathies, e.g. viral, diabetic cardiomyopathy, amyloidosis.
- Cor pulmonale, e.g. COPD, PE, 1° pulmonary hypertension.
- Endocarditis.
- 'Diastolic' heart failure.
- High output failure, e.g. severe anaemia, Paget's disease, (wet) beri beri (rare).

Investigations
Routine
- 12-lead ECG.
- CXR.
- Echocardiogram (essential for accurate diagnosis).
- FBC.
- U&E.
- TFTs.
- LFTs (including albumin; remember haemochromatosis).
- Serum lipid profile.

As indicated in selected patients
- ESR.
- CRP.
- ANF.
- Viral serology.
- Blood cultures (multiple if endocarditis suspected).
- Venous plasma glucose.
- CK.
- Troponin I or T.
- 24h cardiac tape.
- Radionuclide cardiac imaging.
- Exercise test.
- Coronary angiography/ventriculography.
- Myocardial biopsy.
- Rectal biopsy (2° amyloidosis).

OHCM pp120–122.

Hepatomegaly

Measure liver edge below the (R) costal margin after percussing out the upper and lower borders. Bruits may be heard in hepatoma and a friction rub may occur with malignant deposits. Other signs may suggest the underlying diagnosis (*see below*).

Common causes
- CCF.
- Malignant deposits.
- Hepatitis/cirrhosis (usually alcoholic or infectious, e.g. EBV, viral hepatitis).

Foreign residence?
If so, consider amoebic and hydatid cysts, schistosomiasis, malaria.

Investigations
- FBC, film, LDH (leukaemia, lymphoma).
- ESR.
- Virology (EBV, CMV, hepatitis A, B, C antibody serology).
- LFTs—transaminases.
- Serum albumin.
- Prothrombin time (hepatocellular damage).
- γ-glutamyl transpeptidase, MCV (alcohol).
- Alkaline phosphatase (obstructive causes; malignant deposits if isolated ↑).
- Serum Igs may be polyclonal ↑ in IgG (autoimmune hepatitis), IgA (alcoholic liver disease) or IgM (PBC).
- Serum protein electrophoresis (myeloma, amyloid).
- Reticulocytes, bilirubin (if ↑ suggests haemolysis).
- Haemoglobinopathy screen (thalassaemia/sickle disorders).
- USS to assess liver texture, splenomegaly, lymphadenopathy.
- CXR and cardiac investigations (cardiomyopathies, sarcoid).
- α-fetoprotein (primary hepatocellular carcinoma).
- Serum ferritin, transferrin saturation, DNA analysis (haemochromatosis).
- Mitochondrial antibodies and autoimmune markers, e.g. ANA (autoimmune hepatitis), ANCA (primary sclerosing cholangitis).
- Caeruloplasmin, urinary copper (Wilson's disease).
- α1-antitrypsin (α1-antitrypsin deficiency).
- Porphyria screen.

Pitfalls

Hepatomegaly is a common sign but may not necessarily implicate liver pathology.

📖OHCM pp60, 502.

Herpes zoster

The pattern of the eruption varies from mild to dense with the involvement of several dermatomes. Complications may occur if involvement of the eye, motor nerves, autonomic nerves (bladder), or when disease presents as an encephalomyelitis or purpura fulminans.

▶▶**In the immunocompromised host, zoster is both more likely to occur and to disseminate.**

Investigations
- Confirm diagnosis by isolation of virus from vesicular fluid.
- Consider underlying disorders if recurrent or severe attacks.
- Look for lymphadenopathy (Hodgkin's or other lymphoma).
- FBC, film, LDH (↑ in lymphoma).
- Serum protein electrophoresis (myeloma, amyloid).
- Serology for HIV (zoster is common in adult HIV individuals).
- Immunodeficiency work-up.

Pitfalls

The rash is not always unilateral: it may be bilateral.

📖OHCM p570.

Hypertension

Hypertension is very common; the diagnosis is arbitrary and requires repeated measurements using a reliable method. Thresholds for therapeutic intervention vary according to:
- The presence of other risk factors for CVD.
- Hypertension is common in patients with type 2 DM (up to 70%) in which it is regarded as part of the insulin resistance syndrome (syndrome X) of ↑ CVD risk.
- Evidence of 'target' organ damage (myocardium, kidneys, etc.). *Note* that in assessment, the sensitivity of tests should be borne in mind. Thus, sensitivity for detection of left ventricular hypertrophy (LVH) = echocardiogram > 12 lead ECG > clinical examination.
- The prevalence of hypertension ↑ with age. Obesity, excessive etOH and a high salt, low K^+ diet are associated with higher BP. Racial associations (e.g. higher prevalence in African-Caribbeans, African-Americans *cf*. white Europeans) are well recognised. A family history of *hypertension* and *premature CHD* should be sought.
- Some uncommon causes of hypertension, e.g. Conn's syndrome, are potentially curable. Others, e.g. phaeochromocytoma, are potentially lethal if unrecognised.
- Accelerated or malignant hypertension is uncommon, but may cause severe target organ damage. A detailed history and thorough physical examination are mandatory in all patients.
- ▶▶Numerous pitfalls in the simple process of measuring BP!

Causes

Essential hypertension—by far the most common cause (>90% of cases).

Secondary causes
- Acute or, more commonly, chronic renal disease.
- Coarctation of the aorta.
- Eclampsia (acute).
- Endocrine disease (Cushing's syndrome, Conn's syndrome, phaeochromocytoma, acromegaly, diabetic nephropathy, primary hypothyroidism, hyperthyroidism, primary hyperparathyroidism).
- Inherited syndromes (rare), e.g. Liddle's syndrome, some forms of congenital adrenal hyperplasia, glucocorticoid suppressible hyperaldosteronism.
- Drugs—corticosteroids, NSAIDs, combined contraceptive pill, erythropoietin, liquorice, carbenoxolone.

Investigations may be required in the following
- Confirming the diagnosis of sustained hypertension.
- Determining the cause of hypertension.
- Assessing the severity of target organ damage.
- Calculating risk of CVD for the individual (this guides the need for pharmacological intervention). Published tables are available.
- If endocrine or renal cause suspected seek an expert opinion at an early stage before embarking upon detailed investigations.

Routine investigations
- ECG (LVH, ischaemia, hypokalaemia of Conn's, diuretic Rx).
- CXR (cardiac size, LVF, rib notching of coarctation).
- Echocardiography (more sensitive in detecting LVH).
- U&E.
- Venous plasma glucose; fasting or casual. Unsuspected type 2 DM is relatively common in middle-aged/elderly. Degrees of glucose intolerance more common if a sensitive diagnostic test, i.e. OGTT used.
- ESR (e.g. autoimmune renal disease).
- Serum lipid profile.
- Serum uric acid (may be elevated in hypertension, renal impairment. Hyperuricaemia is a putative CVD risk factor).
- Urinalysis (protein, glucose—less sensitive in detecting glucose intolerance than blood glucose testing, microscopic haematuria).
- MSU (exclude infection if there is proteinuria).
- Urine microscopy (casts—hyaline or granular).
- 24h urinary protein *or*
- Urinary albumin/creatine ratio (📖p442) if proteinuria on dipstick testing.

Confirmation of diagnosis or attainment of BP targets
- 24h ambulatory BP monitoring (ABPM) in selected cases, e.g. suspected 'white coat' hypertension. The evidence base for ABPM is less robust than for conventional BP measurements using the sphygmomanometer.
- Self-monitoring of BP by patients at home—this is becoming more popular and may provide useful complementary information.

Endocrine hypertension
- Renin/aldosterone studies (consult local endocrine laboratory).
- Investigations for Cushing's syndrome (📖p111).
- Investigations for acromegaly.
- Urinary catecholamines/metabolites.

- TFTs.
- Serum Ca^{2+}.

Renal studies
- Renal USS (renal size, scarring, polycystic kidneys, etc.).
- Renal doppler studies (renovascular disease).
- IVU.
- Captopril renogram (if RAS suspected).
- Renal vein renin determinations (may aid lateralisation).
- Renal angiogram (if angioplasty for RAS contemplated).

Others
- Urinary glucocorticoid metabolites (glucocorticoid suppressible hyperaldosteronism). Very rare.

OHCM pp124, 126, 272.

Beevers DG, Lip G, O'Brien E. (2001) *ABC of Hypertension*, 4th edition, British Medical Association, London; Guidelines Subcommittee. (1999) World Health Organization – International Society of Hypertension guidelines for the management of hypertension. Journal **17**, 151–183; Stewart PM. (1997) Endocrine hypertension. *Medicine* **25**, 17–19.

49

Incontinence: faecal

Alteration of bowel habit, Constipation, Diarrhoea (p8, 26, 28).

Causes include
- Any cause of diarrhoea (OHCM section 7).
- Overflow diarrhoea from severe constipation.
- Inflammatory bowel disease (acute or chronic).
- Coeliac disease (diarrhoea is a variable feature).
- Infectious diarrhoea (OHCM section 1).
- Hyperthyroidism (may cause diarrhoea; rare cause of incontinence).
- Carcinoma of colon (stricture).
- Diverticular disease of colon (acute attack, chronic stricture).
- Neurological (multiple CVAS, MS, spina bifida, post-childbirth neuropathy) may often be associated with sphincter disturbances.
- Drugs, e.g. laxatives, orlistat (causes fat malabsorption).
- Causes of steatorrhoea (OHCM section 7).
- Intestinal hurry, e.g post-gastrectomy (OHCM section 7).
- Diabetic diarrhoea (autonomic neuropathy—rare; diagnosis of exclusion but may cause nocturnal faecal incontinence).
- VIPoma (very rare).

Investigations
Non-invasive tests
- Stool cultures (ova cysts, parasites). *Note: Clostridium difficile*—relatively common in patients who have received recent antibiotic therapy.

- FBC (anaemia, especially iron deficiency).
- CRP.
- ESR.
- U&E.
- TFTs.

Imaging
- Pelvic/abdominal XR.
- Barium enema.
- CT abdomen.

Procedures
- Colonoscopy.
- Sigmoidoscopy ± biopsy.

OHCM p204.

Incontinence: urinary

 Anuria (p12).

Consider

- Common causes of polyuria (OHCM section 4); these may present as, or aggravate, urinary incontinence.
- Acute or chronic confusional state (common; loss of voluntary sphincter control).
- Urinary tract infection (very common—always exclude).
- Drug induced, e.g. thiazide or loop diuretics; α-adrenergic blockade, e.g. doxazosin (uncommon).
- Psychological, e.g. severe depression.
- Immobility, e.g. Parkinson's disease (Shy-Drager syndrome is uncommon).
- Other causes of autonomic neuropathy (OHCM section 10).
- Detrusor muscle instability.
- Urethral incompetence.
- Stool impaction.
- Spinal cord compression.
- Tabes dorsalis.

Investigations
- U&E.
- Urinalysis for blood, protein, glucose, nitrates, nitrites.
- MSU for C&S.
- Plasma glucose (if glycosuria).
- Serum Ca^{2+}.

In selected patients, consider referral to urology or gynaecology services for consideration of
- Bladder manometry studies.
- Post-voiding USS of bladder.
- Pelvic imaging, e.g. CT scan.

OHCM p532.

Indigestion

This term is often loosely used by patients to describe a variety of symptoms. These are often regarded as representing relatively minor and usually intermittent pathology. However, serious pathology, e.g. carcinoma of the stomach, may present as a vague complaint of 'indigestion'. The symptoms may be retrosternal or abdominal. A detailed history is essential, focusing on features that raise the probability of serious pathology, e.g. dysphagia and weight loss.

Examination should include a search for the following signs, particularly in the middle-aged and elderly patients
- Anaemia (especially iron deficiency—common).
- Ascites.
- Troissier's sign (malignant involvement of left supraclavicular lymph nodes due to carcinoma of the stomach—rare).

Note: The presence of associated pathologies, e.g. pernicious anaemia (📖OHCM section 7)—↑ risk of stomach cancer—will alter the threshold for more detailed, expert investigation. Carcinoma of stomach is more common in Japanese.

51

Peptic ulceration may have classic elements that point to the diagnosis. Non-ulcer dyspepsia is very common and is often treated empirically with antacids, H_2 receptor antagonists or H^+ pump inhibitor drugs. The clinical challenge is to identify the patient for whom more detailed, and often invasive, investigation is indicated.

Alternative causes, e.g. cardiac ischaemia, should be considered in the differential diagnosis; similarity of the symptoms between cardiac and upper gastrointestinal disorders are well recognised and sometimes pose considerable diagnostic difficulties.

Causes include
- Oesophageal acid reflux.
- Hiatus hernia.
- Inflammatory disease.
- Peptic ulcer disease of duodenum or stomach.
- Biliary colic (usually distinctive clinical features).
- Malignancy of oesophagus, stomach or rarely small intestine.
- Cardiac symptoms, usually ischaemia.
- Irritable bowel syndrome.
- Symptoms arising from other structures within the chest or abdomen.

Investigations
- FBC.
- U&E.
- ESR.
- Upper GI endoscopy ± tissue biopsy.
- LFTs.

- Creatine kinase (CK) if MI/ACS suspected.
- Troponin (T or I) if MI/ACS suspected.
- Serum amylase (normal in chronic pancreatitis; may be ↑ by duodenal ulcer eroding posterior wall).
- Barium swallow and meal (for oesophageal disease).
- CLO test for *Helicobacter. pylori*.
- Urea ^{13}C breath test for *H. pylori*.
- USS of biliary tract (📖p520).
- Cholecystogram.

If diagnosis remains uncertain consider
- CT abdomen (discuss with radiologist).
- Serum gastrin (Zollinger-Ellison syndrome, 📖OHCM p738).
- 24h ambulatory oesophageal pH monitoring.
- Oesophageal manometry (oesophageal motility disorders).

Irregular pulse

An irregular pulse may be detected by the patient (perceived as 'palpitations' or 'dropped beats'), more commonly, by a health care professional. It may be symptomatic or asymptomatic, acute, intermittent or chronic. An irregular pulse may arise from a variety of pathological causes, most frequently coronary heart disease (CHD), or be an isolated finding, e.g. so-called 'lone' atrial fibrillation (AF) for which no cause can be identified.

Investigations are directed towards
- Determining the nature of the arrhythmia.
- Elucidating its cause.
- Identifying associated pathologies that:
  - Might influence treatment, e.g. presence of left atrial hypertrophy (may reduce chances of long-term restoration of sinus rhythm after DC cardioversion for AF; contraindications to anticoagulation).
  - May exacerbate the symptoms, e.g. anaemia.
- Establishing global risk of CVD (lipids, presence of DM, hypertension, as indicated).

Note: AF is very common, especially in the elderly (prevalence approaches 10% in over 80s in UK).

Causes
- Multiple ventricular or atrial ectopic beats (very common—often asymptomatic).
- AF (common but may be paroxysmal).
- Atrial flutter with variable atrioventricular block (common).
- Complete heart block (uncommon—may be transient following inferior MI).

Note: Remember drugs as a cause or aggravating factor, e.g. theophylline or other β-adrenergic stimulants (ectopic beats).

Initial investigations
- 12-lead ECG.
- U&E.

- FBC.

Consider
- Continuous inpatient cardiac monitoring (e.g. if acute or associated with MI, heart failure).
- CXR (heart size, valvular calcification, etc., (📖p497–503).
- 24h cardiac tape.
- Echocardiography (to identify predisposing or associated structural lesions of valves and myocardium, LV function, etc.).
- Investigations for CHD if indicated, e.g treadmill test for suspected CHD.
- Elucidate cause of AF (TFTs, γGT, etc.).

Jaundice

This defines the yellow discoloration of the sclerae, mucous membranes and skin that occurs when bilirubin accumulates. Bilirubin is the major bile pigment in humans, and is produced as an end-product of haem catabolism. Jaundice usually only becomes noticeable when the serum bilirubin >30–60µmol/L.

Causes
- Can be pre-hepatic, hepatic or post-hepatic.
- Haemolysis.
- Hepatitis (viral, drugs, alcohol).
- Pregnancy.
- Recurrent cholestasis.
- Hepatic infiltration.
- Stones in the common bile duct.
- Carcinoma of the bile duct, head of pancreas or ampulla.
- Biliary strictures.
- Sclerosing cholangitis.
- Pancreatitis.

Investigations
- FBC (?haemolysis).
- Clotting screen (often deranged in liver disease).
- LFTs.
- Viral serology for HAV, HBV and HCV.
- USS abdomen.
- Consider ERCP.
- Liver biopsy may be indicated depending on history, examination and laboratory findings. Discuss with gastroenterology team before embarking on this.

📖OHCM pp206, 556.

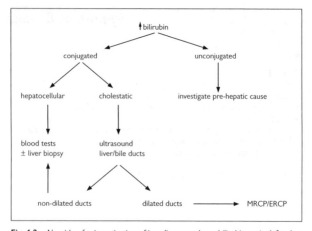

Fig. 1.2 Algorithm for investigation of jaundice, once hyperbilirubinaemia defined as conjugated or unconjugated

Joint pain/swelling

Covers a multitude of disorders including
- Osteoarthritis.
- Rheumatoid arthritis.
- Tendinitis.
- Bursitis.
- Trigger finger.
- Mechanical low back pain.
- Fibromyalgia.
- Other arthropathies.

History and examination
- Ask about affected joints, site of origin, mono- or polyarticular, oligoarticular (e.g. 2–4 joints involved), migratory features, arthralgia (joint pain without swelling).
- Is pain constant or intermittent?
- Aggravating or precipitating factors?
- Any associated neurological features?
- Is there swelling?
- Associated redness or excessive warmth?
- Drug history (e.g. diuretic induced).
- Race (e.g. sickle).
- Past history.
- Family history.
- Occupational history.
- Social history.

Investigations
- FBC—a normochromic normocytic anaemia is common in chronic inflammatory disorders. May be microcytic if long-standing inflammation or associated iron deficiency (e.g. induced by NSAIDs).
- ESR—non-specific marker of inflammation.
- CRP—as for ESR.
- Biochemistry screen, especially looking at bone profile and LFTs.
- Consider serum Igs and protein electrophoresis (myeloma).
- Uric acid levels (gout).
- X-ray affected joint(s).
- Consider USS, especially if soft-tissue swelling.
- MRI can be useful to help visualise intra-articular structures.
- CT scan.
- Bone scintigraphy (helps identify abnormal bone turnover).
- DEXA scan (useful for diagnosis and monitoring of osteoporosis).
- Arthroscopy may help in selected cases.
- Joint aspiration (allows culture and examination of fluid for crystals).

Loin pain

Definition: Pain located in the renal angle.

Causes
- Ureteric colic.
- Renal or ureteric obstruction.
- Acute pyelonephritis.
- Renal infarction or papillary necrosis.
- Acute nephritis (uncommon).
- IgA nephropathy—pain caused by extension of the renal capsule.
- Musculoskeletal causes.
- Shingles at T10–12 (obvious if a rash is seen on examination or be suspected if pain is in a dermatomal distribution).
- Infection or bleeding into a cyst in polycystic kidneys.
- Vesico-ureteric reflux—pain occurs when the bladder is full, this worsens at the initiation of micturition and then is rapidly relieved on voiding.
- Loin pain-haematuria syndrome—this is recurrent pain which occurs in young women. Angiography reveals tortuous vessels.

Investigations
- U&E.
- Serum creatinine.
- Creatinine clearance (if renal impairment).
- FBC.
- ESR.
- Urine dipstick for protein, blood, nitrites, leucocytes.
- Urine microscopy (for casts).

- MSU for culture and sensitivity testing.
- Blood cultures (if bacteraemia suspected).
- Plain x-ray (KUB view).
- IVU (e.g. if +ve urine dipstick for haematuria).
- Renal USS (useful for rapid non-invasive exclusion of obstruction).
- CT of urinary tract.
- Angiogram (if suspicion of thrombus, embolus or loin pain-haematuria syndrome).
- Serum IgA concentration.
- Cystoscopy (specialist procedure).
- Retrograde pyelography.
- Renal biopsy (*only after specialist advice*).

Lymphadenopathy

Lymph node enlargement may be localised or generalised.

Localised cervical lymphadenopathy
- Local causes in mouth (pharyngitis, dental abscess).
- Scalp (skin malignancies or disease).
- Nose (nasopharyngeal carcinoma).

Enlargement of left supraclavicular nodes
- May suggest carcinoma of stomach.

Isolated posterior cervical node enlargement
- Is less often due to malignancy.

Other causes
- Sometimes drugs may be associated with lymph node enlargement (phenytoin, antithyroid).

Investigations
- FBC, film, LDH (leukaemia, lymphoma, Hodgkin's).
- Serology/virology/microbiology/other antigen detection tests:
  - Viral (EBV, hepatitis, CMV, HIV).
  - Bacterial (tuberculosis, bacterial endocarditis, syphilis).
  - Fungal (histoplasmosis).
  - Protozoal (toxoplasmosis).
- ANA (collagen disorder, lupus).
- TFT (hyperthyroidism).
- CXR (sarcoid, tuberculosis).
- USS/CT scan (to assess intra-abdominal, mediastinal/hilar lymphadenopathy).
- LFT/hepatomegaly (↑alkaline phosphatase suggests malignant deposits).
- Lymph node biopsy (groin nodes should usually be avoided because commonly enlarged due to skin and infectious disorder).
- BM (may confirm haematological malignancy).

Note: Fine-needle aspiration, although easier to perform may not be diagnostic and lymph node biopsy should be considered for microbiology and histology.

OHCM p580.

Infection	
Viral	Infectious hepatitis, EBV syndromes, HIV, rubella, varicella, herpes zoster.
Bacterial	Streptococcal, staphylococcal, salmonella, brucellosis, Listeria, cat-scratch (Bartonella).
Fungal	Histoplasmosis, coccidioidomycosis.
Chlamydial	
Mycobacterial	
Parasites	Trypanosomiasis, microfilaria, toxoplasmosis.
Spirochaetes	Syphilis, yaws, leptospirosis.
Connective tissue	Rheumatoid arthritis, SLE, dermatomyositis, serum sickness, drugs, e.g. phenytoin.
Malignancy	
Haematological	Hodgkin's lymphoma, non-Hodgkin's lymphoma, acute and chronic lymphoid malignancies (CLL, ALL), AML.
Non-haematological	Metastases from carcinomas (breast, bowel, lung, prostate, kidney, head & neck).
Endocrine	Thyrotoxicosis.
Miscellaneous	Sarcoidosis, amyloidosis.

57

Although we have provided a large list of possibilities common sense should be used in determining the cause. For example, an 80-year-old woman with axillary lymphadenopathy is unlikely to have cat-scratch disease! *Common things are common.*

Myocardial infarction

Classically, the presentation is with severe, acute, central crushing chest pain that may radiate into the arm (especially →left) and/or the neck; associated with systemic features including sweating, nausea (p59) and dyspnoea (if LVF).

Note: Occasionally, an acute MI may be clinically 'silent', e.g. in patients with long duration DM. Atypical symptoms, e.g. non-classic pain or presentation as collapse or acute confusional state in the elderly.

Classic 12-lead ECG changes (OHCM section 5) comprise ST elevation of 2mm in consecutive lateral leads or 1mm elevation in the limb leads). Less commonly, a 'posterior' MI is evident as an R wave in V1 and V2 leads and deep ST depression in the anterior leads. Sometimes ECG changes are absent at presentation or presentation is 'late' and an MI is diagnosed by a raised serum makers of myocardial damage, notably troponin I and/or LDH (remains for 2–3 weeks). Check for pathological Q waves.

Other causes of cardiac chest pain must be excluded
- Aortic dissection (📖OHCM section 5) may mimic an MI especially if the dissection involves the right coronary artery (leading to ST elevation in the inferior leads, II, II and AVF). Severe tearing pain radiating to the inter-scapular area is suggestive. If the diagnosis is considered likely perform urgent echocardiography and consider:

1. Spiral CT of thorax
2. MRI of thorax

- Acute pericarditis may need to be excluded by the history, the ECG classically demonstrating 'saddle'-shaped ST elevation. T wave inversion and low voltages (if pericardial effusion) are also recognised; the ESR may be markedly raised.

Note: Transient pericarditis is a complication of acute MI within days; Dressler's syndrome may occur several weeks later (may be associated with systemic symptoms and positive serum antimyocardial antibodies).

Additional investigations

These are required after the diagnosis has been made and thrombolysis started if the criteria for treatment are met
- CXR (pulmonary oedema, cardiac size, mediastinal width).
- FBC (exclude anaemia; transient leucocytosis following MI).
- U&E (hypokalaemia 2° to prior diuretics; acute ↓ K⁺ reflects sympathetic activation following MI).
- Serum CK (rises within ~3–6h of acute MI).
- Serum troponin I or T (cardiac-specific proteins, 📖p307).
- ABGs (if LVF or cardiogenic shock).
- Echocardiogram (if LVF, chordae tendinae rupture, aortic dissection or acute VSD suspected).
- Early angiography with view to 1° angioplasty or CABG in selected patients (specialist cardiology opinion required—may be indicated if response to thrombolysis is inadequate).
- Risk factors for an MI should be assessed to guide 2° prevention measures.
- Serum lipid profile (📖p153).
- Venous plasma glucose (*Note*: acute MI may be associated with transient hyperglycaemia (📖p144 for investigations and management)).
- Vasculitis screen, if the history suggestive (rare cause of MI).
- Echocardiogram—to assess LV function.

Tests that are usually done as an outpatient are
- Exercise tolerance test—if significant ST changes occur during exercise or in recovery, or if the time tolerated on the treadmill is limited, referral to a cardiologist for consideration of angiography might be appropriate (📖p529). Assess the BP response to exercise (a fall is a poor prognostic sign).
- Adenosine stress tests may be performed if physical disability limits exercise. Radioisotope scanning can help identify any reversible ischaemia (📖p561). Discuss indications with nuclear medicine department.
- Coronary angiography is the 'gold standard' and will demonstrate coronary artery architecture, plaque distribution and LV function (📖OHCM p92).

OHCM pp104–105, 780.

Nausea

The so-called *vomiting centre* is located in the medulla oblongata and is stimulated by the chemoreceptor trigger zone in the 4th ventricle. There are many causes of acute and chronic nausea. These can be divided into gastrointestinal (GI) causes and non-GI causes.

GI causes of nausea
- Food poisoning (viral, bacterial—common).
- Acute and chronic gastritis (remember *Helicobacter pylori*).
- Peptic ulceration.
- Biliary and renal colic.
- Inflammatory bowel disease.
- Cholecystitis.
- Appendicitis.
- Pancreatitis.
- Gastric outflow obstruction.
- Post-gastrectomy syndrome.
- Acute liver failure.
- Pseudo-obstruction of bowel.

Investigations
- U&E.
- LFTs.
- ESR.
- CRP.
- Serum or urinary amylase.
- Abdominal x-ray (erect and supine—beware perforated viscus).
- Abdominal ultrasound.

Consider
- OGD.
- Barium swallow and meal.
- Isotopic gastric emptying studies.
- Oesophageal manometry.
- Oesophageal muscle biopsy (rarely indicated).

Non-GI causes
- Acute infections, e.g. UTI.
- Metabolic disorders including:
  - Hypercalcaemia.
  - Ketoacidosis (diabetic, alcoholic).
  - Uraemia.
- Pregnancy. NB hyperemesis gravidarum may be associated with ↑ FT4, ↓ TSH.
- Many drugs, notably opiates and digoxin toxicity (check serum levels).
- MI (nausea common; exacerbated by opiates).

59

- Acute glaucoma.

Investigations
- FBC.
- ESR.
- Venous plasma glucose.
- Urine dipstick (UTI).
- Serum Ca^{2+}.
- Serum drug levels, e.g. digoxin, theophylline.
- 12-lead ECG.
- CK.
- Troponin I.

Neurological causes
- Acute migraine.
- ↑ intracranial pressure.
- Acute labyrinthine lesions.
- Meniere's disease.
- Cerebellar lesions (e.g. infarct, haemorrhage, metastases, demyelination).

Investigations
- Cranial CT.
- MRI if cerebellar lesion suspected.
- Tilt table test (□p322).
- Audiometry (specialist technique).

□OHCM p426.

Neck stiffness

The main concern in a patient with neck stiffness is that he or she may have **meningitis** which may result from infection or may reflect infiltration by a disease such as acute leukaemia.

Causes
- Bacterial infection.
- Viral infection.
- Fungal infection.
- Tuberculosis.
- Infiltration by malignancy (e.g. acute lymphoblastic leukaemia, high grade lymphoma, or sometimes acute myeloid leukaemia).
- Drug-induced.
- Contrast media (myelogram).
- Blood (e.g. post-subarachnoid haemorrhage).
- Mechanical/trauma.
- Connective tissue disease, e.g. rheumatoid arthritis.

Investigations
- CT scan of brain ± contrast.
- Lumbar puncture if no ↑ intracranial pressure:
  - Glucose.
  - Protein.

- MC&S ± TB culture.
- Xanthochromia if SAH suspected.
- If patient immunocompromised consider:
  - PCR for viruses, e.g. HSV.
  - Toxoplasma serology.
  - India ink stain for *Cryptococcus*.
- If considering malignancy, send CSF for cytospin.

📖 OHCM, pp358, 360, 806.

Nystagmus

An involuntary oscillatory or (more commonly) rapid jerking movement of the eyes that is rhythmic and repetitive. It results from acute or chronic lesions of the eight cranial nerves, brainstem or cerebellum. The 'slow' phase is pathological, the rapid rhythmic jerking phase (used arbitrarily to define the direction of nystagmus) being a corrective response. Nystagmus 'to the right' describes the direction of the quick phase. Such 'saw tooth' nystagmus may be evident in the horizontal or vertical plane (including 'downbeat' nystagmus of foramen magnum lesions) or as oscillations around a central point (e.g. in albinism).

Jerk nystagmus may be graded in severity depending on whether it occurs
- Only in the direction of directed gaze.
- When eyes are in the midline *or*
- Is present even on looking in direction contralateral to the rapid movement.

Note: Nystagmus (or more correctly, nystagmoid jerks) may be induced by inappropriate testing, often being present at the extremes of gaze. Do not ask patient to follow visual target beyond ~30° of midline when testing at the bedside.

In unilateral causes

Cerebellar nystagmus
Greatest when gaze directed towards the side of the destructive lesion.

Vestibular nystagmus
Greatest away from the side of the lesion.

Pathological nystagmus
May be due to labyrinthine and vestibular lesions—occurs in one direction only. If visual fixation is removed, nystagmus becomes worse.

Central lesions
Including brainstem lesions caused by e.g. tumour, MS; cerebellar lesions or medial longitudinal fasciculus lesions leading to internuclear ophthalmoplegia (📖 OHCM section 10) with ataxic nystagmus.

Investigations

- Positional nystagmus may be investigated by using the Hallpike manoeuvre (☐OHCM section 10). Abrupt alteration of the spatial position of the head (from supine, with head below the bed, rapidly to a sitting position) will induce nystagmus. This will demonstrate benign positional vertigo (common), vestibular disorders or brainstem lesions.
- Audiometry (specialised investigation).
- Auditory and visual evoked potentials (VEPs) may be pathologically reduced in MS. Examination of CSF may reveal oligoclonal bands.
- MRI to include brainstem. (Upbeat nystagmus will suggest a midbrain lesion and downbeat nystagmus will suggest a foramen magnum lesion.) MRI is superior to CT for demonstrating cerebellopontine angle lesions. Gadolinium enhancement is used to investigate acoustic neuromas.
- Ototoxicity can be caused by some drugs such as gentamicin and phenytoin. Acute poisoning with alcohol or barbiturates may cause transient nystagmus. Chronic alcoholism can lead to permanent cerebellar damage. Excessive doses of anticonvulsant drugs, e.g. phenytoin, are a common cause—measure serum concentrations of drug.

☐OHCM p45.

Obesity

The World Health Organisation defines obesity as a body mass index (BMI) greater than $30kg/m^2$.

	BMI (kg/m^2)
Underweight	<18.5
Normal	18.5–24.9
Overweight	>25.0–29.9
Obesity	
Class I	30.0–34.9
II	35.0–39.3
III	>40

Note: Central (abdominal) fat distribution—commoner in men—is associated with greater health risks. Waist to hip ratio or simply waist girth can be used to identify levels at which long-term health risks warrant intervention:

Men	>102cm
Women	>88cm

Aetiology

The great majority of obese subjects have no identifiable metabolic or hormonal defects and detailed investigation is rarely indicated. A chronic imbalance of the equation with energy intake (dietary calories) on the one hand and expenditure (resting metabolic rate + physical activity) on the other is thought to be responsible. Reduced levels of habitual activity allied to an abundance of energy-dense foods appears to account for the current pandemic of obesity and related disorders:

- Impaired glucose regulation.
- Type 2 DM.
- Dyslipidaemia.
- Hypertension.
- CVD.
- Osteoarthritis.
- Impaired physical functioning.
- Gout.
- ↑ Surgical risk.
- Depression.
- Certain cancers, e.g. bowel, breast.

Weight gain tends to occur in middle age; ♀ are more at risk than ♂. Socioeconomic factors are also important.

Specific causes

Genetic
E.g. Prader-Willi syndrome, Laurence-Moon (Biedl-Bardet) syndrome.

Single gene defects
E.g. mutations of leptin (provides feedback from adipocytes to hypothalamus about body fat stores) or its hypothalamic receptor (very rare).

Hypothalamic lesions
Lesions which damage the ventromedial nucleus (the 'satiety' area) may lead to obesity.

Lesions include
- Trauma.
- Tumours—craniopharyngiomas and astrocytomas.
- Inflammation—such as TB and meningitis.
- Infiltration—histiocytosis and sarcoidosis.

Cushing's syndrome
With 'buffalo' hump and central obesity.

Hypothyroidism
Disputed unless severe myxoedema, but hyperthyroidism is associated with unphysiological weight loss.

Insulinoma
Often associated with moderate weight gain; rare.

Marked ↓ motor inactivity
E.g. severe mental retardation or physical disability.

Investigations
- Weight (calibrated scales).
- Height (stadiometer).
- Waist circumference (maximal).
- BP (large cuff required).
- Venous plasma glucose (or OGTT).
- TFTs.
- LFTs (↑ non-alcoholic steatohepatitis in obese subjects).
- Fasting lipid profile ($\square$p153).
- Serum urate.

Additional investigations
These may occasionally be indicated if clinical features give cause for suspicion of organic cause:
- Cranial CT or MRI of pituitary and hypothalamus.
- Investigations for Cushing's syndrome ($\square$p111).
- Genetic testing (seek advice of genetics service).

Lean MEJ, Han TS, Seidell JC. (1998) Impairment of health and quality of life in men and women with a larger waist. *Lancet* **351**, 853–856.

Oliguria

Causes
Acute renal failure: distinguish pre-renal from renal and post-renal causes.

Pre-renal
- Severe sepsis.
- Hypovolaemia, e.g. GI haemorrhage, diuretics.
- Burn injury.
- CCF.
- Addison's disease.
- Acute pancreatitis.

Renal
- Acute tubular necrosis (ATN, e.g. 2° to nephrotoxins such as aminoglycosides and radiological contrast media).
- Acute cortical necrosis.
- Renal infarction.
- Accelerated hypertension.
- Salicylate overdose.
- Hepatorenal syndrome.

Post-renal
- Renal calculi.
- Retroperitoneal calcinosis.
- Papillary necrosis.
- Bladder, prostate and cervical tumours.
- Blocked urinary catheter (common!).

Investigations
- U&E.
- Serum creatinine.
- Creatinine clearance.
- FBC.
- ESR.
- Autoimmune profile.
- LFTs.
- Urinary Na^+ excretion (<20 pre-renal, >40 ATN).
- Urine osmolality (>500mOsmol/L=pre-renal, <350mOsmol/L=ATN).
- Urine dipstick for blood, protein, nitrites, leucocytes.
- Urine microscopy for casts.
- Renal ultrasound (± biopsy in selected cases).
- IV urogram.
- CT pelvis.
- Investigation of renal stones:
  - Serum calcium, phosphorus.
  - 24h excretion of oxalate, calcium, creatinine.

OHCM pp64, 245, 260, 440.

Palpitations

Definition: an unpleasant awareness of the forceful or rapid beating of the heart.

This is, of course, a physiological response to strenuous exercise and is part of the *flight-or-flight* reaction.

Pathological causes include
- Ectopic beats—supraventricular or ventricular (common).
- Heart failure (p44).
- Atrial fibrillation (p52).
- Severe anaemia (p9).
- Hyperthyroidism (especially in bed).
- Severe aortic regurgitation (forceful heart beat and throbbing sensation in the neck).
- Anxiety—especially if associated with a lump in the throat or tingling in the hands (*Paraesthesiae* p67).
- Associated with angina (esp. if nitrates taken).
- Cocaine or amphetamine abuse.
- Phaeochromocytoma (rare).

Investigations
- FBC.
- U&E.
- TFTs.

- 12-lead ECG to (ischaemia, Wolff-Parkinson-White syndrome, AF. etc.).
- Echocardiogram.
- 24h cardiac tape.
- Toxicology screen if drug abuse suspected (&Poisoning Ch11).
- 24h urine collection for catecholamines and metabolites (phaeochromocytoma).

&OHCM p64.

Pancytopenia

Pancytopenia (↓Hb, ↓WBC and ↓platelets) may occur because of bone marrow failure (hypoplasia) or inefficient production (MDS) or peripheral destruction of cells or sequestration (splenomegaly/hypersplenism).

▶▶Pancytopenia usually means something is seriously wrong.

Bone marrow assessment is necessary to establish whether the marrow is hypocellular or hypercellular in the face of peripheral blood pancytopenia. If hypercellular, the cause may be an infiltrative process (due to leukaemia/carcinoma, granulomatous disease, fibrosis-myelofibrosis, osteosclerotic-osteopetrosis, increased macrophages-haemophagocytic syndromes due to viral infections). Causes of hypoplastic bone marrow failure may be hereditary (e.g. Fanconi's anaemia) or acquired (e.g. drugs). Critically ill patients may develop pancytopenia for multiple reasons (sepsis, haemorrhage, DIC).

Investigations
- FBC, film (aplastic anaemia usually presents with ↓ lymphocyte count but minor morphological changes).
- Reticulocytes (↓ if production failure).
- Serum vitamin B_{12}, folate (megaloblastic anaemia can be associated with pancytopenia).
- Serology for EBV, hepatitis A, B, C, HIV (associated with aplastic anaemia).
- Serology for parvovirus infection (if pure red cell aplasia also consider lymphoma, thymoma).
- ANA (lupus).
- NAP score (↑ in aplastic anaemia).
- Check for lymphadenopathy, hepatomegaly, splenomegaly.
- CXR (bronchial carcinoma, sarcoid, tuberculosis, lymphoma).
- USS/CTS to assess lymphadenopathy/splenomegaly (pancytopenia may be due to hypersplenism and portal hypertension).
- Ham's test for paroxysmal nocturnal haemoglobinuria (PNH) or cell marker analysis of CD55 and CD59.
- BM aspirate and cytogenetics (myelodysplasia is a clonal disorder).

&OHCM p664.

Paraesthesiae

This may be described by the patient as an abnormal sensation of aching, pricking, tickling or tingling commonly in the extremities or face. Often described as feeling like 'pins and needles'.

The selection of investigations will be determined largely by the history (transient? chronic?), the surface anatomical site of the abnormal sensation and associated symptoms or precipitating factors (e.g. clear history of hyperventilation).

The common causes include the numbness or tingling associated with pressure on the peripheral nerves such as caused by sleeping awkwardly on an arm ('Saturday night palsy' of the radial nerve), or chronic or recurrent pressure, e.g. on the ulnar nerve at the elbow.

If paraesthesiae is persistent, consider the following conditions, depending on the distribution of the symptoms
- Carpal tunnel syndrome (with radiation proximally along forearm; worse at night).
- Peripheral neuropathy (DM, alcohol, drug-induced, 📖OHCM section 10).
- Sciatica (reduced straight leg raising).
- Meralgia paraesthetica (lateral cutaneous nerve of the thigh).
- Lateral popliteal palsy (common peroneal nerve).

Other less common causes include

Peripheral neuropathy due to
- DM.
- Vitamin B_1 or B_{12} deficiencies.
- Chronic renal failure.
- Chronic hepatic failure.
- Malignancy.
- Neurotoxic drugs:
  - Vinca alkaloids.
  - Metronidazole.
  - Nitrofurantoin.
  - Isoniazid (pyridoxine-dependent).
- Environmental toxins.
- Hypothyroidism.
- Guillain-Barré syndrome (acute).
- Certain porphyrias.
- Multiple sclerosis.

Acute hypocalcaemia causes a characteristic perioral paraesthesia and can be due to many causes including 1° and 2° hypoparathyroidism and alkalosis.

General investigations
- ABGs (acute or chronic acid-base disturbances leading to alterations in ionised Ca^{2+}).
- Serum calcium (not all laboratories measure ionised Ca^{2+}).
- Serum PTH (uncuffed sample).
- Serum magnesium (see below).
- Venous plasma glucose.
- Vitamin B_{12} (and other investigations in suspected chronic peripheral neuropathy).

If serum calcium or magnesium concentration is low, identify cause
- Chronic GI loss (fistula, excessive diarrhoea, bowel obstruction).
- Chronic renal loss (diuretic drugs, intrinsic renal disease).
- Diabetic ketoacidosis (DKA); total body magnesium may be low but this very rarely causes symptoms.

Additional investigations
- Urinary $[Mg^{2+}]$.

Consider
- USS abdomen/renal tract and subsequent GI investigations.
- U&E.
- Nerve conduction studies.
- TFTs.
- IGF-1, GH response during 75g OGTT (if features of acromegaly present; 🕮p104).

Peripheral neuropathy

The patient will complain of numbness in the hands and feet that progresses proximally in a distribution classically termed 'glove and stocking'. Different aetiologies lead to a motor, sensory or mixed sensorimotor picture.

Common causes
- Idiopathic (50%, most common).
- Diabetes mellitus.
- Vitamin B_{12} deficiency (may occur in absence of anaemia).
- Vitamin B deficiency (e.g. alcoholics).
- Vitamin E deficiency.
- Carcinomatous neuropathy.
- Drugs, e.g. isoniazid, vinca alkaloids, cisplatin, dapsone, gold, metronidazole.
- Paraproteinaemias (e.g. MGUS or myeloma).

Rarer causes
- Amyloidosis.
- Uraemia.
- Collagen vascular diseases, e.g. rheumatoid, SLE, PAN.
- Endocrine disease, e.g. myxoedema, acromegaly.
- Guillain–Barré syndrome.
- Infections, e.g. tetanus, leprosy, diphtheria, botulism.
- Sarcoidosis.
- Hereditary, e.g. Charcot-Marie-Tooth disease.

- Acute intermittent porphyria.
- Toxins, e.g. lead (predominantly motor), arsenic (mixed sensory and motor), mercury (sensory) and thallium (mixed sensory and motor).
- Chronic inflammatory demyelinating polyneuropathy.
- Hereditary motor and sensory neuropathy types I or II.

Investigations
- Nerve conduction studies to confirm the diagnosis.

Further investigations
- In order to determine the underlying cause.
- Discuss with neurology staff.

OHCM pp326, 378.

Petechiae and thrombocytopenia

Spontaneous bleeding in the absence of trauma is uncommon with platelet counts >20 × 10^9/L. However, bleeding is much more likely if the thrombocytopenia is not immune in origin (e.g. aplastic anaemia, acute leukaemia, drug-induced, chemotherapy, myelodysplasia).

Thrombocytopenia may be *inherited* or *acquired* (e.g. DIC). As for pancytopenia, these may be classified as due to a failure of production, increased consumption in the peripheries (DIC, ITP) or due to abnormal tissue distribution (splenomegaly).

Idiopathic thrombocytopenic purpura (ITP) may be 1° or 2° (e.g. lymphoma, lupus, HIV).

Drugs (e.g. heparin) and blood transfusion (post-transfusion purpura) may cause severe thrombocytopenia.

Investigations
- FBC, film:
  - Inherited causes may be associated with giant platelets.
  - Morphological abnormalities may suggest MDS.
  - Red cell fragments suggest thrombotic microangiopathies, e.g. TTP.
- LDH (↑ in TTP and lymphoproliferative disorders).
- Serum vitamin B$_{12}$, folate (megaloblastic anaemia can be associated with ↓ platelets).
- ANA, autoimmune screen, immunoglobulins (lupus, hyperthyroidism).
- Virology (HIV, EBV, viral hepatitis, CMV).
- Clotting screen (DIC).
- Lupus anticoagulant, cardiolipin antibodies (antiphospholipid antibody syndromes).
- Platelet serology for drug- or transfusion-related causes.
- Bone marrow assessment to establish whether thrombocytopenia is due to a bone marrow production problem or due to peripheral con-

sumption (discuss with haematology team: depending on degree of thrombocytopenia, other haematological findings and age of patient, a marrow may not be required).

Pitfalls

Thrombocytopenia due to HIV infection must be considered especially in all younger adults. Not worth checking platelet-associated IgG or IgM since these are elevated in thrombocytopenia caused by immune *and* non-immune mechanisms, so add no useful information.

Plethora

A plethoric appearance is typically seen in association with polycythaemia but may also be mistaken for a normal outdoors complexion or cyanosis. Patients with haematocrits above the normal reference range may or may not have an increased red cell mass (real or relative polycythaemia respectively).

Investigations

- FBC, film (repeat FBC as sampling errors can falsely cause elevations of Hb; PRV may be associated with neutrophilia, basophilia or ↑ platelets).
- Measurement of red cell mass may be necessary to confirm true polycythaemia.
  - Investigations are then aimed at establishing whether real polycythaemia, if documented, is due to a 1° bone marrow abnormality (PRV) or a 2° disorder (e.g. respiratory disease).
- Neutrophil alkaline phosphatase score (may be raised in PRV). Seldom used now (📖 *NAP score* (p216)).
- Cobalamin and urate (may be raised in PRV).
- ESR/CRP (acute phase reactants may suggest secondary causes).
- Blood gas analysis, oxygen saturation, carboxyhaemoglobin levels (2° polycythaemia due to respiratory disease, smoking).
- Biochemistry (urea, creatinine; renal disease).
- Erythropoietin (↑ in 2° causes).
- USS abdomen (renal cysts, liver disease, uterine fibroids and other malignancies may 'inappropriately' secrete erythropoietin; also check for splenomegaly in PRV).
- Sleep studies (obstructive sleep apnoea, supine desaturation).

Polycythaemia		
↑ red cell count	>6.0 × 10^{12}/L >5.5 × 10^{12}/L	♂ ♀
↑ PCV	>50% >45%	♂ ♀
↑ Hb	>18.0g/dL >16.0g/dL	♂ ♀

- O_2-dissociation studies (polycythaemia due to abnormal, high affinity Hb variant).
- Bone marrow aspirate and chromosomal studies/cytogenetics (PRV is a clonal disorder).

Polyuria

Polyuria (the passage of an excessive volume of urine, which may be associated with frequency of micturition and nocturia) must be differentiated from urinary symptoms associated with prostatic disease and urinary infections. The latter are also characterised by frequency, urgency and nocturia, but usually small amounts of urine are passed at each void.

Causes include
- DM.
- Cranial DI, (📖OHCM section 9):
  - Familial (autosomal dominant).
  - Secondary to posterior pituitary or hypothalamic disease, e.g. surgery, tumours, especially metastases, neurosarcoidosis.
- Nephrogenic DI:
  - Familial (X-linked recessive).
  - Chronic intrinsic renal disease, e.g. pyelonephritis.
  - Hypokalaemia.
  - Hypercalcaemia.
  - Sickle cell crisis.
  - Lithium, colchicine, amphotericin B.
  - Post-obstructive uropathy.
- Primary polydipsia (psychogenic).

Investigations
- 24h urinary volume.
- Venous plasma glucose.
- U&E.
- TFTs.
- LH.
- FSH (?panhypopituitarism).
- Serum calcium and PTH.
- Sickle cell test.
- CXR (?mediastinal lymphadenopathy in TB, sarcoidosis).

If no obvious cause found consider detailed investigations for cranial or nephrogenic DI (📖p105).

📖OHCM p64.

Pruritus

Implies generalised itching and may be associated with many disorders including
- Iron deficiency.
- Malignant disease, e.g. lymphoma.
- Diabetes mellitus.
- Chronic renal failure.
- Liver disease, e.g. primary biliary cirrhosis.
- Thyroid disease.
- Polycythaemia rubra vera.
- HIV infection.

Investigations
- Aim to exclude the above diseases.
- FBC.
- Biochemistry screen, including LFTs and renal function.
- Glucose.
- TFTs.

📖OHCM pp62, 426.

Ptosis

Ptosis can be unilateral and bilateral. Bilateral ptosis can be more difficult to recognise. Ptosis must be considered in association with other signs and symptoms. Ptosis may be long-standing, of recent onset, progressive or intermittent, especially at the end of the day—myasthenia gravis (MG).

Unilateral ptosis
Causes
- Constitutional (congenital).
- Oculomotor (III) nerve palsy—levator palpebrae. 'Down and out' pupil with loss of light reflex (e.g. DM, SOL, demyelination).
- Aneurysm (basilar or posterior communicating arteries).
- Cavernous sinus disease.
- Meningitis.
- Horner's syndrome—superior tarsal muscle (brainstem infarction, syringobulbia, SOL, MS).
- Encephalitis.

If abnormal (reduced) sweating on ipsilateral side face (damage to cervical sympathetic chain)
- Pancoast's tumour.
- Aortic arch aneurysm.
- Cervical injuries.

No disorder of sweating
- Cluster headache.
- Parasellar tumours.
- Carotid artery aneurysm or dissection.
- Nasopharyngeal tumours.

Investigations
- Venous plasma glucose.
- CXR (Pancoast's syndrome).
- Cranial CT or MRI.
- Cerebral angiography (aneurysm).

Bilateral ptosis

Causes
- Guillain-Barré syndrome (Miller-Fisher syndrome).
- Myotonic dystrophy (MD).
- Myasthenia gravis (MG).
- Neurosyphilis (bilateral; Argyll Robertson pupils).

Investigations
- Syphilis serology.
- EMG ('dive-bomber' in MD).
- Serum anti-acetylcholine receptor antibodies (MG).
- Intravenous edrophonium (Tensilon) test (MG, 📖p413).

📖OHCM p66.

Pulmonary embolism

Occurs when thrombus in systemic veins or the right side of the heart embolises into the pulmonary arterial system. Impaired gas exchange occurs because of a mismatch between ventilation and perfusion.

Investigations
- FBC (may be leucocytosis, neutrophilia most likely).
- ESR (often ↑).
- Plasma D-dimers: ↑ with fresh thrombus.
- ABGs: hypoxia and hypocapnia.
- ECG: look for AF. Usually sinus tachycardia, may be evidence of RV 'strain'. In massive PE there may be $S_1Q_3T_3$.
- CXR: often normal but may show signs of pulmonary infarction or effusion.
- V/Q scan (may be useful for detection of areas of the lungs that are being ventilated but not perfused).
- Spiral CT scan: useful for detection of medium-sized pulmonary emboli but does not exclude small PEs.

📖OHCM pp180, 800.

Purpura

Implies bleeding of varying degrees into the skin. Includes petechial haemorrhages (pinpoint) and ecchymoses (bruises). There are many causes including disorders of platelets and blood vessels.

Causes
- Congenital, e.g. Osler–Weber–Rendu syndrome (= hereditary haemorrhagic telangiectasia), connective tissue (Ehlers-Danlos), osteogenesis imperfecta, Marfan's.
- Severe infection (septic, meningococcal, measles, typhoid).
- Allergic, e.g. Henoch–Schönlein purpura.
- Drugs, e.g steroids.
- Miscellaneous, e.g. senile purpura, scurvy, factitious.
- Thrombocytopenia—any cause (immune, marrow infiltration, deficiency of vitamin B_{12} or folate, myelofibrosis, DIC, TTP/HUS).

Investigations
- FBC (looking for platelet abnormalities and presence of leukaemic cells or other signs of infiltration).
- Coagulation screen (looking for factor deficiencies, DIC, etc.).
- Bleeding time using template device (good test of platelet function, but discuss with haematology registrar first).

OHCM pp42, 272, 646, 726.

74

Recurrent thrombosis

The pathogenesis (and hence causes) of thrombosis reflect abnormalities in the dynamics of the circulation, the blood vessel walls or the blood constituents (Virchov's triad). A hypercoaguable or thrombophilic risk factor is an inherited or acquired disorder of the haemostatic mechanisms, which may be associated with an increased likelihood of a thrombotic event (venous or arterial) or recurrent thrombosis. This concept of risk factors for thrombosis is analogous to that for heart disease, and similarly for most patients *multiple causal factors operate*.

Hereditary thrombotic disease may be suggested by a positive family history but should be tested for if the venous thrombotic events occur in the absence of acquired causes, at a younger age, at unusual sites (e.g. mesenteric) or as recurrent thromboses.

Investigations in recurrent thrombosis (including if on warfarin)

Inherited thrombophilia screening
- Deficiency of factors, e.g. protein C, protein S or antithrombin.
- Abnormal protein (FVL).
- Increased procoagulant (PT, VIII); others (homocysteinuria).
- Consider occult malignancy (PSA in ♂, pelvic USS in ♀).
- FBC (myeloproliferative disorder, PNH).
- Biochemistry (cardiac disease, liver disease, nephrotic syndrome).
- ESR/CRP (ulcerative colitis).

Thromboembolic risk factors

Acquired	
Cardiac disease	MI, AF, cardiomyopathy, CCF
Post-op	Especially abdominal, pelvic or orthopaedic surgery
Pregnancy	
Malignancy	Any
Polycythaemia	
Immobilisation	Prolonged
Fractures	Especially hip and pelvis
Obesity	
Varicose veins	
Drugs	E.g. oestrogen-containing oral contraceptive
Inherited	
Activated protein C resistance, e.g. factor V Leiden mutation	
Protein C or S deficiency	
Dysfibrinogenaemias	

75

- ANA/lupus anticoagulant/cardiolipin antibodies (antiphospholipid antibody syndromes, lupus).

Pitfalls

Thrombophilia testing may be complicated if the patient is on warfarin/heparin: discuss with lab before sending samples.

📖OHCM p674.

Retinal haemorrhage

May be
- Flame-shaped (e.g. hypertension).
- Dot & blot (e.g. diabetes mellitus, vein occlusion or haematological disease).
- Pre-retinal haemorrhage, suggests new vessel formation, e.g. diabetes or post-retinal vascular occlusion.
- Hyperviscosity syndromes.

- Severe anaemia.
- Severe thrombocytopenia.
- Haemoglobinopathy, e.g HbSC.

Investigations
- Check BP.
- Renal function.
- FBC (↑↑Hb or platelets).
- ESR or plasma viscosity (hyperviscosity syndromes such as myeloma or Waldenström's).
- Serum Igs and protein electrophoresis.
- Hb electrophoresis.

Rigors

Fever is due to a resetting of the anterior hypothalamic thermostat, is mediated by prostaglandins (hence aspirin is beneficial), and is most commonly caused by infection. Large variations in temperature may be accompanied by sweats, chills and rigors. An undulant fever may suggest Hodgkin's disease or brucellosis. 'B' symptoms define fever (>38°C), night sweats (drenching), weight loss (>10%) and suggest a diagnosis of lymphoma. (Fever is unusual in CLL in the absence of infection.)

Investigations
- FBC, film (Hodgkin's disease is associated with anaemia, neutrophilia, eosinophilia, lymphopenia).
- LDH (↑ in lymphoma, non-specific test).
- Microbiological tests, blood/urine cultures (also consider pyogenic infection and abscesses in more unusual sites, e.g. renal).
- Antigen detection tests for specific pathogens.
- CXR (tuberculosis, lymphoma).
- ANA (connective tissue disease).
- BM aspirate/trephine may be necessary as part of leukaemia and lymphoma work-up.

Pitfalls

Not all fever is caused by infection.

📖OHCM pp58, 550, 554, 556.

Short stature

The assessment of short stature can be a long and difficult process. Constitutional short stature is the most common cause. Psychosocial disease must be considered, but extensive investigation is required to rule out organic disease. If no cause is found, a period of observation may make the underlying cause apparent. Specialist evaluation should be undertaken in all cases.

Causes

Endocrine
- Growth hormone (GH) deficiency.
- GH resistance (very rare).
- Hypothyroidism (readily treatable).
- Cushing's syndrome (rare in children—*Note*: corticosteroid treatment for chronic asthma).
- Rickets.
- Pseudohypoparathyroidism.
- Type 1 DM—Mauriac's syndrome, now rare.

Non-endocrine
- Constitutional short stature (short parents).
- Emotional deprivation.
- Intrauterine growth retardation.
- Achondroplasia.
- Mucopolysaccharidoses (rare).
- Turner's syndrome (46 XO and variants).
- Noonan's syndrome (46 XY but features of Turner's in a male).
- Congenital cardiac disease, e.g. left-to-right shunt, cardiac failure.
- Cystic fibrosis.
- Other causes of malabsorption, e.g. coeliac disease, Crohn's colitis.
- Chronic liver disease.
- Haematological disease, e.g. sickle cell disease.
- Chronic renal disease.

77

Investigations
- Current height + weight (compare to any previous data available; plot on growth charts).
- Growth velocity—normal if prior problem, e.g intrauterine growth retardation.
- Physical stigmata of physical disease. *Note*: CNS examination mandatory.
- FBC.
- ESR.
- U&E.
- LFTs.
- TFTs.
- Serum albumin (?nutritional status).
- Venous plasma glucose.
- Serum calcium.
- Serum alkaline phosphatase (bone isoenzyme).
- Serum phosphate (reduced in rickets).
- X-ray pelvis (Looser's zones), epiphyses (wide, irregular in rickets), ribs (multiple fractures).
- Serum antigliadin and antiendomysial antibodies (coeliac).
- Testosterone or oestradiol, LH, FSH, PRL (if puberty delayed—panhypopituitarism?).
- X-ray of wrist for bone age. If delayed, measure serum IGF-1 (if IGF-1 normal, then GH deficiency unlikely; if IGF-1 low, consider nutritional

and general health status before diagnosing GH deficiency—stimulation tests required, 🕮p136). If normal—constitutional short stature.
- Karyotype (Turner's and Noonan's syndromes).
- 24h urinary free cortisol (as screen for Cushing's syndrome, 🕮p111).
- CT or MRI of pituitary (if GH deficiency or panhypopituitarism).

Skin pigmentation

Skin pigmentation can be due to increased melanin deposition, such as racial differences in skin pigmentation or due to increased melanin deposition seen in sun exposure. Lentigines and freckles are common. Haemosiderin and other substances can increase skin pigmentation.

Increased pigmentation can be seen in various dermatological conditions, chronic inflammation and fungal infection can result in increased skin pigmentation. Lichen planus and fixed drug eruptions are associated with increased pigmentation.

Increased pigmentation may also be found in association with chronic systemic disease
- Addison's disease (palmar creases, buccal pigmentation, recent scars).
- Porphyria cutanea tarda (especially exposed areas—dorsum of hands).
- Chronic malabsorption syndromes.
- Drugs, e.g. amiodarone, psoralens, mepacrine, minocycline, chloroquine.
- Chronic uraemia.
- Haemochromatosis (so-called 'bronzed diabetes').
- Primary biliary cirrhosis (deep green-yellow jaundice, chronic pruritus).
- Ectopic ACTH syndrome, e.g. bronchial carcinoma.
- Nelson's syndrome (excessive ACTH secretion from pituitary basophil adenoma in patients with Cushing's disease treated by bilateral adrenalectomy).
- Carotenaemia (orange discoloration does not involve sclerae *cf.* jaundice).
- Chloasma (pregnancy, ostrogen-containing oral contraceptive pill).
- Acanthosis nigricans—most often a marker of insulin resistance in obese patients with type 2 DM. Rarely in association with underlying carcinoma.
- Peutz-Jegher's syndrome (fingers, lips in association with small intestine polyposis).

Contrast with hypopigmentation
- Localised acquired depigmentation (vitiligo) is a marker of autoimmune disease.
- Oculocutaneous albinism (autosomal recessive).
- Chronic hypopituitarism (🕮p103).
- Phenylketonuria.

Investigations
- FBC.
- U&E.
- Venous plasma glucose.

- Antigliadin and antiendomysial antibodies.
- Short synacthen test (if 1° hypoadrenalism suspected, 🕮p162).
- Urinary porphyrins.
- LFTs, serum albumin and prothrombin time (INR).
- Fe/TIBC/ferritin + genetic markers for haemochromatosis + liver biopsy.
- ESR and/or CRP.
- Autoimmune profile (🕮Ch4).
- Testosterone (or oestradiol) + LH, FSH.
- Antimitochondrial antibodies, liver Bx (1° biliary cirrhosis).
- Investigations for Cushing's syndrome (🕮p111).
- Investigations for causes of chronic renal failure.

Splenomegaly

A palpable spleen is at least twice its normal size, when its length >14cm. Enlargement may represent changes in the *white pulp* (lymphoid tissue expansion, inflammation), *red pulp* (blood congestion, extramedullary haemopoiesis) or occasionally supporting structures (cysts).

79

Cause in Western societies
- Leukaemias.
- Lymphomas.
- Myeloproliferative disorders.
- Haemolytic anaemias.
- Portal hypertension.
- Infections, e.g. infective endocarditis, typhoid, TB, brucellosis, viral (EBV, viral hepatitis).

Less common causes
- Storage disorders (e.g. Gaucher's).
- Collagen diseases.
- Sarcoid.
- Amyloid.

If foreign residence, consider infectious causes (malaria, leishmaniasis, schistosomiasis) and haemoglobinopathies (HbC, HbE, thalassaemia).

Massive splenomegaly (>8cm palpable below LCM)
- Myelofibrosis.
- CML.
- Gaucher's.
- Malaria.
- Leishmaniasis.

Investigations
Thorough history and physical examination.
- FBC, blood film, LDH (leukaemia, lymphoma, pernicious anaemia).
- Reticulocytes, bilirubin (if ↑ suggests haemolysis).

- Virology/microbiology (sepsis, bacterial endocarditis, EBV, CMV).
- Serum protein electrophoresis (myeloma, amyloid).
- Autoantibody screen, ANA (collagen disease, lupus, RA).
- Haemoglobinopathy screen.
- LFTs (splenomegaly may be associated with hepatomegaly, or due to portal hypertension).
- Peripheral blood cell markers (immunophenotype—may show leukaemia or lymphoma).
- BM aspirate/trephine/cell markers/cytogenetics.
- Leucocyte glucocerebrosidase activity (Gaucher's disease).
- USS to assess liver texture, splenomegaly, lymphadenopathy.

OHCM pp502, 673.

Steatorrhoea

Implies that the patient is passing pale, bulky stools that are offensive (contain fat and tend to float) and are difficult to flush away.

Causes
- Any disorder that prevents absorption of micellar fat from the small bowel.
- Ileal disease.
- Ileal resection.
- Parenchymal liver disease.
- Obstructive jaundice.
- Pancreatic disease, including cystic fibrosis.
- ↓ bile salt concentration.
- Bile salt deconjugation by bacteria.
- Cholestyramine.
- β-lipoprotein deficiency.
- Lymphatic obstruction.

Investigations
Blood tests
- LFTs.
- Bone profile.
- Vitamin B_{12} and serum (or red cell) folate.
- Autoantibody profile.
- Serum amylase.

Pancreatic investigations
- Pancreatic function tests.
- CT scan.

Small bowel
- Small bowel follow-through.
- Jejunal biopsy (?villus atrophy).
- Bacterial overgrowth (^{14}C glycocholate breath test).

Parasites
- Stool culture (e.g. *Giardia*).

Ileal disease
● Consider Crohn's.

📖OHCM p240.

Stridor

Stridor denotes a harsh respiratory added sound during inspiration. It may be a high-pitched musical sound similar to wheeze but arises from constriction of the larynx or trachea. Stridor may be aggravated by coughing.

Note: Progressive breathlessness accompanied by indrawing of intercostal spaces and cyanosis indicates severe laryngeal obstruction with risk of sudden death.

In young children

Because of the smaller size of the larynx and trachea in children, stridor may occur in a variety of conditions.
● Postural stridor (laryngomalacia).
● Allergy, e.g. nut allergy, insect stings; common. *Note:* Emergency Rx with IM or SC adrenaline (epinephrine) (self-administered or by parent), and parenteral hydrocortisone.
● Vocal cord palsy.
● Croup (acute laryngitis—often coryza).
● Acute epiglottitis.
● Inhaled foreign body, e.g. peanut (common—inhalation further down the respiratory tract, usually into the right main bronchus, may produce localised wheeze or distal collapse, 📖p503–504).

Investigations
● Pulse oximetry (non-invasive measurement of PO_2).
● Plain lateral x-ray of neck (for radio-opaque foreign body).
● Endoscopic nasolaryngoscopy.

Adults
● Infection especially *Haemophilus influenzae*.
● Inflammatory or allergic laryngeal oedema, e.g. penicillin allergy (see *above*); may be accompanied by anaphylactic shock.
● Pharyngeal pouch (may be recurrent lower respiratory tract infection).
● Inhaled vomitus or blood in unconscious patient.
● Tetany (due to low serum calcium or alkalosis, 📖OHCM section 17).
● Large multinodular goitre, carcinoma or lymphoma of thyroid (uncommon).
● Laryngeal tumours.
● Bronchogenic tumour with bilateral cord paralysis (subcarinal and para-tracheal gland involvement. *Note:* 'Bovine' cough of right recurrent laryngeal nerve palsy).
● Shy–Drager syndrome (of autonomic neuropathy).

Investigations
- CXR.
- Lateral x-ray of neck.
- Ultrasound of thyroid.
- Endoscopic nasolaryngoscopy.
- Bronchoscopy.
- Barium swallow (pharyngeal pouch).
- CT neck and mediastinum.

📖 OHCM p70.

Suspected bleeding disorder

Bleeding problems present a considerable challenge. Patients may present with simple easy bruising—a common problem—or catastrophic post-traumatic bleeding. The best predictors of bleeding risk are found in taking an accurate history, focusing on past haemostatic challenges (e.g. tonsillectomy, teeth extraction, menses—especially at time of menarche), and current drug history (e.g. aspirin). The history may also help delineate the type of defect. Platelet bleeding (e.g. thrombocytopenia) starts at the time of the (even minor) haemostatic insult but if controlled by local pressure tends not to recur. Bleeding due to coagulation factor deficiency tends to be associated with internal/deep muscle haematomas as the bleeding typically occurs in a delayed fashion after initial trauma and then persists.

Inappropriate bleeding or bruising may be due to a local factor or an underlying systemic haemostatic abnormality.

▶*Acquired causes of bleeding are much more common than inherited causes.*

Causes of bleeding include
- Surgical.
- Trauma.
- Non-accidental injury.
- Coagulation disorders.
- Platelet dysfunction.
- Vascular disorders.

Clinical features
History and presenting complaint. Is this an isolated symptom? What type of bleeding does the patient have—e.g. mucocutaneous, easy bruising, spontaneous, post-traumatic. Duration and time of onset—?recent or present in childhood. Menstrual and obstetrical history are important.

Systemic enquiry
Do the patient's symptoms suggest a systemic disorder, bone marrow failure, infection, liver disease, renal disease?

Past medical history
Previous episodes of bleeding, recurrent—?ITP, congenital disorder. Exposure to trauma, surgery, dental extraction or pregnancies.

Family history
First degree relatives. Pattern of inheritance (e.g. autosomal, sex-linked). If family history is negative this could be a new mutation (one-third of new haemophilia is due to new mutations).

Drugs
All drugs cause some side effects in some patients. Bleeding may result from thrombocytopenia, platelet dysfunction. Don't forget to ask about aspirin and warfarin.

Physical examination

Signs of systemic disease
Is there any evidence of septicaemia, anaemia, lymphadenopathy ± hepatosplenomegaly?

Assess bleeding site
Check palate and fundi. Could this be self-inflicted? Check size—petechiae (pin head); purpura (larger ≤1 cm); bruises (ecchymoses; ≥1 cm).

Joints
Swelling or other signs of chronic arthritis.

Vascular lesions
Purpura—allergic, Henoch-Schönlein, senile, steroid-related, hypergammaglobulinaemic, HHT—capillary dilatations (blanches on pressure), vasculitic lesions, autoimmune disorders, hypersensitivity reactions.

Investigations
- FBC, film, platelet count, biochemistry screen, ESR, coagulation screen.
- Special tests, e.g. BM for 1° haematological disorders; radiology, USS.
- Family studies.

Suspected stroke

A stroke denotes an acute neurological deficit. Strokes may vary in presentation, from a rapidly resolving neurological deficit to a severe permanent or progressive neurological defect (e.g. multi-infarct disease). Neurological deficits persisting >24h are referred to as a *completed stroke* cf. transient ischaemic attack (TIA). With a suspected stroke, a full history and general physical examination are mandatory. Risk factors for cerebrovascular disease should be sought, including a history of hypertension (common—major risk factor), DM (common—major risk factor) and dyslipidaemia. Ask about recent falls or trauma. Hemiparesis can occur as a post-ictal phenomenon or a result of migraine or hypoglycaemia (see below). Hysterical or functional paralysis is also seen but should not be confidently assumed at presentation. Neuroanatomical localisation of the deficit and the nature of the lesion(s) requires appropriate imaging. Clinical hunches may sometimes be misleading.

Note: The post-ictal state may be associated with temporary (<24h) limb paresis (Todd's paralysis) in focal epilepsy (suggests structural lesion—cranial imaging is mandatory)

General investigations
- FBC (polycythaemia, anaemia).
- U&E.
- ESR.
- Protein electrophoresis (if hyperviscosity syndrome suspected, e.g. ⬆⬆ESR).
- ECG (atrial fibrillation, IHD—statins reduce risk of stroke in patients with previous MI).
- CXR (cerebral metastases from bronchogenic carcinoma?).

Specific risk factors
- Venous plasma glucose. *Note*: Severe hypoglycaemia, e.g. insulin-induced or 2° to sulphonylureas, may mimic acute stroke. Always check capillary fingerprick glucose concentration to exclude this possibility—even if there is no history of DM. Take venous sample in fluoride-oxalate tube (+ serum for insulin concentration) if hypoglycaemia confirmed. (See 🔲p144 for further details of investigation and treatment.) Hyperosmolar non-ketotic diabetic coma may also be misdiagnosed as stroke (plasma glucose usually >50mmol/L with pre-renal uraemia).
- Thrombophilia screen (if indicated by clinical or haematological features).
- Lipid profile (not an immediate investigation; secondary prevention, *see above*).
- Blood cultures (if SBE or other sepsis suspected. *Note*: cerebral abscess).

Imaging
- Cranial CT scan (± IV contrast).
- Echocardiogram (if mural thrombus, endocarditis suspected).
- Carotid doppler studies—may not be indicated if surgical intervention (endarterectomy) is unlikely because of poor prognosis, e.g. dense hemiplegia or coma.

Consider alternative diagnoses including
- Primary or secondary brain tumour (may present as acute stroke; search for primary).
- Cerebral abscess (usually clear evidence of sepsis).
- Cerebral lupus (ESR, autoantibodies).

🔲OHCM pp346, 348, 526.

Sweating

Fairly non-specific symptom, but one which may indicate serious underlying disease.

Causes
- Excess heat (physiological).

- Exercise (physiological).
- Fever—any cause.
- Anxiety.
- Thyrotoxicosis.
- Acromegaly.
- Diabetes mellitus.
- Lymphoproliferative disease, e.g. lymphomas.
- Cancer (any).
- Hypoglycaemia.
- Alcohol.
- Nausea.
- Gustatory.
- Neurological disease, e.g. lesions of sympathetic nervous system, cortex, basal ganglia or spinal cord.

Investigations
- FBC.
- ESR.
- Biochemistry screen including LFTs.
- Glucose.
- TFTs.
- Urinalysis and culture.
- Blood cultures.
- CXR.
- Further investigation depending on results of above.

Tachycardia

Patients with tachycardia (heart rate >100 beats/min) may be asymptomatic. Tachyarrhythmias may, however, present with palpitations, chest pain, breathlessness or collapse. When investigating the causes of tachycardia, others causes should be sought apart from cardiac disease. Anxiety, certain drugs and infection may cause tachycardia. Ventricular tachycardias are usually more serious than supraventricular tachycardias. However, cardiac decompensation may occur with either if there is already a compromised myocardium, e.g. due to ischaemic myopathy, or structural lesions, e.g. severe aortic valve disease.

Causes of tachycardia
- Physiological—exercise, pregnancy.
- Drug-induced—β-adrenergic agonists, amphetamines.
- Hyperthyroidism.
- Coronary artery disease (MI, unstable angina, paroxysmal tachyarrhymias).
- Cardiac failure (an early clinical sign).
- Myocarditis.
- Pulmonary embolism.
- Severe anaemia.

- Systemic effects of infection.

Investigations
- 12-lead ECG (📖OHCM pp84–90)
- Look at the QRS complex:
    >120ms—broad complex (probably ventricular) tachycardia.

If narrow QRS and regular
Sinus tachycardia.
Atrial tachycardia (may be 2° to digoxin toxicity).
Junctional tachycardia.
Atrial flutter (flutter waves seen best in inferior leads, 2:1, 3:1 block, etc.).

If narrow and irregular
Atrial fibrillation.

If broad and regular
Ventricular tachycardia (VT) 120–200/min, may cause hypotension.
Bundle branch block (with atrial tachycardia).

If broad and irregular
Atrial fibrillation with bundle branch block.

- Continuous ECG monitoring (on coronary care unit).
- 24h cardiac tape.

Blood investigations
- FBC.
- ESR.
- U&E (especially K^+ level).
- TFTs.
- Cardiac enzymes (if MI suspected, e.g. creatinine kinase, troponin I).
- ABGs.
- Blood D-Dimers (usually ↑ in thromboembolic disease, but rather non-specific, e.g. may also be ↑ in sepsis).

Further investigations
- Infection screen.
- Urine for C&S.
- CXR.
- Sputum culture.
- Blood cultures.
- Look for evidence of underlying heart disease.
- Echocardiogram.
- Exercise tolerance test.
- Cardiac isotope scan.
- Coronary angiography (discuss with cardiologist).

Diagnostic manoeuvres
- Carotid sinus massage (unilateral—increases AV block—care in elderly with carotid bruits).

Zipes DP. (1997) Specific arrhythmias: diagnosis and treatment, in *Heart Disease*, 5th edition, ed Braunwald E, WB Saunders, Philadelphia.

- Valsalva manoeuvre (increases vagal tone).
- IV adenosine (often terminates atrial tachycardia).
- Electrophysiological studies (invasive—specialist procedure).

📖OHCM pp88, 112, 116, 788, 790.

Tinnitus

Tinnitus is a common symptom in which the patient perceives a sound, often chronic and distressing, in the absence of aural stimulation. It usually manifests as a 'ringing' or 'buzzing' in the ears. Tinnitus may occur as a symptom of nearly all disorders of the auditory apparatus. Psychological stresses may be relevant in some cases.

Causes include
- Acoustic trauma (prolonged exposure to loud noise, e.g. gun shots, amplified music).
- Barotrauma (blast injury, perforated tympanic membrane).
- Obstruction of the external auditory meatus (wax, foreign body, infection).
- Otosclerosis.
- Menière's disease.
- Drug-induced ototoxicity.
- Gentamicin—may be irreversible.
- Acute salicylate toxicity.
- Quinine toxicity.
- Acute alcohol poisoning.
- Hypothyroidism.
- Hypertension (rare symptom).
- Intra- or extracranial aneurysm (typically cause 'pulsatile' tinnitus).
- Glomus jugulare tumours.

Note: Consider acoustic neuroma in unilateral tinnitus (📖OHCM section 10).

Investigations
- FBC.
- Serum concentrations of e.g. salicylates, gentamicin (►mandatory during systemic therapy).
- TFTs.
- BP.

Audiological assessment
Specialist investigations include
- Assess air and bone conduction thresholds.
- Tympanometry and acoustic reflex testing.
- Speech perception thresholds.

Consider
- CT temporal bone (acoustic neuroma).
- Cranial MRI (following specialist advice).

📖OHCM p338.

Unstable angina

Unstable angina is characterised by a sudden change in the pattern of exertional angina. Angina may be experienced with minimal physical activity. Rest pain or pain awakening the patient from sleep (decubitus angina) or prolonged or recurrent pain at rest may be a warning of impending myocardial infarction (MI).

Features supporting the diagnosis
- Known coronary heart disease (CHD).
- History of premature CHD in a 1° relative.
- Presence of risk factors for coronary heart disease.
- Smoking.
- Hypertension.
- DM.
- Hyperlipidaemia.
- Premature menopause.

If the 12-lead ECG does not show typical features of ischaemia, consider other causes of chest pain
- Pulmonary embolism.
- Aortic dissection.
- Pneumothorax.
- Oesophageal spasm.
- Acute pericarditis.
- Pleurisy.
- Costochondritis.

Note: A normal 12-lead ECG does not exclude the presence of severe CHD. The patient's history should not be dismissed. Minor degrees of myocardial damage can be detected by specific serum protein markers (troponins, 📖p306). If raised, this places the patient in a higher-risk category.

General investigations
- 12-lead ECG—look for ST segment depression or T wave inversion.
- Serum markers of myocardial damage:
    - CK may be elevated >6h after the onset of myocardial damage.
    - Troponin I (or T) is elevated 8h after onset of myocardial damage. Particularly helpful if ECG is normal and CK is not elevated but strong suspicion of acute coronary event.
- FBC.
- Venous plasma glucose.
- Serum lipid profile.

Patient should be considered at high risk of an MI if
- Anginal chest pain not resolving with nitrates and additional prophy-lactic anti-anginal medication.
- Recent MI (within previous 6 weeks).
- Haemodynamic instability.
- Elevated serum markers of myocardial necrosis (*see above*).
- Changing ST segments of T waves on ECG.

Note: Urgent coronary angiography may be required—a cardiology opinion should be sought.

Patient may be considered at relatively low risk of MI if
- New onset angina, no symptoms for preceding two weeks.
- Normal 12-lead ECG.
- No increase in concentration of serum markers of myocardial necrosis.

Consider further investigation with
- Exercise ECG (□OHCM pp84–90).
- Thallium scan of the myocardium.

If diagnosis of unstable angina unlikely consider other tests to establish cause of chest pain

89

Pulmonary embolism
- ABGs.
- D-dimers.
- V/Q scan.

Pleurisy
- FBC.
- ESR.
- CXR.

Pericarditis
- ESR.
- Serum viral titres.
- Echocardiogram (may reveal pericardial fluid).

Aortic dissection
- PA CXR.
- CT thorax.
- MRI scan thorax.

□OHCM p782.

Urgency

Urgency of micturition denotes a strong desire to void and the patient often has to rush to the toilet because of an acute call to micturate. Urinary incontinence may result, especially if physical mobility is impaired.

Urgency forms part of a cluster of symptoms which include frequency of micturition (📖p71), nocturia and hesitancy of micturition.

Men
- Prostatic disease.
- Urinary tract infection.
- Bladder irritability.
- Urethritis.
- States of polyuria (📖p71); may lead to urinary incontinence (📖p50).

Investigations to consider
- Urinalysis—stick test for glucose, protein, blood, nitrites.
- MSU for microscopy and culture.
- FBC.
- U&E.
- Venous plasma glucose.
- ESR.
- Serum PSA.
- PSA is increased in 30–50% of patients with benign prostatic hyperplasia, and in 25–92% of those with prostate cancer (depending on tumour volume), i.e. a normal PSA does not exclude prostatic disease. Check reference range with local laboratory.
- Transrectal USS of prostate.
- Prostatic biopsy (specialist procedure).

Women
- Urinary tract infection.
- Gynaecological disease, e.g. pelvic floor instability, uterine prolapse.
- Bladder irritability.
- Urethritis.
- States of polyuria; may lead to urinary incontinence (📖p50).

Investigations to consider
- FBC.
- U&E.
- MSU for microscopy and culture.
- Urodynamic studies.

📖OHCM pp42, 532–533.

Vasculitis

Definition
Disease caused by inflammatory destructive changes of blood vessel walls.

Presentation
Wide variety of clinical presentations affecting one or more organ systems.

Skin: splinter haemorrhages, nail fold infarcts, petechiae, purpura, livedo reticularis.

Respiratory: cough, haemoptysis, breathlessness, pulmonary infiltration, sinusitis.

Renal: haematuria, proteinuria, hypertension, acute renal failure.

Neurological: mononeuritis multiplex, sensorimotor polyneuropathy, confusion, fits, hemiplegia, meningoencephalitis.

Musculoskeletal: arthralgia, arthritis, myalgia.

Generalised: pyrexia of unknown origin, weight loss, malaise.

Causes of primary vasculitis

	Granulomatous	Non-granulomatous
Large vessel	Giant cell arteritis	Takayasu's arteritis
Medium vessel	Churg-Strauss disease	Polyarteritis nodosa
Small vessel	Wegener's arteritis	Microscopic arteritis

Causes of secondary vasculitis

91

- Infective endocarditis.
- Meningococcal septicaemia.
- Malignancy.
- Rheumatoid arthritis.
- Henoch-Schönlein purpura.
- SLE.
- Cryoglobulinaemia.
- Drug reaction.

Investigations

- FBC.
- U&E.
- LFTs.
- ESR.
- CRP.
- Protein electrophoresis.
- ANA.
- RHF.
- ANCAs.
- CXR.
- Biopsy of artery and/or skin lesions.
- Urine dipstick and microscopy.

📖 OHCM pp410, 412.

Visual loss

Total loss of vision may be bilateral or unilateral. Unilateral blindness is due to a lesion either of the eye itself or between the eye and the optic chiasm. Determine whether the visual loss is gradual or sudden. Gradual loss of vision occurs in conditions such as optic atrophy or glaucoma. In the elderly, cataract and macular degeneration are common. Remember tobacco amblyopia and methanol toxicity. Trachoma is a common cause worldwide.

Causes of sudden blindness include

- Optic neuritis, e.g. MS.
- Central retinal artery occlusion.
- Central retinal vein occlusion.
- Vitreous haemorrhage (*Note*: proliferative diabetic retinopathy).
- Acute glaucoma.
- Retinal detachment.
- Temporal (giant cell) cell arteritis (TA). *Note*: Visual loss is potentially preventable with early high-dose corticosteroid therapy (☐OHCM section 11).
- Migraine (scotomata).
- Occipital cortex infarction.
- Acute severe quinine poisoning (consider stellate ganglion block).
- Hysteria (rare) Is blindness:
  - Complete? No pupil response or opticokinetic nystagmus.
  - Cortical? Normal papillary light reflex, no opticokinetic nystagmus.
  - Hysterical? Normal papillary light reflex, normal opticokinetic nystagmus.
- HELLP syndrome (haemolysis, elevated liver enzymes and low platelet count syndrome) complicating pre-eclampsia—rare.

Investigations will be determined by history and examination findings; a specialist opinion should be sought without delay.

If TA suspected

- ESR/C-reactive protein.
- Autoimmune profile including cANCA/pANCA.
- Temporal artery biopsy (within days—do not withhold steroid therapy).

Investigations in sudden onset of visual loss

- Visual acuity (Snellen chart).
- Goldmann perimetry.
- Intraocular pressure measurement (tonometry).
- Fluorescein angiography (specialist investigation—may delineate diabetic retinopathy in more detail. Risk of anaphylaxis).
- Cranial CT scan.
- Cranial MRI scan.
- LP (CSF protein and oligoclonal bands if MS suspected).

Screen for risk factors and causes of cerebrovascular thromboembolic disease

- Venous plasma glucose.
- Serum lipid profile.
- Carotid doppler studies.
- 12-lead ECG.
- Echocardiogram.

Jurgensen JS et al. (2001) Postpartum blindness. *Lancet* **358**, 1338.

Wasting of the small hand muscles

Wasting of the small muscles of the hand may be found in isolation or may be associated with other neurological signs. If found in isolation this suggests a spinal lesion at the level of C8/T1 or distally in the brachial plexus, or upper limb motor nerves.

Unilateral wasting of the small muscles of the hand may occur in association with
- Cervical rib.
- Brachial plexus trauma (Klumpke's palsy).
- Pancoast's tumour (may be associated with a Horner's syndrome).
- Cervical cord tumour.
- Malignant infiltration of brachial plexus.

Bilateral wasting of the small muscles of the hand occurs in
- Carpal tunnel syndrome (common).
- Rheumatoid arthritis (common).
- Cervical spondylosis (common).
- Bilateral cervical ribs.
- Motor neurone disease.
- Syringomyelia.
- Charcot-Marie-Tooth disease.
- Guillain-Barré syndrome.
- Combined median and ulnar nerve lesions.
- Cachexia.
- Advanced age.
- Peripheral neuropathies.

93

Investigations
- ESR.
- C-reactive protein.
- Rheumatoid factor.
- CXR.
- X-ray cervical spine.
- Nerve conduction studies (📖p397).
- Electromyography (📖p399).
- LP, CSF protein, etc. (📖p384).
- CT thorax.
- MRI of cervical cord/brachial plexus.

Weight loss

Causes
- Diet.
- Anorexia.
- Diabetes mellitus.
- Malnutrition.

- Small intestinal disease (coeliac, bacterial overgrowth).
- Malignant disease (carcinoma and haematological malignancies).
- HIV/AIDS.
- Chronic pancreatitis.
- Chronic respiratory failure.
- Cirrhosis.
- Diuretic therapy.
- Hyperthyroidism.
- Addison's disease.

Investigations

May well need extensive investigation before determining the cause but start with
- FBC.
- ESR or CRP.
- Biochemistry screen.
- TFTs.
- MSU including C&S.
- CXR.
- Stool culture (if appropriate).
- Blood culture.
- Other endocrine tests as appropriate.
- Consider HIV testing.

📖 OHCM p72.

Wheeze

Wheezes (rhonchi) are continuous high-, medium- or low-pitched added sounds audible during respiration. Typically they are loudest on expiration in asthma and may on occasion be heard without a stethoscope. The implication is reversible or irreversible airway obstruction. If wheeze is audible only during inspiration this is termed stridor, implying upper respiratory obstruction. An important distinction must be made between monophonic and polyphonic wheezes and whether wheeze is localised to a single area or is heard throughout the thorax.

Polyphonic wheeze

Wheezes with multiple tones and pitch. The commonest causes of wheeze (usually recurrent) are:
- Asthma.
- Chronic obstructive pulmonary disease (COPD; often audible during both phases of respiration).

Fixed monophonic wheeze

A wheeze with a single constant pitch. Implies local bronchial obstruction, usually due to:
- Bronchogenic carcinoma
- Foreign body.

Note: Stridor is a harsh form of monophonic wheeze arising from upper airway obstruction (📖 *Stridor* (p81)).

Investigations
- ABGs (*Note*: inspired O_2 concentration should be recorded).
- Pulse oximetry at bedside (does not provide information about PCO_2).
- Spirometry (PFR, pre- and post-bronchodilator therapy).
- Pulmonary function tests (FEV$_1$, FVC, total lung capacity; 📖p365).
- CXR (PA and lateral).
- Sputum cytology (if tumour suspected).
- CT thorax.
- Bronchoscopy and biopsy (specialist procedure—especially if foreign body or suspected tumour).

📖OHCM pp40, 150.

Part 2
Investigations

Chapter 2

Endocrinology & metabolism

Guiding principles of endocrine investigation

Investigations for endocrine disease have caused a lot of confusion in the minds of clinicians (many still do!). Tests have come and gone over the years and have been adopted with varying degrees of enthusiasm by specialist centres. In particular, there is often confusion over which tests to do, what procedures to follow and how to interpret the results. In some areas (e.g. Cushing's syndrome), controversy persists among the experts. In others, a clear consensus approach exists.

Here are some useful general principles:
1. *Use dynamic tests*—rather than random (untimed) sampling where the hormone under investigation is secreted in infrequent pulses (e.g. growth hormone, GH) or levels are easily influenced by other factors (e.g. cortisol varies markedly with stress levels and has a marked circadian rhythm)—*see table* (pxx).

In general

> If you are suspecting a **LOW** level—do a **STIMULATION** test (*to see if it stays LOW*)
>
> If you are suspecting a **HIGH** level—do a **SUPPRESSION** test (*to see if it stays HIGH*)

2. *Use the correct collection method*—e.g. ACTH OR insulin levels require rapid separation of the sample and prompt freezing (–20°C); urinary catecholamines require a specific acid preservative in the collection container. Timing of sampling may also be critical. Label samples carefully, including time of collection! Check procedures with the local laboratory. Many units will have protocols for endocrine investigations.
3. *Do tests in the right sequence*—e.g. ACTH levels can only be interpreted once the cortisol status is known. In many cases simultaneous samples are required for interpretation, e.g. PTH with calcium for hypo/hyperparathyroidism, glucose with insulin for insulinoma.
4. *'Normal' results may be 'abnormal'* depending on the activity of the hormone axis under investigation. Interpretation of the absolute levels of hormones in isolation may be highly misleading. For example, a serum PTH within the normal range *in the presence of hypocalcaemia* suggests hypoparathyroidism; 'normal' LH AND FSH levels in the presence of a very low serum testosterone concentration suggest pituitary failure. In both instances, the regulatory hormone concentration is inappropriately low. Thus, the level of the regulatory hormone (or releasing factor) must be considered in the light of the simultaneous level of the 'target' hormone or metabolite.
5. *Results may vary according to the lab assay*—e.g. different prolactin assays cross-react very differently with macroprolactin (📖 *Galactorrhoea* (p132)). Reference ranges also vary between labs—interpret your tests according to your local lab's 'normal range'. Some individuals have a heterophile interfering antibody that affects the results

of many radioimmunoassays. Resist 'discarding clinical evidence in favour of a numerical value'.

6. *Beware of interfering medication*—e.g. inhaled beclomethasone can suppress serum cortisol levels, administered hydrocortisone (cortisol) is detected by the cortisol assay, synthetic androgens and oestrogens can appear to cause low serum testosterone/oestrogen (not detected in the testostrone/oestrogen assay); some anti-emetics and antipsychotics can raise circulating prolactin levels; carbenoxolone or liquorice may cause hypokalaemia. Always ask patient for a full medication list (including herbal remedies and other self-medication).

7. *Take a family history*—familial forms of many common endocrine problems exist which require important changes in management approach, e.g. familial hypercalcaemia may suggest MEN-1 or MEN-2 requiring a different form of parathyroid surgery and a risk of phaeochomocytoma (MEN-2).

Endocrine tests are generally expensive and should not be performed unnecessarily or outside of standard protocols. Dynamic tests may have cautions and contraindications and *can be hazardous* if used inappropriately. A high degree of organisation and close liaison with the lab is required to perform these tests in a way that can be clearly interpreted. Dynamic tests should ideally be performed in an endocrine investigation unit. Chemical pathologists (clinical biochemists) and other lab staff generally have great experience with performing and interpreting endocrine tests—seek their advice wherever possible—*before* embarking on tests with which you are unfamiliar.

Ismail AAA, & Bart JH. (2001) Wrong biochemistry results. *BMJ* **232**, 705–706.

Random sampling vs. dynamic testing	
Hormone	**Random or dynamic sampling?**
GH	Glucose tolerance test Insulin stress test or alternative if suspect low
IGF-1	Random
LH, FSH	Random in males, post-menopausal females Timed with menstrual cycle in pre-menopausal females Random or stimulated in pre-pubertal children
Testosterone	Random
Oestrogen (*oestradiol*)	Random in males, post-menopausal females Timed with menstrual cycle in pre-menopausal females
ACTH	Random
Cortisol	Dexamethasone suppression test for excess Synacthen stimulation test if suspect low
TSH	Random
T4 & T3	Random
Prolactin	Random
ADH/vasopressin	Don't normally measure directly
Osmolality	Water deprivation test if suspect diabetes insipidus
Parathyroid hormone	Random, but need simultaneous calcium value
Insulin	Fasting, plus simultaneous glucose value
Calcitonin	Random
Renin/aldosterone	Upright usually, off medication
Catecholamines 5HIAAs	Measure in urine, 24h sample Measure in urine, 24h sample

Hypothalamus/pituitary function

Hypothalamic dysfunction

Causes
- Familial syndromes (Laurence-Moon-Biedl, Prader-Willi).
- Tumours (esp. craniopharyngiomas, dysgerminomas, optic gliomas, meningioma—rarely pituitary tumours).
- Pituitary surgery.
- Infiltration (histiocytosis X, sarcoidosis).
- Trauma.

- Meningitis.
- Encephaltitis.
- TB.

Symptoms & signs
- Obesity/hyperphagia.
- Somnolence.
- Thermodysregulation.
- Diabetes insipidus.
- Hypogonadism.
- Precocious puberty.

Investigations
- MRI.
- Water deprivation test for diabetes insipidus (📖 *Polydypsia/polyuria* (p105)), (tests of pituitary function).

Hypopituitarism
Definition
- Failure of one or more pituitary hormones (usually multiple).

Causes
- Congenital.
- Pituitary tumour (including infarction of tumour 'apoplexy').
- Craniopharyngioma.
- Post-cranial irradiation.
- Following pituitary irradiation.
- Metastases to pituitary (especially breast).
- Post-surgery.
- Empty sella syndrome (occasionally).
- Sheehan's syndrome (infarction with post-partum haemorrhage).

Symptoms & signs
Often very vague, e.g. tiredness, normocytic anaemia (easily missed). Combined with impotence or ammonorrhoea—very suggestive. Other clues, loss of body hair (especially axilliary), reduced shaving, hyponatraemia, growth failure in children. Diabetes insipidus is not a feature as ADH can be secreted directly from the hypothalamus. Also signs of space-occupying lesion: bitemporal hemianopia (rarely optic nerve compression, homonymous hemianopia), headache (esp. following apoplexy), III, IV, V_1, V_2 or VI cranial nerve lesions, CSF rhinorrhoea. Occasionally galactorrhoea following pituitary stalk compression by tumour ('disconnection').
Note: Generally GH is lost first, then LH/FSH, and ACTH/TSH last. With any degree of hypopituirism, GH secretion is usually affected.

Investigations
See flow chart. Note that the short synacthen test (📖*Protocols* (p162)) is only suitable for testing the hypothalmo-pituitary adrenal axis if pituitary failure is of long standing (>6 weeks) allowing time for adrenal atrophy to occur.

Alternative investigations

GH stimulation tests including GHRH administration, GHRH + synthetic GH-releasing peptides, IV arginine test, IV glucagon test (causes nausea), oral L-dopa test (also causes nausea) and IV/oral clonidine test in children. However, the reliability of these tests has not been confirmed and the ITT (📖*Protocols* (p155)) remains the gold standard. Combined anterior pituitary testing—giving LHRH, TRH, ACTH and GHRH (📖*Protocols* (p158))—no clear advantage of this approach has been demonstrated and the results of the LHRH test in particular are difficult to intepret in pre-pubertal children. Long (depot) synacthen test—rarely required (📖 *Hypoadrenalism* (p127)).

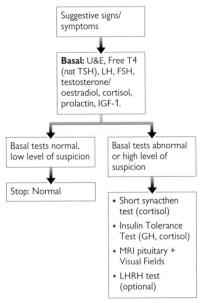

Fig. 2.1 Investigation of suspected hypopituitarism

Bouloux P-MG, Rees LH. (1994) *Diagnostic Tests in Endocrinology and Diabetes.* Chapman & Hall Medical, London; Mahajan T, Lightman SL. (2000) A simple test for growth hormone deficiency in adults. *J Clin Endocrinol Metab* **85**, 1473–1476.

Acromegaly

Clinical features
- Often insidious over many years.
- Enlarging hands and feet with rings having to be resized.
- Increase in shoe size.
- Coarsening of facial features especially enlargement and broadening of the nose.
- Sweating.

- Headache.
- Malocclusion (protruberance of lower jaw) and splaying of teeth.
- Skin tags.
- Hypertension.
- Cardiac failure.
- Renal stones.
- Arthritis.
- Colonic polyps.
- Sleep apnoea.
- Carpal tunnel syndrome.
- Diabetes mellitus.
- May be local symptoms from the pituitary tumour and symptoms/signs of loss of other pituitary hormones (📖*Hypopituitarism* (p103)).
- Growth hormone excess commencing before puberty results in gigantism.

Investigations

- A random growth hormone is not helpful—may be high in normal people.
- Perform a standard 75g oral GTT with glucose and growth hormone measurements at 0, 30, 60, 90 and 120min.
- If no growth hormone values are <2mU/L then the diagnosis of acromegaly is confirmed.
- A random insulin-like growth factor 1 (IGF-1) level should be measured and compared to laboratory normal ranges corrected for age. This can be used as a screening test but IGF-1 assays vary in reliability. IGF-1 levels should be raised in all cases of acromegaly but levels can be affected (reduced) by fasting and systemic illness.
- The vast majority (99%) of cases of acromegaly are due to pituitary tumours. If a pituitary tumour is not seen on MRI scanning yet acromegaly is confirmed, a GHRH level should be requested to exclude ectopic production of this polypeptide by non-pituitary tumours stimulating the release of growth hormone from the pituitary.
- For follow-up of treated cases of acromegaly, IGF-1 levels (more sensitive) and nadir of growth hormone in a series of 4 estimations over 2h is a reasonable approach.
- Life expectancy appears to return to normality when the nadir of GH values is <5mU/L.

Polydipsia & polyuria: diabetes insipidus

'First line tests'

It is relatively common for patients to report excess thirst or increase need to pass urine. The flow chart and table summarise the causes. Prostatism and urge incontinence resulting in urinary frequency should be distinguished by history taking as the patients do not have thirst. Then the first step is to identify straightforward causes such as drugs (diuretics), diabetes mellitus, hypercalcaemia, hypokalaemia and chronic renal failure. A glucose tolerance test should not be required to diagnose diabetes mellitus as the renal threshold for glucose needs to be exceeded (~10mmol/L) to cause polyuria and there should be glucose in the urine.

Causes of polyuria/polydipsia
• Diabetes mellitus
• Diabetes insipidus (cranial or nephrogenic)
• High Ca^{2+}
• Low K^+
• Chronic renal failure
• Primary polydipsia (including dry mouth, e.g. Sjögren's)

'Second line tests'

Subsequent tests aim to distinguish diabetes insipidus from primary polydypsia (compulsive water drinking). A carefully supervised water derpivation test should be performed (□Protocols (p159)). However, it is not always easy to arrive at a conclusive diagnosis. Serum sodium levels are helpful as diabetes insipidus is unlikely if Na^+ <140mmol/L. Morning spot urine osmolality after overnight water restriction (not shown on chart) is occasionally useful: values >600mOsmol/L make significant degrees of diabetes insipidus unlikely. Measuring 24h urine volume is also useful as volumes over 3L are likely to be pathological. However, obligate urine volumes as low as 2L could still cause the patient to complain of polyuria. In such borderline cases, the distinction between partial diabetes insipidus, normality and primary polydipsia can be very difficult. Guidance on interpretation of the second line tests including the water deprivation test is given in the table. Note that primary polydipisa may be a psychiatric condition but can also occur in patients with a dry mouth (e.g. Sjögren's syndrome, anticholinergic drugs) or who have been previously encouraged to drink regularly 'to help their kidneys'.

Distinction between partial cranial diabetes insipidus and habitual (psychogenic) water drinking is complicated by the fact that drinking very high volumes over time may 'wash out' the renal medullary concentrating gradient. In this situation a plasma vasopressin level at the end of the water deprivation test may be very helpful to distinguish lack of vasopressin from a lack of vasopressin action. 24h urine volume is also helpful as volumes of less than 3L/day are unlikely to cause renal 'wash-out'. Clues to primary polydipsia include an initial plasma osmolality (and serum Na^+) that is low, plasma osmolality rises to >295mOsmol/L and thirst is not abolished by DDAVP despite a rise in urine osmolality. Note that 'full blown' cranial diabetes insipidus results in urine volumes around 500mL/h (12L/day).

Interpretation of second line tests for polyuria/polydipsia

	Normal	Partial diabetes insipidus : cranial (C) or nephrogenic (N)	Primary polydipsia
Random serum Na$^+$	Normal	>140mmol/L	<140mmol/L
Random serum osmolality**	Variable	>290mOsmol/L	<290mOsmol/L
Morning urine mOsm**	Variable	Unlikely if >600 (C) Excluded if >600 (N)	
End of water deprivation test *before* DDAVP**	Urine >600 Plasma 280–295	Urine <600 Plasma >295	Urine >600* Plasma 280–295
Urine osmolality after DDAVP SC:**	>600	Rises to >600 or >50% increase (C) Rises to <600 or <50% increase (N)	Rises to >600 or >than 50% increase
Plasma vasopressin at end of water deprivation test	Normal for plasma osmolality	Low for plasma osmolality (C) Normal for plasma osmolality (N)	Normal for plasma osmolality

*With longstanding large volume polyuria (>3L/day), these values may not be achieved due to wash-out of the renal medullary concentrating gradient—if results equivocal, see text.

**Osmolalities are all expressed in mmol/L.

'If all else fails'

In cases of doubt, a carefully supervised therapeutic trial of DDAVP (desmopressin) can be useful to distinguish diabetes insipidus from primary polydypsia (📖*Protocols* (p160)). This should be done as an inpatient as there is a risk of significant hyponatraemia in habitual water drinkers. The principle is that patients able to regulate water intake according to their thirst (diabetes insipidus) should not develop a hypo-osmolar plasma. In primary polydipsia, the urine volume will fall and the urine concentrating gradient will gradually recover. However, if the patient continues to drink due to their psychological drive rather than their thirst, they will become water overloaded and hypo-osmolar.

An additional valuable test to distinguish partial diabetes insipidus from primary polydypisa is hypertonic saline infusion testing, which usually requires access to a plasma vasopressin assay but has been used with urinary vasopressin levels (*see references*). MRI scanning typically shows

Robertson GL. (1995) Diabetes insipidus. Endocr Metab Clin N Am **24**, 549–572; Thompson CJ, Edwards CR & Baylis PH. (1991) Osmotic and non-osmotic regulation of thirst and vasopressin secretion in patients with compulsive water drinking. Clin Endocrinol (Oxf) **35**, 221–228; Diederich S, Eckmanns T, Exner P et al. (2001) Differential diagnosis of polyuric/polydispic syndromes with the aid of urinary vasopressin measurements in adults. Clin Endocrinol (Oxf) **54**, 665–671.

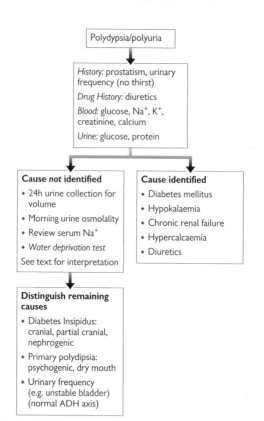

Fig. 2.2 Investigation of polydipsia/polyuria.

an increased signal in the posterior pituitary which is lost in cranial diabetes insipidus. However, this sign is not helpful in distinguishing more subtle degree of diabetes insipidus from other causes.

Hyponatraemia (including SIADH)

Hyponatraemia is a very common clinical problem. Figure 2.3 shows a flow chart for investigation. If patients are on diuretics, further evaluation is usually not possible. The diuretic will need to be discontinued. If this is not possible, the hyponatraemia is likely to be attributable to an underlying condition (cardiac, renal or liver failure). Pseudo- or dilutional hyponatraemia is important to exclude at an early stage (*see table below*). A careful clinical assessment should be made of volume status including identification of oedema, fluid loss (e.g. diarrhoea, fistula leakage) and signs of dehydration including postural drop in blood pressure. A urine sodium and TSH estimation is useful at this stage (see Fig. 2.3). Note that the most important diagnosis not to miss is hypoadrenalism as this can be fatal if untreated. Clinicians should have a low threshold for performing a short synacthen test (see *Protocols* (p162)). Hypoadrenalism due to pituitary failure may not be accompanied by hyperkalaemia, hypotension or hyperpigmentation and can easily be missed.

Causes of pseudohyponatraemia

- With normal serum osmolality
  - Hyperproteinaemia (e.g. myeloma)
  - Hyperlipidaemia (hypertriglyceridaemia)
  - Glycine or sorbitol (from bladder irrigant)
- With ↑ serum osmolality
  - Hyperglycaemia
  - Mannitol
  - Glycerol

The syndrome of inappropriate ADH (SIADH) is a diagnosis of exclusion.

Criteria for diagnosing SIADH

- Hyponatraemia present
- No diuretics
- No oedema
- Normal renal function
- Normal adrenal function
- Normal thyroid function
- Urine Na$^+$ >20mmol/L
- Euvolaemic

109

The diagnosis can be made if hyponatraemia persists in patients not on diuretics, without oedema who have normal renal, adrenal and thyroid function. Volume status should be normal and urine Na$^+$ is normally >20mmol/L. A specific cause is frequently not found or there may be a combination of precipitating factors (see *table below*). In the elderly, a state of chronic SIADH is relatively common and usually explains hyponatraemia persisting for many years without any other apparent cause. Affected individuals should be encouraged to drink less than a litre a day ('5 cups or less'), to only drink if they are thirsty and avoid exacerbating factors (see *table*).

Causes of SIADH	
Cause	**Examples**
Drugs	Carbamazepine, chlorpropamide, opiates, psychotropics, cytotoxics
CNS disorders	Head trauma, post-pituitary surgery (transient), stroke, cerebral haemorrhage, Guillain–Barré, meningitis, encephalitis, fits
Malignancy	Small-cell lung cancer, pancreas, prostate
Chest disease	Pneumonia, TB, abscess, aspergillosis
General stimuli	Nausea, pain, smoking
Other	Acute intermittent porphyria

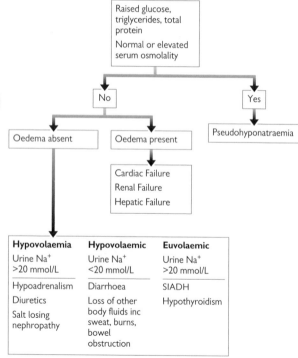

Fig. 2.3 Diagnosis of hyponatraemia

2 Endocrinology & metabolism

The following features of SIADH/hyponatraemia are often underappreciated

1. Other than a chest x-ray, there is no requirement to search for an underlying malignant cause. If there is underlying malignancy it is usually extensive, very apparent and incurable (e.g. extensive small-cell carcinoma of the lung).
2. The urine osmolality does not have to be high. In individuals drinking large volumes of fluid, a urine osmolality as low as 250mOsmol/L (i.e. less than plasma) may be inappropriately concentrated reflecting true SIADH.
3. Conditions previously diagnosed as 'sick cell syndrome' are now thought to represent SIADH in ill patients.
4. 'Water intoxication' is usually the combination of SIADH and excessive fluid intake. Healthy patients drinking to excess can rarely exceed the renal capacity to excrete a water load (~12L/day) and hence do not become hyponatraemic. A degree of SIADH is required for potomaniacs (excess water drinkers) to become hyponatraemic.
5. The post-operative state contains many precipitants to SIADH (nausea, pain, opiates, pneumonia) and ADH secretion is promoted by hypovolaemia from blood loss. The administration of '3L of intravenous fluid a day' post-operatively therefore frequently results in hyponatraemia.
6. Symptoms of hyponatraemia such as drowsiness, coma or fits are dependent on the rate of fall of serum Na^+ not the absolute value. Patients who are alert with Na^+ <125mmol/L have clearly been chronically hyponatraemic and their serum sodium requires only gentle correction. However, a very rapid fall in serum Na^+ to <130mmol/L (typically due to massive infusion of hypotonic fluid into the bladder) may cause coma and needs to be corrected as a medical emergency with hypertonic saline.

111

Obesity/hypercortisolism

Endocrinologists are frequently asked to determine whether there is an underlying cause in patients who are obese. Secondary causes of obesity are listed in the table. A long history of obesity typically going back to childhood is characteristic of constitutional obesity and further investigation other than thyroid function is rarely necessary. However, obesity may result in effects suggestive of hypercortisolism, e.g. striae, central obesity, rounded facial features, mild hyperandrogenism in women, buffalo hump, hypertension and hyperglycaemia. Rapidly progressive obesity, marked hypertension, hypokalaemia, proximal muscle weakness, poor sleep, osteoporosis/vertebral collapse and marked hirsutism or acne are more suggestive of hypercortisolism and require further investigation. Hypothalamic damage is usually apparent from the history.

Secondary causes of obesity
• Constitutional
• Hypothyroidism
• Cushing's syndrome
• Hypothalamic damage (extreme hyperphagia)
• Genetic, e.g. Prader-Willi
• Growth hormone deficiency
• Drugs, e.g. antidepressants

The optimal approach to the diagnosis of hypercortisolism (Cushing's syndrome) is probably the most controversial subject in endocrinology. Endocrinologists who have seen many cases of Cushing's syndrome have seen exceptions to every rule, and the episodic nature of ACTH and cortisol secretion means that low values can occur even in disease. True cyclical Cushing's disease also occurs but is rare.

Diagnosis consists of two phases
1. Does the patient have hypercortisolism or not?
2. What is the cause of the hypercortisolism? Phase 1 must be completed first as phase 2 tests can only be interpreted if hypercortisolism is present.

Investigation of hypercortisolism phase 1

Does the patient have hypercortisolism?

Patients being investigated for hypercortisolism should look Cushingoid. Depression and alcoholism may cause abnormal tests for hypercortisolism without representing a true hypercortisolaemic state and hence are termed 'pseudo-Cushing's syndrome'. Such depressed patients often do not appear cushingoid and alcoholism should be identifiable clinically and biochemically. If there is a high degree of suspicion of hypercortisolism in a depressed patient, midnight cortisol levels <140nmol/L or a negative result on dexamethasone-CRH testing (⊞*Protocols* (p161)) may be helpful in excluding the diagnosis. Note that iatrogenic or factitious Cushing's syndrome is usually due to a steroid other than hydrocortisone and characteristically results in a suppressed hypothalamo-pituitary-adrenal axis.

Four tests are used to determine whether a patients does have hypercortisolism
1. **24h urinary free cortisol collections (UFC).** Three collections with simultaneous creatinine excretion estimation are ideal. If the creatinine excretion varies >10% between collections, the samples are not true 24h collections and should be repeated. If two or more collections have a value >3 times the laboratory upper limit of normal (e.g. >800nmol/24h), then the diagnosis of hypercortisolism is secure. Patients with intermediate values should have repeat sampling after several weeks or additional tests. Steroids, adrenal enzyme inhibitors, statins and carbamazepine must be discontinued prior to testing. False positives can be caused by pregnancy, anorexia, exercise, psychoses, alcohol and alcohol withdrawal.
2. **Low dose dexamethasone suppression test (LDST).** This can be preformed overnight or over 2 days (⊞*Protocols* (p161)), the latter having less false-positives. Some authorities believe it adds little to UFCs as

when cortisol secretion is high, the UFC is clearly raised, but in times when it is intermediate, the LDST may be normal. It is a useful outpatient screening test (📖Overnight protocol (p161)) in individuals who cannot reliably collect 24h urine samples.

3. **Midnight cortisol levels**. High serum cortisol levels (>200nmol/L) measured between 2300 and 0100h indicate loss of diurnal rhythm and although inconvenient, are one of the best tests of hypercortisolism. Samples should be taken via an indwelling cannula in as relaxed state as possibly, preferably during sleep. Values <140nmol/L make hypercortisolism very unlikely. Late evening salivary cortisol levels in an outpatient setting can be used where the assay is available.

4. **Dexamethasone-suppressed CRH test** (📖Protocols (p161)). This is a modification of the LDST which has been said to have a specificity of 100% for hypercortisolism. Experience suggests that exceptions still occur.

Summary
In patients who appear Cushingoid, 3 x UFCs should be performed (note causes of false +ves). If these give equivocal results additional tests are required including further UFCs, midnight cortisols and a formal 2-day LDST followed by CRH.

Investigation of hypercortisolism phase 2: what is the cause of the hypercortisolism?

The common and rare causes of hypercortisolism are summarised in the tables below, along with useful clinical features. Approximately 65% of cases are due to a pituitary adenoma (Cushing's disease), 20% are due to an adrenal adenoma or carcinoma and 10% to ectopic ACTH production.

113

Yanovski JA, Cutler GB, Chrousos G et al. (1993. Corticotrophin-releasing hormone stimulation following low-dose dexamethasone administration: a new test to distinguish Cushing's syndrome from pseudo-Cushing's states. *JAMA* **269**, 2232–2238.

Common causes of hypercortisolism (Cushing's syndrome)		
Cause	Pathology	Characteristic features
ACTH-secreting pituitary adenoma (Cushing's disease)—65%	Pituitary adenoma	Typical features of hypercortisolism with little virilisation
Ectopic ACTH secretion —10%	*Malignant*: small cell lung cancer, thymic carcinoid, medullary thyroid cancer	*Malignant*: rapid progression marked hyperkalaemia, proximal muscle weakness, ↑BP, tumour clinically apparent, few Cushingoid signs
	Indolent/benign: bronchial, pancreatic carcinoids, phaeo	*Indolent*: indistinguishable from Cushing's disease, tumour not easily detected
Adrenal tumour—20%	Adrenal adenoma	Adenomas: typical Cushingoid signs, sometimes virilisation
	Adrenal carcinoma	Carcinomas: rapid progression (months) with virilisation, poor prognosis

These are the 3 main causes to be distinguished using a combination of the tests shown below. Distinction between a pituitary adenoma (which may not be visualisable on MRI) and a small indolent tumour (typically lung carcinoid) represents the greatest challenge. Despite extensive investigation, the cause will remain uncertain in some of these cases.

Investigations

1. **Plasma ACTH level** (separate and freeze immediately). Undetectable plasma ACTH levels are strongly suggestive of an adrenal tumour. However, ACTH secretion is intermittent and two suppressed values with simultaneous high cortisol levels (>400nmol/L) are preferable and should prompt adrenal CT scanning.

2. **High dose dexamethasone suppression test** (📖*Protocols* (p162)). Greater than 90% suppression of basal urine free cortisol levels is strongly suggestive of a pituitary adenoma. Lesser degrees of suppression are seen with ectopic ACTH.

3. **Inferior petrosal sinus sampling (IPSS)**. This is an excellent diagnostic tool but requires expert radiological support and should only be performed in tertiary referral centres. 100mg IV of CRH is also given via a peripheral vein while sampling to ensure active secretion of ACTH during the test. ACTH levels are compared between the inferior petrosal sinus on both sides, and a peripheral vein. Sampling is performed at −15, 0, +15 and +30 min after CRH injection. Ratios >2 (ideally >3) post-CRH are strongly suggestive of pituitary-dependent disease. Risks include failure to enter the sinus, and sinus thrombosis.

4. **Imaging**. Pituitary and adrenal imaging should not be performed without biochemical testing as non-functioning tumours of the pituitary and adrenal are common (false +ves) and conversely functioning pituitary tumours are often be too small to be visualised by MRI (false −ve). However, if the findings are consistent with the biochemical tests this is useful supportive evidence. Patients with findings suggestive of ectopic

ACTH production should have thin-slice CTs of the chest looking for a bronchial adenoma and MRI scanning of the pancreas for an islet tumour. [111]Indium-labelled octreotide scanning may also be useful in locating small tumours.

5. **Plasma CRH levels.** Very rarely 'ectopic ACTH' syndrome is actually due to ectopic CRH production stimulating ACTH from the pituitary (*see table*). Raised plasma CRH levels may be diagnostic in this condition.

Additional tests include

- *Metryapone test.* Here the adrenal enzyme blocker metyrapone is used to lower cortisol levels. Pituitary adenomas respond by increasing ACTH production but ectopic sources of ACTH do not. The test can also be used to confirm that ACTH levels are truly suppressed in adrenal tumours (rarely nececssary).
- *Peripheral CRH test.* ACTH levels are measured before (−30, −15min) and +15 and +30min after injection of 100mg IV of CRH into a peripheral vein. A rise in ACTH levels of >34% is suggestive of a pituitary adenoma. The addition of 5mg IV of desmopression improves the response rate and reduces false negatives.

Summary
See Fig. 2.4.

Boscaro M, Barzon L, Fallo F, Sonino N. (2001) Cushing's syndrome. *Lancet* **357**, 783–791;

Findling JW, Raff H. (2001) Diagnosis and differential diagnosis of Cushing's syndrome. *Endocrinol Metab Clin North Am* **30**, 729–747.

Rare causes of hypercortisolism (Cushing's syndrome)

Cause	Pathology	Characteristic features
Ectopic CRH secretion	Variety of tumours, mostly carcinoids	Clinical features indistinguishable from Cushing's disease but no pituitary tumour, ↑ serum CRH and may fail to suppress with high dose dexamethasone
Ectopic gastrin-releasing peptide secretion	Medullary thyroid cancer	Very rare, resembles ectopic CRH
Factitious ACTH administration	Injections of ACTH	Very difficult to distinguish from ectopic CRH secretion or Cushing's disease, but if isolated from their ACTH source, become adrenally insufficient in days
Cyclical Cushing's disease	Cyclical secretion from pituitary adenoma	Cushing's disease with intermittently negative tests
Pseudo-Cushing's syndromes	Depression or alcoholism	Clinical evidence of Cushing's disease may be limited; evidence of depression or alcoholism
Bilateral micronodular adrenal hyperplasia	Often associated with Carney complex	Investigation suggestive of adrenal tumour (ACTH suppressed) but adrenals normal or slightly enlarged and contain pigmented nodules
Bilateral macronodular adrenal hyperplasia	Sporadic or familial	Investigation suggestive of adrenal tumour (ACTH suppressed) but marked or very marked bilateral nodular enlragment of adrenals on CT scanning

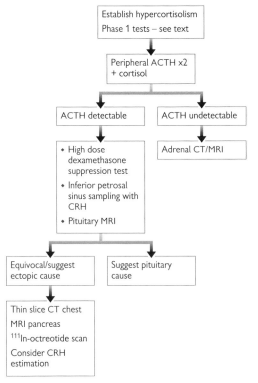

Fig. 2.4 Hypercortisolism. Flow chart for diagnosing the cause once hypercortisolism is established.

Endocrine hypertension

95% of cases of hypertension are 'essential hypertension' with no specific underlying cause. If hypertension is very marked, occurring in younger patients, difficult to control with drugs, episodic/fluctuating, recent-onset, familial, associated with recurrent hypokalaemia or has associated features (see table) then an underlying cause should be excluded.

History and examination should include features of conditions in the table below, with particular attention to paroxysmal attacks, drugs (e.g. liquorice) and family history.

117

Secondary causes of hypertension	
Physical features absent:	
Phaeochromocytoma	Esp. familial, in MEN-2 (may have mucosal neuromas), von Hippel-Lindau syndrome, neurofibromatosis; paroxysmal in only 60% cases with headache, sweating and palpitations
Hyperaldosteronism	Multiple syndromes including Conn's syndrome (*see table*)
Renal artery stenosis	Congenital or acquired (atheroma)
Renal disease	Any cause, including polycystic kidneys
Hyper/hypothyroidism	Diastolic hypertension with hypothyroidism, systolic hypertension with hyperthyroidism
Hyperparathyroidism	Does not usually improve after surgical care
Drugs	Erythropoietin, cyclosporin, cocaine, amphetamines, steroids, liquorice, oestrogens and androgens
Physical features present:	
Coarctation of the aorta	
Cushing's syndrome	
Acromegaly Pregnancy-induced	

Figure 2.5 provides a flow chart for further investigation. At least 3 separate blood pressure readings should be obtained—24h BP monitoring may be useful where 'white coat hypertension' is suspected.

The majority of secondary causes of hypertension can be rapidly excluded by the investigations shown in the first box Fig. 2.5. If the results are normal or the only abnormality is a low potassium, then the possibilities of hyperaldosteronism or renal artery stenosis remain to be distinguished from essential hypertension. Further investigation should be driven by the severity of the hypertension, the (young) age of the patient and the difficulty in obtaining control with drugs.

Investigation of renal artery stenosis/high renin levels
Selective renal angiography remains the gold standard for diagnosing renal artery stenosis—other imaging methods can miss the diagnosis. Renal duplex scanning in experienced hands is a useful non-invasive test. Isotope renography (± captopril) and digital subtraction angiography can generate false negatives. 3D MR angiography is a promising non-invasive alternative. High renin levels associated with hypertension (off drugs) in the absence of renal artery stenosis should prompt a search for juxtaglomerular cell tumour of one kidney. Note that the presence of hypertension is essential, as many conditions associated with low or normal blood pressure can result in 'appropriate' hyper-reninaemia (e.g. diuretics, cardiac, renal or

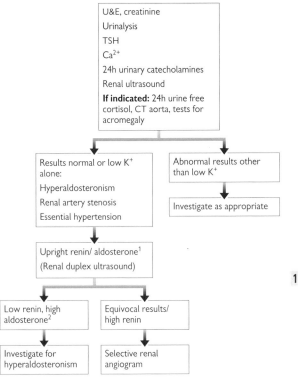

U&E, creatinine

Urinalysis

TSH

Ca^{2+}

24h urinary catecholamines

Renal ultrasound

If indicated: 24h urine free cortisol, CT aorta, tests for acromegaly

---

Results normal or low K^+ alone:

Hyperaldosteronism

Renal artery stenosis

Essential hypertension

Abnormal results other than low K^+

Investigate as appropriate

Upright renin/ aldosterone[1]
(Renal duplex ultrasound)

Low renin, high aldosterone[2]

Investigate for hyperaldosteronism

Equivocal results/ high renin

Selective renal angiogram

Notes

[1] Ideally, this test should be performed off all antihypertensive drugs for 2 weeks (6 weeks for spironolactone) except alpha blockers.

[2] Low renin and very low aldosterone should prompt investigations for 'apparent mineralocorticoid excess'.

Fig. 2.5 Investigation of cause of hypertension.

liver failure, hypocortisolism, hypovolaemia). High renin levels can also occur in essential hypertension.

Investigation of hyperaldosteronism

Hypertension with persistent hypokalaemia, raises the possibility of hyperaldosteronism which may be due to a variety of causes (*see table below*). Note that investigation for hyperaldosteronism is also appropriate with K^+

levels in the normal range, if other investigations are negative and hypertension is marked, difficult to control or in a younger patient. The optimal approach to investigation remains controversial and equivocal cases frequently occur. If there is marked hypokalaemia of recent onset, a 24h urinary free cortisol (and review of medication) is indicated to exclude recent-onset hypercortisolism (usually due to ectopic ACTH production) in which Cushingoid features have not yet become apparent. True hyperaldosteronism is never due to a malignant lesion, so that if hypertension can be medically controlled, it is not always necessary to establish a definitive diagnosis of aetiology. Published guidelines for investigation are often ambiguous. A detailed practical scheme is therefore provided here (Fig. 2.6).

Establishing hyperaldosteronism

The initial investigation is an upright renin/aldosterone ratio, performed when the patient has been upright or sitting (not lying) for at least 2h. The sample needs to be taken to the laboratory and frozen immediately. Ideally, the patient should be on no antihypertensives other than α-blockers (e.g. doxazosin) as most drugs can affect interpretation of the test results (see table, p121). This is difficult to achieve in subjects with very marked hypertension. Combination antihypertensive therapy and spironolactone cause most confusion. An undetectable renin with an unequivocally high aldosterone level makes the diagnosis very likely. A normal or raised upright renin excludes hyperaldosteronism. Borderline results should be repeated off interfering medication and after potassium

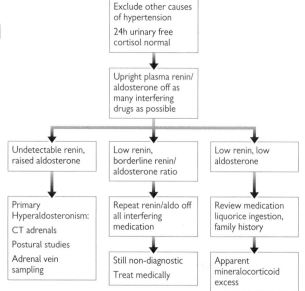

Fig. 2.6 Investigation of hyperaldosteronism/mineralocorticoid excess in patients with hypertension.

replacement (hypokalaemia can inappropriately lower aldosterone). A low renin with a normal aldosterone can be seen in essential ('low renin') hypertension. Refer to the laboratory for normal and diagnostic ranges. Additional tests (e.g. renin after sodium restruction/frusemide, aldosterone after captopril, sodium loading or IV saline) are used in specialist centres but their exact role in testing remains unresolved.

Causes of hyperaldosteronism/apparent mineralocorticoid excess

Primary hyperaldosteronism ($\downarrow$ renin $\uparrow$ aldosterone)
- Aldosterone-producing adenoma (Conn's syndrome)
- Renin-responsive adenoma
- Idiopathic unilateral hyperplasia
- Idiopathic bilateral hyperplasia
- Glucocorticoid-remediable hyperaldosteronism

Apparent mineralocorticoid excess ($\downarrow$ renin $\downarrow$ aldosterone)
- Liquorice ingestion, carbenoxolone, fludrocortisone
- Congenital 11β hydroxysteroid dehydrogenase deficiency
- Liddle's syndrome
- Congenital adrenal hyperplasia (11β hydroxylase or 17α hydroxylase def.)
- Hypercortisolism

121

Renin/aldosterone testing and drugs

Drug	Effect on PRA	Effect on aldosterone
Drugs that $\uparrow$ PRA		
Spironolactone	$\uparrow$	Variable
Ca^{2+} channel blockers	May $\uparrow$	$\downarrow$
ACE inhibitors*	$\uparrow$	$\downarrow$
Diuretics	$\uparrow$	$\uparrow$
Vasodilators	$\uparrow$	$\uparrow$
Drugs that $\downarrow$ PRA		
β-blockers	$\downarrow$	$\downarrow$
NSAIDs	$\downarrow$	$\downarrow$

PRA, plasma renin activity; * angiotensin II receptor antagonists are likely to have same effects.

Investigating the cause of established primary hyperaldosteronism
There are 5 causes of established primary hyperaldosteronism with suppressed renin and high aldosterone (see *table,* above). Surgery (unilateral adrenalectomy) is indicated for adenoma (65% of cases), the unusual renin-responsive adenoma and the rare cases of unilatral hyperplasia but not for bilateral hyperplasia (idiopathic hyperaldosteronism, 30% of cases) or the rare, familial glucocorticoid-remediable aldosteronism

(GRA). Tests to distinguish these are summarised in the table (p121) and Fig. 2.7.

📖OHCM p304.

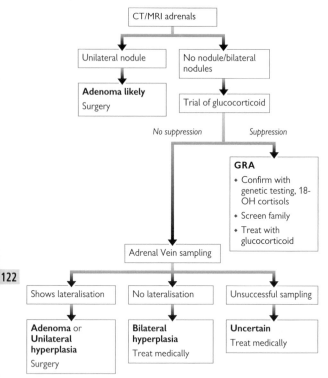

Fig. 2.7 Identifying the cause of established primary hyperaldosteronism.

If hyperaldosteronism is established and a nodule is visible on CT/MRI imaging, it is reasonable to proceed to unilateral adrenalectomy/excision of the nodule. If no nodule or bilateral nodules are seen, then adrenal vein sampling is the most useful test to determine whether surgery should be performed. Aldosterone levels after glucocorticoid administration or genetic testing for the chimeric CYP11B1/CYP11B2 gene should be performed beforehand to exclude GRA (*see table*, pxx—family members may be only mildly hypertensive, making family histories unreliable). Unfortunately, the right adrenal vein cannot be catheterised in up to 25% of cases and **there is a risk of precipitating adrenal haemorrhage**. Postural studies identifying a >50% rise in aldosterone comparing recumbent and 2–4h of standing/walking suggest idiopathic hyperplasia, but a small renin-responsive adenoma not visible on CT could give similar results.

Investigating the cause of apparent mineralocorticoid excess

Rarely, investigation reveals low renin and low aldosterone levels in the presence of hypertension, hypokalaemia and alkalosis. There are 5 causes of this (*see table,* p121). A 24h urinary free cortisol estimation will rapidly exclude recent-onset, aggressive hypercortisolism. Repeated enquiry should be made for drug and liquorice product ingestion. The remaining causes may be diagnosed by urinary cortisol/cortisone ratio (11β OH steroid dehydrogenase deficiency—often referred to alone as 'apparent mineralocorticoid excess') or other appropriate changes in urinary and plasma cortisol metabolites (e.g. raised DOC levels—11β hydroxylase or 17α hydroxylase deficiency) or responsiveness to amiloride (Liddle's syndrome).

Phaeochromocytoma

Phaeochromocytoma is rare but an important diagnosis not to miss—can result in fatal hypertensive crisis especially during surgery or after inadvertent β adrenoreceptor blockade without α blockade. It can be sporadic (90%) or be the first clue to a familial syndrome (*see table,* p121). Approximately 10% of cases are extra-adrenal, 10% multiple and 10% malignant. 90% of cases have sustained or paroxysmal hypertension but paroxysmal attacks of some nature are a feature of only 55% of cases. Pure adrenaline-secreting lesions can occasionally cause hypotension. They are always intra-adrenal. Phaeochromocytoma needs to be excluded in cases of incidentally found adrenal masses.

123

24h urinary catecholamine estimations (collect into an acidified container) have now replaced measures of catecholamine metabolites (VMAS, metanephrines) as they are more sensitive and specific. A single clearly positive estimation in the presence of hypertension is usually sufficient. If non-diagnostic, sampling initiated immediately after an 'attack' should provide the answer. Mild ↑ can be seen in anxiety states, and with very small lesions detected in the follow-up of familial, recurrent disease. Causes of false positive results include methyldopa, levodopa, labetalol, clonidine withdrawal, intracranial events (e.g. subarachnoid haemorrhage, posterior fossa tumour) or metabolic stress (e.g. hypoglycaemia, myocardial infarction). Measurement of plasma catecholamines and stimulation tests are now largely obsolete.

Once the diagnosis is established, α blockade (typically with increasing bd doses of phenoxybenzamine) should be established before invasive investigation. The tumours are usually large (>2cm) and bright on T2-weighted images. CT/MRI scanning therefore identifies virtually all adrenal lesions. Radionuclide scanning with ^{131}I MIBG is useful to confirm activity if more than one adrenal nodule is present and to identify extra-adrenal lesions where no adrenal lesion is seen. Note that extra-adrenal phaeochromocy-

Thakker RB, Oparil S. (2001) Primary aldosteronism: a practical approach to diagnosis and treatment. *J Clin Hypertens* (Greenwich) **3**, 189–195; Stewart PM. (1999) Mineralocorticoid hypertension. *Lancet* **353**, 1341–1347; Dluhy RG, Lifton RP. (1999) Glucocorticoid-remediable hyperaldosteronism. *J Clin Endocrinol Metab* **84**, 4341–4344; Stewart PM. (1999) Mineralocorticoid hypertension. *Lancet* **353**, 1341–1347.

Investigating established primary hyperaldosteronism

	Change in aldosterone with posture	CT findings	Adrenal venous sampling (ratio between sides)	Response to glucocorticoids*	Treatment of choice	Notes
Adenoma (Conn's)	None/fall	Unilateral nodule visible	>10:1 ratio of aldosterone	Absent	Surgery	
Renin-responsive adenoma	Rise	Unilateral nodule	10:1 ratio of aldosterone	Absent	Surgery	
Unilateral hyperplasia	None/fall	Normal	10:1 ratio of aldosterone	Absent	Surgery	
Bilateral hyperplasia	Rise	Normal	No difference	Absent	Medical	
Glucocorticoid	None/fall	Normal	No difference	Present	Steroids	Very raised 18-oxo cortisols. Positive genetic screening**

* Dexamethasone 0.5mg 6-hourly for 2–4 days resulting in suppression of aldosterone levels to nearly undetectable levels (usually associated with a fall in blood pressure also).

** Positive for chimeric CYP11B1/CYP11B2 gene.

tomas (paraganlionomas) are usually in the chest or abdomen but can occur in the neck (including chemodoctomas of the carotid body), pelvis and bladder.

📖OHCM p304.

Hypokalaemia

Persistent hypokalaemia (<2.5mmol/L) can cause muscle weakness, cramps, tetany, polyuria, exacerbate digoxin toxicity and predispose to cardiac arrhythmias. The majority of cases are due to the common causes (see table below) and are relatively easy to diagnose. However, puzzling cases where none of these features are present occur and prompt further investigation. A flow chart is shown below Fig. 2.8.

Common causes of hypokalaemia*

- Diuretics
- Vomiting/diarrhoea
- Intestinal fistula
- Laxative or diuretic abuse
- Steroids (including fludrocortisone), liquorice, ACTH therapy

---
*See text for investigation of rare causes

Note the importance of identifying the presence of acidosis and hypertension. Occult diuretic and purgative use should always be borne in mind. The commonest cause of persistent hypokalaemia with no other cause presenting in adulthood is Gitelman's syndrome, an asymptomatic congential disorder which can usually be separated from the rare, more severe Bartter's syndrome (which usually presents neonatally or in early childhood), by low serum Mg^{2+} levels.

📖OHCM p694.

Schurman SJ, Shoemaker LR. (2000) Bartter and Gitelman syndromes. *Adv Pediatr* **47**, 223–248.

Hyperkalaemia

Artefactual and common causes need to be excluded of which renal failure is the most important (see table below). If these fail to reveal a cause, then hypoadrenalism (which can be life-threatening), isolated mineralocorticoid deficiency and type IV renal tubular acidosis need to be excluded.

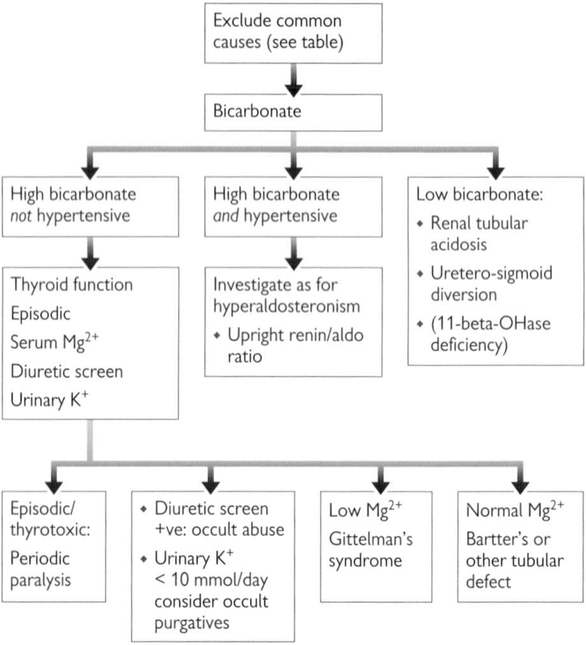

Fig. 2.8 Investigation of hypokalemia.

Causes of hyperkalaemia

Artefactual	Other	Rare but important
Sample left unseparated overnight	Excess K^+ replacement	Hypoadrenalism
Sample haemolysed	K^+-sparing diuretics, ACE inhibitors	Type IV RTA
Myeloproliferative disease (leakage of K^+ from high cell counts)	Renal impairment, esp. acute and after trauma or surgery	Isolated mineralocorticoid deficiency
	Metabolic acidosis (esp. DKA), rhabdo-myolysis, burns, massive blood transfusion	

Hypoadrenalism is suggested by concomitant hyponatraemia, hypotension (including postural), malaise and skin pigmentation. Diagnosis is by short synacthen testing (📖*Adrenal failure* (p127)). Note that hyperkalaemia is not a feature of secondary (pituitary) hypoadrenalism since aldosterone production is maintained by the renin-angiotensin system. Type IV renal tubular acidosis is common in patients with diabetes. It is associated with a renal tubular dysfunction as well as mildly impaired glomerular function. Serum creatinine is usually at or above the upper limit of normal. It is a state of hyporeninaemic hypoaldosteronism. Renin/aldosterone testing is suggestive but there is no definitive test. Isolated mineralocorticoid deficiency is usually congenital (e.g. due to aldosterone synthase deficiency), but can be acquired (e.g. HIV disease) and aldosterone resistance (pseudo-hypoaldosteronism with high aldosterone levels but biochemical mineralocorticoid deficiency) has been described. High renin and low aldosterone levels would be expected.

📖 OHCM pp262, 694

Adrenal failure

Hypoadrenalism is often insiduous in clinical onset. However, it is an important diagnosis to make as it can be life-threatening especially at times of stress. The key is to have a high index of suspicion. Primary adrenal failure is suggested by hyperkalaemia, hyponatraemia, hypotension (including postural), malaise, weight loss, nausea, abdominal pain and skin pigmentation. In pituitary (secondary) adrenal failure, hyperkalaemia, hypotension and pigmentation are absent and malaise may be the only feature. Signs/symptoms of gonadal failure (e.g. loss of libido, reduced shaving or amenorrhoea) are often associated features with pituitary failure. Basal cortisol levels can be misleading as they may be high in the morning and low in the evening. Nonetheless, a random cortisol level >550nmol/L excludes the diagnosis and is a useful test in patients undergoing severe stress/illness (e.g. in ITU).

127

▶Where there is a strong suspicion of adrenal failure, treatment must not be delayed pending investigation. A short synacthen test or random cortisol should be performed immediately and treatment commenced with steroids awaiting results. Alternatively, treatment with dexamethasone, 0.5mg daily (which does not cross-react in the cortisol assay) can be used and then discontinued for the day of testing. Patients on other forms of glucocorticoid therapy should discontinue treatment on the morning of the test and ideally 24h beforehand (12h for hydrocortisone or cortisone acetate). Mineralocorticoid replacement need not be discontinued.

Short ACTH (synacthen) test
The standard test for adrenal failure is the short ACTH test (📖Protocols (p162)). In recent years there has been interest in the low dose (1μg or 0.5μg) test. Although this appears to detect more minor cases of hypoadrenalism, the clinical significance of defining these differences remains uncertain.

For secondary (pituitary) adrenal failure, alternative tests include the insulin stress test (📖Protocols (p155)) and the metyrapone test

(📖(p115)). However, these tests involve applying a stress and carry a risk in patients who are profoundly hypoadrenal. They are only indicated in patients within 6 weeks of pituitary surgery or a pituitary insult, where hypotrophy of the adrenal cortices has yet to develop.

Test to distinguish primary vs. secondary adrenal failure
In the context of known pituitary disease and with failure of other pituitary hormones, adrenal failure can be assumed to be secondary (pituitary) in origin. Where isolated adrenal failure is identified, primary adrenal failure is most likely and suggested by increased skin pigmentation and hyperkalaemia.

Three additional tests can be used to confirm the level of adrenal failure
1. *Anti-adrenal antibodies* (anti-21 hydroxylase antibodies). These antibodies are present in around 70% of patients with autoimmune adrenalitis (Addison's disease), the commonest cause of primary adrenal insufficiency. However, they can also be present without adrenal failure in patients with other autoimmune conditions.
2. *Basal plasma ACTH.* This is usually the only additional test required. High levels are seen in primary adrenal failure, 'normal' or low levels are be seen in secondary adrenal insufficiency. Note that the sample must be taken and separated immediately at least 24h after the last dose of a short-acting glucocorticoid (e.g. hydrocortisone) to avoid pharmacological suppression. Patients on longer acting steroid, may have to have the test repeated more than 24h after cessation of the steroid if the result is equivocal.
3. *Long (depot) ACTH test.* Chronic stimulation with ACTH can recover function in adrenal glands that have have failed because of lack of pituitary ACTH but not in primary adrenal failure. This is given in the form of ACTH in oil on 2 consecutive days (📖 *Protocols* (p163)), or as an infusion over 48h. With the advent of reliable ACTH assays, this test is rarely indicated.

Additional diagnostic tests
While the majority of cases of primary hypoadrenalism are due in developed countries to autoimmune disease, there are multiple other rare causes. These should particularly be considered where adrenal failure occurs in childhood and/or is associated with neurological disease or hypogonadism (*see table*, p129).

Ten S, New M, Maclaren N. (2001) Clinical review 130: Addison's disease 2001. *J Clin Endocrinol Metab* **86**, 2909–2922; Vaidya B, Pearce S, Kendall-Taylor P. (2000) Recent advances in the molecular genetics of congenital and acquired primary adrenocortical failure. *Clin Endocrinol* (Oxf) **53**, 403–418.

Vaidya B, Pearce S, Kendall-Taylor P. (2000). Recent advances in the molecular genetics of congenital and acquired primary adrenocortical failure. *Clin Endocrinol* (Oxf). 2000 **53**:403-18.

Amenorrhoea

Amenorrhoea is often separated into primary (never menstruated) and secondary (cessation of periods after menarche) amenorrhoea, but many causes are shared between the two categories. Structural assessment of the genital tract should be performed earlier in investigation of primary amenorrheoa. Investigation of oligomenorrhoea is similar to secondary

Causes of primary adrenal failure

Cause	Associated features	Diagnostic tests
Autoimmune adrenalitis	Autoimmune damage associated with polyglandular failure types 1 and 2	Anti-adrenal (21-OH-ase) antibodies
Tuberculosis	Extra-adrenal TB	Calcified or enlarged adrenals, extra-adrenal TB, but may only show shrunken glands
Other infections, e.g. histoplasmosis, syphilis	Seen in N and S America	Adrenal glands enlarged
Metastatic malignancy	Common with breast, lung, melanoma or GI cancer though does not always cause adrenal failure	Enlargment/deposits in adrenal glands on CT
Bilateral adrenal haemorrhage	Anticoagulation, adrenal vein sampling	Signs of haemorrhage on CT
AIDS	CMV/TB, cryptococcus adrenalitis	
Adrenaleukodystrophy Adrenomyeloneuropathy	Especially ♂ <15 years, dementia, quadriplegia, neuropathy, blindness—may appear after adrenal failure	
Familial glucocorticoid deficiency	Defective melanocortin 2 receptors including Allgrove's syndrome, hypoadrenalism associated with seizures, achalasia and alacrima from childhood	
Defective cholesterol metabolism Congenital adrenal hypoplasia	Mutation on DAX1 or related genes causing failure of adrenal to develop. Adrenal insufficiency from birth	
Drugs	Ketoconazole, mitotane, etomidate, rifampicin, phenytoin	Exacerbate pre-existing adrenal impairment

129

amenorrhoea. Menorrhagia and intermenstrual bleeding are due to different causes, often gynaecological in origin. 'Irregular periods' can fall into either category, depending on whether it actually refers to intermenstrual bleeding or variably spaced (anovulatory) periods. A plan of investigation is shown in Fig. 2.9.

In secondary amenorrhoea, it is helpful early on to identify primary ovarian failure (e.g. due to Turner's syndrome, premature ovarian failure, radiation, mumps orchitis, radiation, chemotherapy or non-45X gonadal dysgenesis) characterised by high gonadotrophins (LH, FSH). Where the gonadotrophins are equivocal or low, amenorrhoea due to hyperprolactinaemia or thyrotoxicosis should be excluded but the commonest diagnosis is chronic anovulation due to polycystic ovarian syndrome. In this condition, the ovaries still produce oestrogen resulting in a positive progesterone withdrawal test: 10mg of medroxyprogesterone is given daily for 5 days and the test is positive if any menstrual bleeding occurs in the following week. If the test is negative, a pituitary (e.g. pituitary tumour) or hypothalamic (e.g. stress, anorexia nervosa, systemic illness or weight loss) cause resulting in profound oestrogen deficiency must be considered.

Infertility

Detailed assessment of infertility is beyond the scope of this text and is best referred to a specialist in this area. However, the general physician can take the following basic steps, always remembering that the couple should be assessed together as the problem may lie with the man, the woman or a combination of both:

1. Semen analysis of the male and where possible a post-coital test to confirm that live semen are delivered to the vaginal tract.
2. If amenorrhoea is present in the female, investigate as in Fig. 2.9.
3. If female is menstruating, determine if the cycles are ovulatory, e.g. by day 21 progesterone levels or home measurement urinary dipstick of the LH surge.

If live semen are delivered and ovulation is occurring, then structural damage or chlamydial infection in the female genital tract is likely and will require gynaecological assessment.

Hirsutism/virilisation (raised testosterone)

Hirsutism refers to an increase in androgen-dependent terminal hairs in the female, typically over the face/chin, lower abdomen, arms and legs and around the areola of the breast. Virilisation reflects much higher androgen levels and comprises the features shown in the table below. Over 20% of women have more androgen-dependent hair than they consider to be normal. In >95% of cases, this is associated with androgen levels in the female normal range or slightly elevated in association with polycystic ovarian syndrome. Some drugs such as cyclosporin, diazoxide, minoxidil and androgenic steroids can also cause hirsutism. A history of recent onset (<6 months), rapidly progressive hirsutism, particularly when associated with features of virilisation and a testosterone level of >5nmol/L,

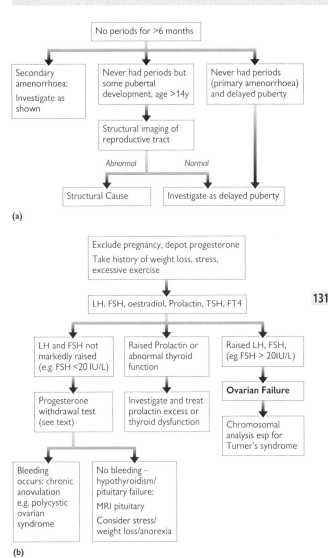

Fig. 2.9 Investigation of amenorrhoea: (a) primary, and (b) secondary.

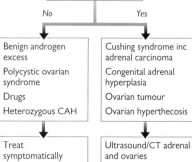

Fig. 2.10 Investigation of hirsutism

should prompt a search for alternative adrenal or ovarian causes (Fig. 2.10).

Features of female virilisation
Clitoral enlargement
Temporal hair loss
Breast atrophy
Deepening of voice

📖 OHCM p306.

Galactorrhoea (hyperprolactinaemia)

Galactorrhoea is always due to prolactin. Rarely, it can occur with prolactin levels in the normal range and regular menses, but usually is associated with mildly raised levels and amenorrhoea in females or very
elevated levels in males. There is no link with breast size—gynaecomastia

in males is associated with excess oestrogen. Once dopamine-blocking drugs (major tranquillisers and antiemetics but not antidepressants), depot progesterone administration and hypothyroidism have been excluded, all patients should have pituitary imaging to exclude a large tumour pressing on the pituitary stalk (Fig. 2.11). Very high prolactin levels (>10,000iu/L) are invariably associated with prolactinomas. Nipple manipulation (e.g. to check if galactorrhoea has ceased) and chest wall trauma (including shingles) can also stimulate prolactin levels.

Asymptomatic raised prolactin

If prolactin is found (accidentally) to be persistently >1000iu/L but menstruation is normal and there is no galactorrhoea, consider the possibility of macroprolactin. This is a circulating complex of prolactin and immunoglobulins of no biological importance but gives a high reading in the prolactin assay and the result often varies widely between assays. If the lab is alerted to a mismatch between prolactin levels and clinical picture, they can easily screen for this with a PEG precipitation. Stress and epileptic fits can result in transiently raised prolactin levels insufficient to cause galactorrhoea.

📖OHCM p312.

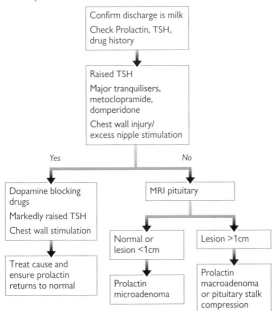

Fig. 2.11 Investigation of galactorrhoea.

Impotence/loss of libido/male hypogonadism

Symptoms and signs of hypogonadism in men (low testosterone levels)
- Reduced shaving.
- Loss of libido.
- Impotence.
- Reduced energy/aggression levels.
- Loss of pubic, chest and axilliary hair.
- Gynaecomastia often results due to a lower testosterone/oestrogen ration.

Impotence alone (without loss of libido) can also be caused by neurovascular and psychological causes (e.g. diabetes, spinal damage, urological surgery, atheroslerosis of the aorta, drugs, stress and psychosexual dysfunction). Note that very low levels of testosterone (at least <5nmol/L, typical normal range 10–30nmol/L) are required to result in symptoms. Mild reductions are common especially in the elderly and are rarely of importance.

After history taking for conditions described above, investigation of suspected male hypogonadism requires
- Prolactin.
- Thyroid function.
- LH & FSH.
- Testosterone.

Hyperprolactinaemia or thyrotoxicosis if present need to be treated on their own merits. If the testosterone level is clearly low, high gonadotrophins point to testicular failure (e.g. testicular surgery, irradiation or trauma, chemotherapy, crypto-orchidism, previous orchitis, gonadal dysgenesis including Klinfelter's syndrome XXY). Low gonadotrophin levels with a clearly low testosterone point to a hypothalamic or pituitary cause (systemic illness, pituitary tumour). If no cause is found for hypogonadotrophic hypogonadism, the likely cause is Kallman's syndrome, especially if associated with anosmia.

📖 OHCM p306.

Gynaecomastia

Gynaecomastia results from an excessive effect of oestrogens or a raised oestrogen/testosterone ration. Causes are summarised in the table below. True gynaecomastia should be associated with palpable breast tissue and distinguished from apparent breast enlargement due to obesity. Though very rare, the most important diagnoses to exclude are hypogonadism, testicular and lung tumours.

Leslie H, Courtney CH, Bell PM et al. (2001) Laboratory and clinical experience in 55 patients with macroprolactinemia identified by a simple polyethylene glycol precipitation method. *J Clin Endocrinol Metab* **86**, 2743–2746.

Causes of gynaecomastia	
Physiological	Newborn, adolescent, elderly
Hypogonadism	e.g. Klinefelter's syndrome, testicular failure
Increased oestrogen	Testicular tumours, lung Ca producing hCG, liver disease, thyrotoxicosis
Drugs	Including oestrogens, spironolactone, cimetidine, digoxin, testosterone administration

Investigations should include
- LFTs.
- Thyroid function.
- LH & FSH.
- Testosterone.
- Oestradiol.
- hCG.
- αFP.
- Chest x-ray.
- Testicular ultrasound.
- Further review of drug history.

Physiological gynaecomastia should only be diagnosed if other causes have been excluded.

135

OHCM p306.

Delayed puberty

Definition
Puberty is considered delayed in girls if there is no breast development by age 13 (or menses by age 15) and in boys if there is no testicular enlargement by age 14. Note that 3% of normal children will fall into these categories.

Clinical features & initial investigations
A detailed history and examination is required for overt systemic disease, psychosocial stress, anorexia nervosa and to assess the child's height, pubertal features (pubic hair, testicular size, breast growth, menses) and any dysmorphic features (e.g. features of Turner's syndrome). Where possible growth rate should be calculated from sequential height measurements over at least 6 months.

If no obvious cause is identified, baseline investigations should include
- LH & FSH.
- TSH, FT4, prolactin.

- FBC, U&E, HCO_3^-, CRP, antigliadin/endomysial antibodies for occult systemic disease.
- Bone age.

This should enable the child to be placed in one of 5 categories

1. Raised LH/FSH (primary gonadal failure).
   Causes: Turner's syndrome, Kleinfelter's syndrome, ovarian/testicular injury. Proceed to karyotyping (should be performed in all girls with delayed puberty as Turner's syndrome may not be apparent).
2. Short, low LH/FSH, overt systemic disease.
   Causes: asthma, anorexia nervosa, social deprivation, generalised illness, treatment for cancer including cranial irradiation, dysmorphic (Noonan's syndrome and others).
3. Short, low LH/FSH, occult systemic disease.
   Causes: hypothyroidism, hyperprolactinaemia, renal failure, renal tubular acidosis, coeliac disease, Crohn's disease.
4. Short, low LH/FSH, no systemic disease.
   Causes: constitutional delay of puberty, hypothalamic/pituitary disease.
5. Not short, low LH/FSH.
   Causes: Kallman's syndrome (if anosmia present) or isolated gonadotrophin deficiency. Cannot reliably distinguish from constitutional delay of puberty. Observe.

The investigation of children who fall into the commonest category, 'short, low LH/FSH, no systemic disease' is summarised in Fig. 2.12. The onset of puberty after a period of observation is reassuring but continued observation is required to ensure the process proceeds to completion including a growth spurt. If not, further investigation for disorders of steroidogenesis, androgen insensitivity, skeletal dysplasia, premature gonadal failure and in the female, genital tract abnormalities and polycystic ovarian syndrome are indicated.

Short stature

Evaluation of children who are below the 3rd growth centile for age or particularly small for their family should include

- Height for age (percentile).
- Mid-parental height (for girls mean of father's height minus 12.6cm + mother's; for boys add 12.6cm to mother's height).
- Bone age (to assess growth potential/height prediction).
- Observation over 3–6 months to determine growth velocity.

Children of short (but normal) parents who are growing normally can be observed. Dysmorphic children require further evaluation/specialist assessment. Children who are short for their parental heights (low predicted height), particularly if growing slowly and short children of pubertal age who have not entered puberty should be investigated as for 'delayed puberty'. Referral for paediatric endocrinological assessment is advised.

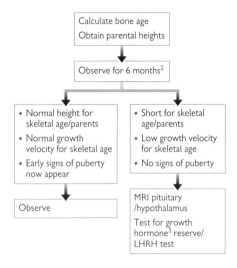

Notes

1. Including normal thyroid function and prolactin.

2. If develops headache, vomiting or visual symptoms proceed immediately to MRI.

3. Refer to paediatric endocrinologist. Tests used vary e.g. gonadotrophin response to LHRH after androgenic priming and insulin tolerance test for growth hormone

Fig. 2.12 Investigation of delayed puberty in children who are short, with no evidence of systemic disease[1] and low LH/FSH levels.

Precocious puberty

Definition

Puberty is considered premature if multiple signs including accelerated growth rate and bone age appear by age 8 in girls or age 9 in boys. Note that isolated breast development (premature thelarche) or pubic hair (premature adrenarche) are benign conditions if no other evidence of puberty appears. True precocious puberty requires urgent investigation to determine the cause and avoid irreparable loss of final adult height. In girls, it is often idiopathic *but not in boys.*

Causes

Causes of precocious puberty	
Central	**Gonadotrophin independent**
Idiopathic (especially girls)	CAH (males)
CNS hamartoma (esp. pinealoma)	Adrenal/ovarian/hCG-secreting tumour
Other CNS diseases, e.g. hydrocephalus, trauma	McCune-Albright syndrome, hypothyroidism, follicular cyst (female) familial testitoxicosis (male)

Investigations

Precocious puberty is confirmed by pubertal levels of sex steroids (oestradiol, testosterone). Testicular enlargement (or ovarian enlargement on ultrasound) and detectable LH/FSH levels suggest central precocious puberty and CT/MRI scan of the brain is indicated. Gonadal enlargement can also be seen with testitoxicosis, hCG-producing tumours, hypothyroidism and McCune-Albright syndrome. Further investigation should be performed in combination with a paediatric endocrinologist.

Thyroid function testing—general

In the majority of cases, thyroid function testing and interpretation is straightforward. However, the following points should be borne in mind.

Which first line test?—TSH

TSH levels are the most sensitive indicator of thyroid dysfunction but cannot be used in patients with pituitary disease. TSH used alone as a first line test will miss (levels 'normal') unsuspected cases of secondary hypothyroidism and some laboratories therefore combine TSH and T4 as first line tests.

Which tests?—T4/T3

Free T3 and T4 tests (FT3, FT4) are now more reliable and preferred (though more expensive) to total T3 or T4 measurements. Interference in the assays does occur but is increasingly rare. Total thyroid hormone levels are markedly influenced by changes in binding proteins (e.g. due to pregnancy, oestrogen-containing contraceptives).

Thyroid autoantibodies

These are markers of autoimmune thyroid disease. Antithyroid microsomal antibodies have been identified as antithyroid peroxidase (ANTI-TPO) antibodies. Antimicrosomal antibodies are much more sensitive than antithyroglobulin antibodies and are present in around 45–80% of Graves' disease and 80–95% of Hashimoto's disease/atrophic thyroiditis. Increasingly, labs are measuring anti-TPO directly as their only antibody test. Note that anti-TSH receptor antibodies—*the cause of Graves' disease*—are difficult to measure and not routinely assayed. Although they are the most reliable test for diagnosing Graves' disease, currently their

Dayan CM. (2001) Interpretation of thyroid function tests. *Lancet* **357**, 619–624.

only definite indications are to determine the cause of thyroid disease in pregnancy and the post-partum period and assess the risk of neonatal thyrotoxicosis.

Tests should agree
To confirm thyroid dysfunction at least two thyroid function tests and in cases of doubt all three (TSH, FT3, FT4) should be performed. The results of the tests should be in agreement—if not, assay interference (heterophile antibodies, anti-T4 or anti-T3 antibodies present in the serum) or unusual causes should be suspected.

Avoid thyroid function testing in systemically unwell patients
In very ill patients, especially in intensive care, a pattern of 'sick euthyroidism' is often seen, with low TSH levels, low free T3 levels and sometimes low free T4 levels. Accurate interpretation of true thyroid status is impossible. A raised free T3 level in a very ill patient suggests significant hyperthyroidism and a very raised TSH (>20mU/L) with undetectable free T4 levels suggests profound hypothyroidism. Other changes should be interpreted with extreme caution and the tests repeated after recovery.

📖 OHCM pp292, 294.

Hyperthyroidism (thyrotoxicosis)

Clinical features
Hyperthyroidism is rare in childhood but affects all adult age groups. Classic features include weight loss despite increased appetite, palpitations, atrial fibrillation, heat intolerance, anxiety, agitation, tremor and proximal weakness. Lid-retraction and lid-lag can be seen in any cause of hyperthyroidism but proptosis, periorbital oedema, chemosis, diplopia and optic nerve compression only occur in association with Graves' disease (thyroid eye disease), or occasionally associated with pretibial myxoedema and thyroid acropachy. In the elderly, presentation with isolated weight loss or atrial fibrillation is common. Raised alkaline phosphatase and sex hormone-binding globulin, leucopenia and rarely hypercalcaemia are recognised associations.

Thyroid function testing
An undetectable TSH level and a ↑ free T3 level are required to diagnose hyperthyroidism. In milder cases, T4 levels may be in the normal range ('T3 toxicosis'). Normal TSH levels with ↑ T4 and T3 are seen in TSH-secreting pituitary tumours (very rare) or in patients with thyroid hormone resistance (also very rare).

Investigation of cause (see Fig. 2.13)
Under the age of 40, Graves' disease is the commonest cause. After this age, Graves' disease, toxic nodular goitre and toxic nodule all occur. However, a short history (≤1 month) of symptoms raises the possibility of

self-resolving (transient) thyroiditis, a diagnosis supported by neck pain and raised ESR (viral/subacute/De Quervain's) or occurrence in the first 9 months post-partum (post-partum thyroiditis). Transient thyrotoxicosis can also occur in patients with subclinical autoimmune thyroiditis ('silent thyroiditis'). When thyroid eye disease is present, no further tests are required to diagnose Graves' disease. If not, antithyroid antibodies (e.g. anti-TPO antibodies) and isotope thyroid scanning can be useful to distinguish possible causes. No uptake is seen in transient thyroiditis. Excess thyroid hormone ingestion rarely causes very marked thyrotoxicosis unless the active form (T3) is taken (T3 tablets or dessicated thyroid extract).

Iodine

Iodine has multiple and conflicting effects on the thyroid. Potassium iodide inhibits release of thyroid hormones from the gland and thyroid hormone biosynthesis (Wolff-Chaikoff effect) promoting hypothyroidism. However, escape from these effects occurs in most individuals in a few weeks. In patients with a multinodular goitre, excess iodine (e.g. in amiodarone or radiographic contrast media) can result in thyrotoxicosis by excess provision of substrate (Jod-Basedow effect).

Amiodarone

Has 3 main effects on the thyroid hormone axis: (1) inhibits T4→T3 conversion, which in the pituitary can result in a mild rise in TSH (reduced thyroid hormone action), (2) can induce hypothyroidism, usually in the first year of treatment, (3) can induce hyperthyroidism either via the Jod-Basedow effect in patients with multinodular goitre or by a destructive thyroiditis in healthy glands. Thyrotoxicosis can occur at any time after commencing therapy and can be very difficult to treat.

Hyperthyroidism in pregnancy

Significant hyperthyroidism in pregnancy is generally due to Graves' disease. Mild hyperthyoidism, particularly in association with hyperemesis gravidarum in the first trimester, is often due to a cross-reaction by the very high hCG levels with the TSH receptor ('gestational thyrotoxicosis'). In the post-partum period, thyrotoxicosis may be due to post-partum thyroiditis (self-resolving) or a recurrence of Graves' disease (requires treatment). Measurement of anti-TSH receptor antibody levels may be indicated to distinguish these possibilities.

Thyroid storm

This is defined as severe thyrotoxicosis with confusion/delirium not explained by other factors. There is no definitive test and levels of thyroid hormone are not higher than in other individuals with no features of storm. Severe agitation, tachycardia and hyperpyrexia are usually seen. Usually precipitated by infection, trauma or surgery, especially to the thyroid gland. Very rare but tends to occur in individuals who have been poorly compliant in the first few weeks of drug therapy for thyrotoxicosis.

Anti-TSH receptor antibody testing

This test is not routinely available in most labs. Although it is positive in >90% of cases of Graves' disease, in most cases it does not alter clinical management. Indications include distinguishing gestational thyrotoxicosis or post-partum thyroiditis from Graves' disease, indicating the risk of neonatal thyrotoxicosis and (controversial) predicting recurrence after a course of thionamide drug therapy.

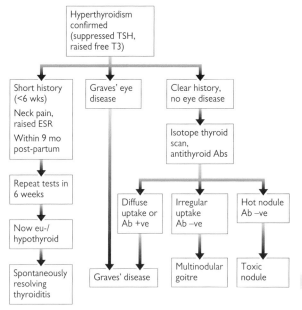

Fig. 2.13 Investigation of the cause of hyperthyroidism.

📖OHCM p294.

Hypothyroidism

Clinical features

Classic clinical features of hypothyroidism include weight gain, cold intolerance, dry skin, constipation, memory loss, lethargy/slow thought/'slowing up', menorrhagia, periorbital/facial oedema, loss of outer two-thirds of eye brows, deafness, chest pain and coma. Rarely seen nowadays as thyroid function tests are easy to perform and detect the disease usually at an earlier stage. Weight gain, dry skin and lethargy are frequently reported, but even in biochemically hypothyroid individuals can only confidently be ascribed to thyroid status if they reverse on treatment.

Biochemical diagnosis

↑ TSH with T4 in the normal range is referred to as subclinical hypothyroidism. ↑ TSH with ↓ T4 is overt hypothyroidism. ↓ T4 with TSH in the normal range may be due to pituitary failure (2° hypothyroidism) and if

141

persistent requires pituitary function testing. See Fig. 2.14 for other patterns of thyroid function tests.

Differential diagnosis (causes)

In iodine sufficient countries, the vast majority of spontaneous hypothyroidism is due to autoimmune thyroiditis (Hashimoto's disease if goitre present, atrophic thyroiditis if goitre absent)—antithyroid antibodies present in 80–90% of cases. Other common causes are post-thyroidectomy, post-radioiodine therapy and side effects of amiodarone or lithium. Rarer causes include treatment with cytokines (e.g. interferons, GM-CSF, interleukin-2), vast excess iodine intake (iodine drops, water purifying tablets), congenital hypothyroidism (caused by a variety of genetic defects, should be detected by neonatal screening programme), iodine deficiency (urinary iodide excretion <45µg/day, commonest cause worldwide esp. mountainous areas, S Germany, Greece, Paraguay—'endemic goitre'), thyroid-blocking substances in the indigenous diet (goitrogens esp. in brassicas and cassava, e.g. in Sheffield, Spain, Bohemia, Kentucky, Virginia, Tasmania—'endogenous goitre' without iodine deficiency), Pendred's syndrome (mild hypothyroidism with sensineural deafness due to Mondini cochlear defect, positive perchlorate discharge test). For transient hypothyroidism—see below.

▶▶Diagnostic catches

↑ TSH and ↓ T4 always represents hypothyroidism. If the TSH alone is ↑ and the T4 is not even slightly low, a heterophile antibody interfering in the TSH assay may be present in the patient's serum. This is especially likely if there is no change in TSH level after thyroxine treatment but the T4 level rises (confirming compliance with tablets). For unusual patterns of thyroid function tests, see Fig. 2.14. Note that within the first 1–3 months (or longer) after treatment of hyperthyroidism, profound hypothyroidism may develop with a ↓ T4 but the TSH may still be suppressed or only mildly raised due to the long period of TSH suppression prior to treatment. Raised TSH alone with disproportionate symptoms of lethargy may be seen in hypoadrenalism. If suspected treat with steroids first as thyroxine may precipitate an Addisonian crisis.

Transient hypothyroidism

Transient or self-resolving hypothyroidism, often preceded by hyperthyroidism, is seen in viral thyroiditis, after pregnancy (post-partum thyroiditis) and in some individuals with autoimmune thyroiditis (positive antithyroid antibodies). Treatment temporarily with thyroxine is only required if the patient is very symptomatic. Thyroid function should return to normal within 6 months. Hypothyroidism may also be transient in the first 6 months after radioiodine therapy.

Subclinical hypothyroidism

A raised TSH (<20mU/L) with normal T4/T3 is very common and seen in 5–10% of women and ~2% of males. It is usually due to subclinical autoimmune thyroid disease and is frequently discovered on routine testing. In randomised trials, ~20% of patients obtain psychological benefit from beginning T4 therapy, in many others it is probably truly asymptomatic. If antithyroid antibodies are detectable, the rate of progression to overt hypothyroidism is ~50% at 20 years, but higher than this with higher initial TSH levels. If the TSH alone is raised with negative antibodies (or the TSH is normal with raised antibodies alone), overt hypothyroidism develops in 25% at 20 years. A reasonable approach is a trial of thyroxine

	Low **TSH**	Normal **TSH**	Raised **TSH**
Raised FT4/FT3	*Low TSH, raised FT4/FT3* Thyrotoxicosis	*Normal TSH, raised FT3/FT4 (rare)* TSH-secreting pituitary tumour Thyroid hormone resistance (receptor defect) Intermittent T4 therapy/acute overdose Interfering anti-T4/T3 antibody Familial dysalbuminaemic hyperthyroxinaemia Acute psychiatric illness	
Normal FT4/FT3	*Low TSH, normal FT4/FT3* Subclinical thyrotoxicosis Thyroxine ingestion Steroid therapy Non-thyroidal illness Dopamine infusion	*Normal*	*Raised TSH, normal FT4/FT3* Subclinical hypothyroidism Poor compliance with T4 therapy Interfering (heterophile) antibody Recovery from non-thyroidal illness Hypoadrenalism
Low FT4/FT3	*Low/normal TSH, low FT4/FT3* Non-thyroidal illness Pituitary failure Recent (excessive) treatment for hyperthyroidism		*Raised TSH, low FT4* Hypothyroidism

143

Note: free thyroid hormone assays are assumed—effects of changes in binding proteins on total thyroid hormone assays are not included.

(adapted from Dayan CM (2001) Interpretation of thyroid function tests. *Lancet* **357**: 619–24)

Fig. 2.14 Patterns of thyroid function tests.

for 6 months in symptomatic patients with subclinical hypothyroidism or TSH >10mU/L, and observing the TSH level at 6–12-monthly intervals in asymptomatic patients with TSH <10mU/L.

Hypothyroidism and pregnancy

Overt hypothyroidism is associated with poor obstetric outcomes. Recent evidence suggests that subclinical hypothyroidism is associated with a slight reduction in the baby's IQ and should be treated. Many authorities advocate screening for hypothyroidism in all antenatal patients as early as possible in pregnancy. Patients on T4 need to increase their dose by 50μg from the first trimester of pregnancy. Maternal thyroxine can compensate for fetal thyroid failure *in utero* but congenital hypothyroidism must be detected at birth (screening test) to avoid mental retardation developing. Where the mother and fetus are both hypothyroid—most commonly due to iodine deficiency—mental retardation can develop *in utero* (cretinisim). Note that mothers with positive antithyroid antibodies and/or subclinical hypothyroidism have a 50% chance of developing (transient) post-partum thyroiditis.

📖OHCM p296.

Diabetes mellitus

Glycosuria

Urine testing is a valuable pointer to diabetes mellitus (DM) but is insufficient to establish the diagnosis. Although modern glucose oxidase test strips are free from interference by other reducing substances, glycosuria does not always indicate DM; the converse also pertains. Thus, glycosuria has low sensitivity and specificity.

Causes of glycosuria
- DM.
- Impaired glucose tolerance (IGT).
- Lowered renal threshold for glucose (esp. pregnancy, children).

Note: Fluid intake, urine concentration and certain drugs may influence results

The diagnosis of DM relies on the demonstration of unequivocally elevated blood glucose levels that can be
- Casual (random)—usually the first line investigation.
- Fasting plasma glucose (FPG)—an alternative to a casual reading.
- 75g oral glucose challenge—if necessary.

▶Neither the confirmation nor exclusion of DM should rest on measurement of longer term indicators of glycaemia such as glycated haemoglobin or fructosamine. Although of high specificity, these tests are not sufficiently standardised nor do they have sufficient sensitivity. False negative results are particularly likely with less marked degrees of hyperglycaemia, especially in subjects with IGT or IFG.

Blood glucose

A blood glucose measurement is the essential investigation in the diagnosis of DM. A glucose-specific assay is required. An appropriate sample must be collected, usually venous plasma (in a tube containing fluoride oxalate as an inhibitor of glycolysis) and the sample tested without undue delay in an accredited laboratory.

Reagent test strips

Although convenient and readily available, reagent test strips for monitoring of capillary glucose (even when used in conjunction with a calibrated reflectance meter) are unsuitable for diagnosing DM; a confirmatory laboratory measurement must therefore always be performed. In the absence of typical symptoms the diagnosis should be confirmed by a repeat measurement on a separate day; this may be either a casual or FPG sample.

▶Confirmation of the diagnosis is especially important in asymptomatic individuals.

An oral glucose tolerance test (OGTT) is rarely required to confirm the diagnosis and should not be regarded as a first line investigation. The OGTT is time consuming, requires trained staff and is less reproducible than FPG.

Revised diagnostic criteria for diagnosis of diabetes mellitus	
Random plasma glucose	>11.1mmol/L
FPG	> 7.0mmol/L

▶The diagnostic FPG is lower than the previous National Diabetes Data Group (1979) and WHO (1980, 1985) criteria which specified a diagnostic fasting plasma glucose >7.8mmol/L.

The 1997 criteria introduced the new intermediate category of impaired fasting glucose (IFG) defined as:

• FPG 6.1–6.9 mmol/L.

False +ve diagnoses may arise if the subject has prepared inadequately (*see table below*). This possibility is more likely following the reduction in the diagnostic threshold for diabetes based on FPG in the 1997 revised criteria.

Preparation for a fasting blood test
Refrain from any food or drink from midnight before the morning of the test.
Water only is permitted.
Regular medication can generally be deferred until the blood sample has been taken.
The appropriate sample is taken between 0800 and 0900h the following morning.

This preparation is also required for a 75g oral OGTT or for measurement of fasting blood lipids. Fasting blood tests should be avoided in insulin-treated patients—risk of hypoglycaemia.

Impaired glucose tolerance

The diagnosis of IGT can only be made using a 75g oral glucose tolerance test; a random blood glucose measurement will often point to the diagnosis when other results are non-diagnostic.

This category denotes a stage intermediate between normal glucose levels and DM (□OHCM, section 9). By definition, plasma glucose levels are not raised to DM levels so typical osmotic symptoms are absent. Although subjects with IGT are not at direct risk of developing chronic microvascular tissue complications, the incidence of macrovascular complications (i.e. CHD, CVD, PAD) is increased. Presentation with one of these conditions should therefore alert the clinician to the possibility of undiagnosed IGT (or type 2 DM). Note that a proportion of individuals who are diagnosed by an OGTT may revert to normal on re-testing.

Impaired fasting glucose

If an OGTT is performed, the 120min glucose concentration must be <7.8mmol/L. This category is also usually asymptomatic. To date, cross-sectional studies suggest that IGT and IFG may not be synonymous in terms of pathophysiology and long-term implications.

Oral glucose tolerance test

The OGTT (see table below) continues to be regarded as the most robust means for establishing the diagnosis of diabetes in equivocal cases. The WHO suggests that only when an OGTT cannot be performed should the diagnosis rely on FPG. OGTTs should be carried out under controlled conditions after an overnight fast.

Oral glucose tolerance test
Anhydrous glucose is dissolved in 250ml water; flavouring with sugar-free lemon and chilling increase palatibility and may reduce nausea. The subjecrt sits quietly throughout the test.
Blood glucose is sampled before (time 0) and at 120min after ingestion of the drink, which should be completed within 5min. Urinalysis may also be performed every 30min although is only of interest if a significant alteration in renal threshold for glucose is suspected.

The interpretation of the 75g glucose tolerance test is shown in the table below. These results apply to venous plasma. Marked carbohydrate depletion can impair glucose tolerance; the subject should have received adequate nutrition in the days preceding the test.

Effect of intercurrent illness on glycaemia

Patients under the physical stress associated with surgery, trauma, acute MI, acute pulmonary oedema or stroke may have transient ↑ of plasma glucose—often settles rapidly without antidiabetic therapy. However, the hormonal stress response in such clinical situations is liable to unmask pre-existing DM or to precipitate DM in predisposed individuals. Blood glucose should be carefully monitored and urine tested for ketones. Sustained hyperglycaemia, particularly with ketonuria, demands vigorous treatment with insulin in an acutely ill patient.

Interpretation of the 75g oral glucose tolerance test

	Venous plasma glucose (mmol/L)		
	Fasting		120min post-glucose load
Normal	<6.0		<7.8
IFG	6.1–6.9		<7.8
IGT	6.1–6.9	and/or	7.8–11.0
DM	>7.0		>11.1

Notes:
1. In the absence of symptoms a diagnosis of diabetes must be confirmed by a second diagnostic test on a separate day. 2. For capillary whole blood, the diagnostic cutoffs for diabetes are >6.1mmol/lL (fasting) and 11.1mmol/L (120min). The range for impaired fasting glucose based on capillary whole blood is >5.6 and <6.1mmo/L.

Acute myocardial infarction (📖*OHCM section 5)*
Hyperglycaemia at presentation is associated with a higher mortality—even in subjects with previously undiagnosed DM; tight metabolic control using an intravenous insulin-dextrose infusion (followed by subcutaneous insulin) significantly reduced mortality in a recent multicentre Swedish study.

Stroke (📖*OHCM section 10)*
Hyperglycaemia on admission may be associated with a poorer outcome; however, there is no clinical trial evidence to date that intensive control of hyperglycaemia improves prognosis.

147

Re-testing is usually indicated following resolution of the acute illness—an OGTT at a 4–6-week interval is recommended if glucose levels are equivocal.

📖OHCM p282.

Diabetes websites

American Diabetes Association
⌕ http://www.diabetes.org

Diabetes UK (formerly British Diabetic Association)
⌕ http://www.diabetes.org.uk

Alberti KGMM, Zimmet PZ for the WHO consultations. (1998) Definition, diagnosis and classification of diabetes mellitus and its complications. Part 1. Diagnosis and classification of diabetes mellitus. Provisional report of a WHO consultation. *Diabetic Med* **15**, 539–553; Davies M. (1999) New diagnostic criteria for diabetes – are they doing what they should? *Lancet* **354**, 610–611;

Wareham NJ, O'Rahilly S. (1998) The changing classification and diagnosis of diabetes. *BMJ* **317**, 359–360; Yudkin JS. (1998) Managing the diabetic patient with acute myocardial infarction. *Diabetic Med* **15**, 276–281.

Potential diagnostic difficulties of DM

Type 1 DM

- This is diagnosed principally on clinical and biochemical features (□OHCM section 12). The presence of serum islet cell antibodies (ICA, in ~30–60% of patients) at diagnosis may confirm the diagnosis. The proportion of patients testing positive for ICA ↓ with increasing duration of type 1 DM. If there is doubt, treat with insulin if indicated on clinical and biochemical criteria; the need for insulin can be considered at a later date. However, discontinuation of insulin can be disastrous in patients with type 1 DM. The decision to stop insulin should be made only by an experienced diabetologist. ▶A –ve test for ICA does *not* necessarily exclude type 1 DM.
- Other humoral markers of autoimmunity, e.g. anti-GAD65 antibodies, anti-insulin antibodies, are generally only available in research laboratories.
- Stiff man syndrome: rare condition presenting as a progressive spastic paraparesis with polyglandular endocrine involvement (□p246). Anti-GAD65 antibodies are present; approximately 30% of patients develop insulin-requiring DM.
- MODY: a small percentage of young patients with relatively minor hyperglycaemia and no ketonuria, will prove to have relatively uncommon inherited forms of DM, e.g. MODY. Such patients often receive insulin therapy from diagnosis, the assumption being that they have type 1 DM. *Prerequisites for the diagnosis include:*
  - A family history with an autosomal dominant inheritance.
  - Diagnosis under the age of 25 years.
  In some subtypes of MODY (glucokinase mutations; MODY 2), good glycaemic control may be maintained life-long without insulin or even oral antidiabetic agents. The exception is pregnancy; insulin may be required temporarily in order to ensure optimal control—oral antidiabetic agents should be avoided. The diagnosis of MODY may be confirmed by molecular genetic testing although presently this is not widely available. Appropriate counselling is required. Seek expert advice through your local hospital diabetes unit.
- Early-onset type 2 diabetes—In recent years there has been a dramatic increase in the incidence of type 2 diabetes in younger patients (children and adolescents) from non-white ethnic minorities. This may present diagnostic difficulties but some pointers suggest the diagnosis:
  - Obesity is usually a prominent feature.
  - Serum autoantibody tests for type 1 DM are negative.
  - A skin marker of insulin resistance (acanthosis nigricans) may be present.

If in doubt, it is usually safer to treat younger patients with insulin; this is especially true if ketosis is present.

Monitoring diabetic control

Self-testing by diabetic patients
Self-testing of urine and/or capillary blood glucose testing can readily be performed by the majority of patients. Measurements of longer term gly-

caemic control are laboratory-based or require specialised techniques generally suitable only for use in a hospital clinic.

Urine testing

Glycosuria: Semiquantitative testing for glucose using reagent-impregnated test strips by patients is of limited value. Urinalysis provides retrospective information over a limited period of time. Other limitations:

- The renal threshold for the reabsorption of glucose in the PCT is ~10mmol/L on average but varies between individuals. Subjects with a low threshold will tend to show glycosuria more readily, even with normal glucose tolerance ('renal glycosuria'). Children are particularly liable to test positive for glucose. The renal threshold is effectively lowered in pregnancy. Conversely, a high threshold, common among the elderly, may give a misleadingly reassuring impression of satisfactory control. Fluid intake and urine concentration may affect glycosuria. Renal impairment may elevate the threshold for glucose reabsorption.
- Delayed bladder emptying, e.g. due to diabetic autonomic neuropathy (OHCM section 9), will reduce the accuracy of the measurements through dilution.
- Hypoglycaemia cannot be detected by urinalysis.

Ketonuria: Semiquantitative test strips for acetocetate (e.g. Ketostix®) are available for patients with type 1 DM. Useful when intercurrent illness leads to disturbance of metabolic control. The presence of ketonuria on dipstick testing in association with hyperglycaemia indicates marked insulin deficiency (absolute, or more commonly, relative). Increased doses of insulin are indicated in such circumstances to avert more severe metabolic decompensation (DKA, *see below* and OHCM section 21). Occasionally, patients with type 2 DM develop ketosis during severe intercurrent illness, e.g. major sepsis. Neither Ketostix® nor Acetest® tablets detect 3-hydroxybutyrate (although acetone is detected by Acetest®). Occasional underestimation of the degree of ketonaemia using these tests is a well-recognized, albeit uncommon caveat of alcoholic ketoacidosis (OHCM section 9).

149

Self-testing of blood glucose

Self-testing of capillary blood glucose obtained by fingerprick has become an established method for monitoring glycaemic control. Frequent testing is a prerequisite for safe intensive insulin therapy such as that employed in the DCCT. Enzyme-impregnated dry strip methods are available which can be used in conjunction with meter devices to improve accuracy. Most are based on the glucose oxidase reaction:

$$\text{Glucose} + O_2 \xrightarrow[\text{oxidase}]{\text{Glucose}} \text{Gluconic acid} + H_2O_2$$

The hydrogen peroxide generated by the reaction reacts with a reduced dye in the test strip producing an oxidised colour proportional to the amount of H_2O_2 formed. This reflects the amount of glucose that was oxidised. In most strips, blood cells are excluded by a layer within the strip. Thus, the glucose concentration in capillary plasma is measured. Adequate training and a system of quality control are important; even when trained health professionals use such systems in clinics or hospitals misleading results are possible, particularly in the lower range of blood glucose results. Where there is doubt, an appropriate sample (in a tube containing the glycolysis inhibitor fluoride oxalate) should be collected immediately for analysis by the clinical chemistry laboratory. However, acute treatment of hypoglycaemia, where indicated, should not be delayed.

Laboratory assessment of glycaemic control

Glycated haemoglobin

HbA$_{1c}$ (comprises 60–80% total glycated haemoglobin, HbA$_1$) is formed by the slow, irreversible, post-translational non-enzymatic glycation of the N-terminal valine residue of the β chain of haemoglobin. In retina and renal glomerulus this process is implicated in the pathogenesis of the long-term complications of diabetes ($\square$OHCM section 9). The proportion of HbA$_{1c}$: total haemoglobin (normal non-diabetic reference range approximately 4–6%) provides a useful index of average glycaemia over the preceding 6–8 weeks. The result is disproportionately affected by the blood glucose levels during the final month before the test (~50% of value). Average HbA$_{1c}$ levels collected over a longer period (i.e. years) provide an estimate of the risk of microvascular complications. Sustained high concentrations identify patients in whom efforts should be made to improve long-term glycaemic control.

In patients with type 1 DM, a landmark randomised, controlled clinical trial (the DCCT) confirmed a causal link between degree of metabolic control and the development and progression of microvascular complications of diabetes (especially retinopathy) and neuropathy. Consensus panels in the USA and Europe have suggested targets for HbA$_{1c}$ of approximately 7–8% for most patients (if circumstances and frequency of hypoglycaemia allow). By contrast, tight glycaemic control may be contraindicated by advanced complications, e.g. clinical nephropathy with renal impairment. It is recommended that HbA$_{1c}$ should be measured every 6 months in younger patients with type 1 DM. Pregnancy requires monthly monitoring of HbA$_{1c}$ concentrations (although other measures may be preferable in pregnancy—see below: *fructosamine*). Blood can be collected by venesection ahead of the clinic visit (in primary care, by the hospital phlebotomy service or even by a nurse in the community if necessary). Alternatives include rapid assays for use in the clinic, or self-collection in advance of a fingerprick sample (in a capillary tube or on filter paper) which is mailed to the laboratory.

Goldstein DE, Little RR, Lorenz RA *et al.* (1995) Tests of glycemia in diabetes *Diabetes Care* **18**, 896–909.

Limitations of HBA$_{1c}$ measurements

Although glycated haemoglobin levels are a reliable indicator of recent average glycaemic control they do not provide information about the daily pattern of blood glucose levels; this supplementary information required for logical adjustment of insulin doses is derived from home blood glucose monitoring (*see below*). More recent changes in glycaemia (i.e. within the preceding 4 weeks or so) will influence HbA$_{1c}$ level more than glucose levels 12 or more weeks ago.

Spurious HbA$_{1c}$ levels may arise in states of
- Blood loss/haemolysis/reduced red cell survival (low HbA$_{1c}$).
- Haemoglobinopathy (□OHCM section 16).
- ↑ levels of HbS.
- ↑ levels of HbF (high HbA$_{1c}$).

Uraemia due to advanced diabetic nephropathy is associated with anaemia and ↓ RBC survival thereby falsely lowering HbA$_{1c}$ levels.

Fructosamine: refers to protein-ketoamine products resulting from the glycation of plasma proteins. The fructosamine assay measures glycated plasma proteins (mainly albumin) reflecting average glycaemia over the preceding 2–3 weeks. This is a shorter period than that assessed using glycated haemoglobin measurements and may be particularly useful when rapid changes in control need to be assessed, e.g. during pregnancy. Levels can be misleading in hypoalbuminaemic states, e.g. nephrotic syndrome (□OHCM section 8). Some fructosamine assays are subject to interference by hyperuricaemia or hyperlipidaemia. Measurements of fructosamine are less expensive than glycated haemoglobin assays; this may be an important consideration for some laboratory services. The methodology is suitable for automation and rapid results can be obtained for use within a clinic attendance obviating the requirement for a prior blood test.

151

►►Diabetic emergencies: diabetic ketoacidosis, hyperosmolar non-ketotic syndrome & lactic acidosis

Diabetic ketoacidosis (DKA) should be considered in any unconscious or hyperventilating patient. The hyperosmolar non-ketotic (HONK) syndrome is characterised by marked hyperglycaemia and dehydration in

The Diabetes Control and Complications Trial Research Group. (1993) The effect of intensive treatment of diabetes on the development and progression of long-term complications in insulin-dependent diabetes mellitus. *NEJM* **329**, 977–986; UK Prospective Diabetes Study Group. (1998) Intensive blood glucose control with sulphonylureas or insulin compared with conventional treatment and the risk of complications in patients with type 2 diabetes mellitus (UKPDS 33). *Lancet* **352**, 837–853.

the absence of significant ketosis or acidosis. Lactic acidosis (LA) associated with metformin is uncommon. A rapid clinical examination and bedside blood and urine tests should allow the diagnosis to be made (📖OHCM, section 12). Treatment (IV rehydration, insulin, electrolyte replacement) of these metabolic emergencies should be commenced without delay (see reference for details).

Confirm diagnosis by bedside measurement of
- Capillary blood glucose (glucose-oxidase reagent test strip; 📖p144).
- Urinary dipstick for glucose and ketones (e.g. Ketostix®). Note: nitro-prusside tests detect acetoacetate, but not 3-hydroxybutyrate. This may be relevant in some circumstances, e.g. alcoholic ketoacidosis (see below). Venous plasma may also be tested for ketones.
- Urine for nitrites and leucocytes (UTI).

Venous blood for urgent laboratory measurement of
- Plasma glucose (fluoride-oxalate; ▶true 'euglycaemic' DKA is rare).
- U&E (arterial K^+ can be measured by some gas analysers). Plasma Na^+ may be depressed as a consequence of hyperglycaemia or marked hyperlipidaemia.
- Plasma creatinine (▶may be falsely elevated in some assays by DKA).
- Plasma lactate (if indicated—can also be measured by some gas analysers). Indicated if acidosis without heavy ketonuria is present. LA is a complication of tissue hypoxia (type A) and is a rare complication of metformin treatment in patients with type 2 DM (type B).
- Plasma osmolality in HONK—either by freezing point depression or calculated: $2 \times$ [plasma Na^+] + [plasma K^+] + [plasma glucose] + [plasma urea].
- FBC (non-specific leucocytosis is common in DKA).
- Blood cultures (signs of infection, e.g. fever, may be absent in DKA).
- ABGs (corrected for hypothermia) for:
  - Arterial pH, bicarbonate, PCO_2 and PO_2 (if shock or hypotension).

Repeat laboratory measurement of blood glucose, electrolytes, urea at 2, 4 and 6h and as indicated thereafter. Electrolyte disturbances, renal impairment or oliguria should prompt more frequent (1–2 hourly) measurements of plasma K^+. Capillary blood glucose is monitored hourly at the bedside.
▶Avoidance of hypokalaemia and hypoglycaemia are most important during therapy.

Other investigations, as indicated
- CXR.
- Microbial culture of urine, sputum, etc.
- ECG (acute MI may precipitate metabolic decompensation; note that serum transaminases and CK may be non-specifically elevated in DKA).
- Sickle cell test (in selected patients; 📖OHCM section 13).
- Venous plasma PO_4^{3-} (if there is respiratory depression).
▶Performance of investigations should not delay initiation of treatment and transfer to a high-dependency or intensive care unit.

A severe metabolic acidosis in the absence of hyperglycaemia (or other obvious cause of acidosis such as renal failure) raises the possibility of
- Lactic acidosis.

• Alcoholic ketoacidosis—this occurs in alcoholics following a binge. Alterations in hepatic redox state may result in a misleading negative or 'trace' Ketostix® reaction. A similar caveat may occasionally be encountered when significant LA coexists with DKA. Venous plasma glucose may be normal or ↑.

▶Anion gap (📖p432) >15mmol/L. Normally, the anion gap (<10mmol/L) results from plasma proteins, SO_4^{2-}, PO_4^{3-} and lactate ions. When the anion gap is increased, measurement of plasma ketones, lactate, etc. usually confirms the aetiology.

Causes of an anion gap acidosis	
Ketoacidosis	Diabetic ketoacidosis
	Alcoholic ketoacidosis
	Lactic acidosis (▶metformin)
Chronic renal failure	
Drug toxicity	Methanol (metabolised ⟶ formic acid)
	Ethylene glycol (metabolised ⟶ oxalic acid)
	Salicylate poisoning

Krentz AJ, Nattrass M. (1997) Acute metabolic complications of diabetes: diabetic ketoacidosis, hyperosmolar non-ketotic syndrome and lactic acidosis, in *Textbook of Diabetes*, eds Pickup J, Williams G, Oxford, Blackwell Science.

Investigation of hyperlipidaemia

Primary dyslipidaemias are relatively common and contribute to an individual's risk of developing atheroma (e.g. CHD, CVD). Prominent examples include familial combined hyperlipidaemia (FCHL, ~2–3% of UK population) and heterozygous familial hypercholesterolaemia (FH, UK incidence 1 in 500). Major hypertriglyceridaemia also predisposes to pancreatitis. The key features of familial FH, FCHL and diabetic dyslipidaemia are considered later.

Investigations
Although many subtle alterations in plasma lipids have been described, therapeutic decisions rest on measurement of some or all of the following in serum or plasma (plasma being preferred since it can be cooled rapidly):
• Total cholesterol (may be measured in non-fasting state in first instance since levels are not greatly influenced by meals).
• Triglycerides (after 12h fast).
• Low-density lipoprotein (LDL)-cholesterol (calculated using the Friedewald formula when triglycerides are <4.5mmol/L):

$$\text{LDL-cholesterol} = \text{total cholesterol} - \text{HDL-cholesterol} - \text{triglycerides}$$
$$2.9$$

- HDL-cholesterol (regarded as the 'cardioprotective' subfraction—HDL particles are synthesised in the gut and liver and thought to be involved in 'reverse transport' of cholesterol from peripheral tissues to the liver where it can be excreted as bile salts.

Notes on sampling in relation to lipoprotein metabolism
- Triglycerides (triacylglycerols) are measured after a ~12h overnight fast in order to clear diet-derived chylomicrons.
- Alcohol should be avoided the evening prior to measurement of triglycerides (can exacerbate hypertriglyceridaemia).
- A weight-maintaining diet is recommended for 2–3 weeks before testing.
- Lipid measurements should be deferred for 2–3 weeks after minor illness and 2–3 months after major illness, surgery or trauma since cholesterol may be temporarily ↓ and triglycerides ↑. Following acute myocardial infarction it is generally accepted that plasma cholesterol is reliable if measured within 24h of the onset of symptoms.
- The effects of certain drugs on lipids should be considered (*see table*).
- Glycaemic control should be optimised wherever possible before measuring plasma lipids in patients with diabetes.

Important additional considerations are
- Day-to-day variability—generally, decisions to treat hyperlipidaemia should be based on more than one measurement over a period of 1–2 weeks.
- Exclusion of secondary hyperlipidaemia—many common conditions, drugs and dietary factors can influence plasma lipids (*see table*).
- Family members should also have their plasma lipids measured if a familial hyperlipidaemia is suspected in a proband.

Both cholesterol and triglycerides may be affected to some degree by these factors, but one often predominates. Pre-existing primary hyperlipidaemias may be exacerbated.

Clinical features
E.g. xanthelasma, tendon xanthomas, etc. should always be sought. A detailed family history, drug history and medical history (for diabetes and other cardiovascular risk factors such as hypertension) should always be obtained. Certain endocrine disorders, impaired hepatic or renal function can influence circulating lipid composition and cardiovascular risk. A classification of the major familial dyslipidaemias is presented in the table below (p.156).

▶ Specialist advice should be sought in the management of major or resistant hyperlipidaemias.

Jialal I. (1994) Dyslipidaemias and their investigation, in *Diagnostic Tests in Endocrinology and Diabetes*, eds Bouloux P-MG, Ree LH, Chapman & Hall Medical, London; Frayn KN. (1996) *Metabolic Regulation – a Human Perspective*, Portland Press, London; (1998) Joint British recommendations on prevention of coronary heart disease in clinical practice. *Heart* **80** (suppl 2), S1–S29; National Cholesterol Education Program (NCEP) expert panel on detection, evaluation and treatment of high blood cholesterol in adults (adult treatment panel III). (2001) Executive summary of the 3rd report. *JAMA* **285**, 2486–2497.

Causes of secondary hyperlipidaemia

Hypercholesterolaemia

Hypothyroidism (even minor degrees of 1° hypothyroidism)

Cholestasis (note: lipoprotein X)

Nephrotic syndrome

Anorexia nervosa

Diuretics

Immunosuppressive agents

Hepatoma

Dysglobulinaemias

Hypertriglyceridaemia

Obesity

Diabetes (esp. type 2 DM)

Lipodytrophic syndromes (of diabetes and HIV-associated)

Alcohol excess (moderate alcohol consumption may raise HDL-cholesterol)

Renal failure

Antiretroviral agents

Oestrogens (esp. oral preparations in some women)

Corticosteroids

Beta-adrenergic blockers

Retinoids

Recommended investigation for exclusion of 2° hyperlipidaemia: ● U&E ● plasma creatinine ● fasting venous glucose ● LFTs ● TFTs. For patients on statins check ● LFTs ● CK periodically (► measure urgently if myositis occurs—a rare but potentially fatal complication).

155

Test protocols

Insulin tolerance test (insulin stress test)

Indication: suspected ACTH or GH deficiency.

Contraindications: patients with epilepsy, coronary heart disease (check ECG).

Children: use no more than 0.1U/kg. Considerable care should be exercised; the test should only be performed in a centre with expertise.

Alternatives: short synacthen test for hypocortisolism; stimulation tests for growth hormone deficiency (☐see p104).

Preparation: patient fasting overnight. Bed required (though day case procedure). Patient must be accompanied home and may not drive. OMIT morning hydrocortisone or other steroid hormone replacement if patient is taking this and previous day's growth hormone. Physician must be present throughout the test. Requires written consent.

Procedure: early morning outpatient test in fasting patient. Indwelling venous cannula and constant medical supervision required throughout. Cannula is kept patent by running saline infusion with three-way tap for

Familial hyperlipoproteinaemias

Genetic disorder	Defect	Presentation	Cholesterol	Triglycerides	Phenotype
Familial LPL deficiency	Absence of LPL activity	Eruptive xanthomata hepatosplenomegaly	↑	↑↑↑	I
Familial apo C-II deficiency	Absence of apo C-II	Pancreatitis	↑	↑↑↑	I or V
Familial hyper-cholesterolaemia	LDL receptor deficiency	Tendon xanthomata premature atheroma	↑↑↑	↑ or N	IIa or IIb
Familial dysbeta-lipoproteinaemia	Abnormal apo E and defect in TG metabolism	Tubo-eruptive and palmar xanthoma; premature atheroma	↑↑↑	↑↑↑	III
Familial combined hyperlipidaemia	Uncertain	Premature atheroma	↑ or N	↑ or N	IIa, IIb or IV
Familial hypertriglyceridaemia	Uncertain Eruptive xanthomata hepatosplenomegaly; pancreatitis		N ↑	↑ ↑↑↑	IV V

↑, ↑↑ and ↑↑↑, mildly, moderately or severely raised; cholesterol and triglycerides refers to concentrations in plasma; phenotype refers to Fredrickson classification (I to V, see table below); apo, apoprotein; LPL, lipoprotein lipase; N, normal; TG, triglycerides.

Phenotypic (Fredrickson) classification of hyperlipidaemias

Type	Cholesterol	Triglycerides	Particle excess	Usual underlying cause
I	↑	↑↑↑	Chylomicrons	LPL or apo C-II deficiency
IIa	↑↑	N	LDL	LDL receptor defect / LDL overproduction
IIb	↑↑	↑↑	VLDL, LDL	VLDL or LDL overproduction or ↓ clearance
III	↑	↑↑↑	Chlyomicron and VLDL remnants	Impaired remnant removal may be due to certain apo E phenotypes or apo E deficiency
IV	N or ↑	↑↑	VLDL	VLDL overproduction or ↓ clearance
V	↑	↑↑↑	Chylomicrons VLDL remnants	LPL defect, apo C-II deficiency

↑, ↑↑ and ↑↑↑, mildly, moderately or severely raised; LDL, low-density lipoprotein; VLDL, very-low-density lipoprotein; LPL, lipoprotein lipase; apo, apoprotein.

sampling. Discard initial 2–3mL when each sample is taken. Label all samples clearly with time and patient details. Near-patient testing glucometer required.

1. Take baseline blood for glucose, cortisol and GH. Check IV access working well. Review test with the patient and explain symptoms he/she is likely to experience (see 5 below).
2. Draw up 25mL of 50% dextrose for immediate administration IF REQUIRED.
3. Give soluble (regular) insulin as an intravenous bolus in a dose of 0.15U/kg after an overnight fast. Consider 0.1U/kg (lower dose) if suspected profound hypocortisolism. ►This appears a very small dose, e.g. typically around 10 units. CHECK DOSE CALCULATION CAREFULLY. Usually an insulin syringe is used to draw it up and then transfer it to a 2mL syringe containing saline.
4. Take blood at 15min intervals (0, 15, 30, 45, 60min) for glucose, cortisol and GH.
5. Observe for symptoms and signs of hypoglycaemia. First sign is usually profuse sweating. Patient may then be aware of symptoms such as palpitations, hunger, paraesthesiae. This typically occurs 30–45min into the test. Check near-patient glucose to confirm <3.5mmol/L. Continue to talk to and reassure patient. If patient becomes very drowsy or unrousable then given 25mL of 50% glucose. This does not invalidate the test as the hypoglycaemic stimulus has already occurred. Continue blood sampling at standard times.
6. If patient has not experienced hypoglycaemia by 45min and near-patient glucose is >4mmol/L, give a further intravenous bolus of 0.15U/kg or 0.3U/kg if patient known to be very insulin resistant (e.g. acromegalic). Repeat sampling at 15min intervals for 60min after this second bolus.
7. At end of procedure (usually 60min), give IV 25mL dextrose if patient still has symptoms of hypoglycaemia.
8. Give patient a meal including complex carbohydrate (e.g. sandwiches or lunch) and observe for a minimum of 1h further before accompanied discharge.

Unwanted effects: severe hypoglycaemia with depressed level of consciousness or convulsion requires immediate termination of test with 25mL of 50% dextrose IV. Repeat if necessary and follow with 5 or 10% dextrose infusion. Continue to collect samples for hormone and glucose measurements.

Interpretation: test is only interpretable if adequate hypoglycaemia is achieved (<2.2mmol/L). Normal maximal cortisol response >550nmol/L. Normal GH response >20mU/L. Impaired responses (if hypoglycaemic stimulus adequate) denote corticotrophin (assuming adrenal glands are normal) or GH deficiency or both. Peak GH response <10mU/L is sufficient to consider GH replacement; peak GH response <5mU/L is severe growth hormone deficiency.

Combined anterior pituitary function testing

Indication: assessment for anterior pituitary hypofunction.

Contraindications: previous reaction to stimulatory hormones.

Alternatives: insulin tolerance testing for GH and adrenal axis; metyrapone test for adrenal axis.

Preparation: test usually performed in morning for basal sampling.

Procedure: IV cannula inserted. Basal blood samples taken for cortisol, oestradiol (♀) or testosterone (♂), free T4 and IGF-1. Hypothalalmic hormones are given sequentially intravenously each as a bolus over around 20s: LHRH 100µg, TRH 200µg and ACTH 250µg. Additionally GHRH (1µg/kg body weight) may be given. (Reduce doses in children.) Samples are drawn at 0, 20, 30, 60 and 120min for LH, FSH, TSH cortisol and prolactin. If GHRH is given, samples are drawn at the same time points for GH.

Interpretation: normal values as follows:

TRH:	Suspect secondary hypothyroidism if peak response (at 20min) <20mU/L (*Note:* low levels also seen in hyperthyroidism—ensure free T4 or total T4 not raised).
ACTH:	Peak cortisol response >550nmol/L at 30 or 60min.
LHRH:	Peak LH/FSH response 2–5 × basal value.
LH:	Peak at 20min, FSH later.
GHRH:	Normal GH peak response >15mU/L.

Water deprivation test

Indication: diagnosis of diabetes insipidus (DI) and to distinguish cranial and nephrogenic diabetes insipidus.

Contraindications: none if carefully supervised. For correct interpretation, thyroid and adrenal deficiency should be replaced first. Interpretation in the presence of diabetes mellitus and uraemia can be difficult.

Alternatives: morning urine osmolality of >600mOsmol excludes significant degrees of DI. *No other definitive test for diabetes insipidus.*

Patient preparation: usually an outpatient procedure. Correct thyroid and adrenal insufficiency in advance. Renal function and blood glucose should have been checked in advance. Steroid and thyroid hormone replacement should be taken as normal on the day of the test. If the patient is on DDAVP, omit the dose on the evening before the test (or if not possible, halve this dose). Free fluids, but not too excess, up to 0730h on the day of the test. No alcohol on the night before the test or in the morning of the test. Light breakfast but no tea, coffee or smoking on the morning of the test. Empty bladder before attending for the test.

If urine volume is <3L/day ('mild cases'), ask patient to have no fluids or food from 1800h on the evening before the test ('*prolonged water deprivation test*').

Requirements for test: accurate weighing scales. Supervision for the whole test (up to 8h). DDAVP for injection (2µg). Immediate access to serum electrolyte, plasma and urinary osmolality assays. Access to a plasma AVP (ADH) assay desirable.

Procedure: 0730h
1. Weigh patient and calculate 97% of body weight.
2. Mark this target on the chart.
3. No food or fluid for next 8h.
4. Insert cannula for repeated blood sampling and flush.

0800h
5. Obtain plasma for Na^+ and osmolality and urine for osmolality.
6. Then collect urine hourly for volume and osmolality and plasma every 2h for Na^+ and osmolality.
7. Weigh patient before and after passing water if unobserved.
8. If patient loses 3% body weight, order urgent plasma osmolality and Na^+.
9. If plasma osmolality >300mOsmol (Na^+ >140mmol/L) stop test, allow patient to drink and give DDAVP (*see below*).
10. If plasma osmolality <300mOsmol, patient may have been fluid over-loaded before test and water deprivation can continue.
11. Stop test at 8h (4pm) and take final recordings of urine and plasma.
12. Save an aliquot of plasma for vaspressin levels in case of difficulties in test interpretation.
13. Ideally urine osmolalities will have reached a plateau (<30mOsmol rise between samples).
14. Now give 2µg DDAVP IM (or 20µg intranasally) and collect urine samples only for a further 2h. Allow free fluids at this stage.

Interpretation: normal response: plasma osmolality remains in the range 280–295mmol, urine osmolality rises to >2 × plasma (>600mOsmol). If urine volumes during water deprivation do not reduce and yet the plasma does not become more concentrated (rising osmolality) and weight does not fall, suspect surreptitious drinking during test. For interpretation of abnormal results see table (p107).

Diagnostic trial of DDAVP

Indication: distinction of partial diabetes insipidus from primary polydipsia.

Contraindications: cardiac failure. Current diuretic use (test uninterpretable). Note that this test may precipitate severe hyponatraemia in primary polydipsia and should be preformed in an inpatient unit with clinical and biochemical regular review.

Preparation: admission to assessment unit. First line tests for polydipsia/polyuria should have been performed (*see text*).

Procedure:
1. 24h urine volume, morning urine osmolality, weight, fluid intake (as far as possible), serum osmolality, Na^+, urea and creatinine should all be performed daily and the results reviewed the same day.
2. Subjects should have access to fluid *ad libitum* but should be reminded that they should only drink if they are thirsty.
3. After an initial 24h period of observation, desmopressin (DDAVP) is administered at a dose of 2mg bd SC for 3 days.

4. Stop test if serum Na$^+$ falls to <130mmol/L.

Interpretation: reduction in urine volume to <2L/day, ↑ in urine osmolality to >600mOsmol/L without fall in serum Na$^+$ to <140mmol/L suggests central diabetes insipidus. Reduction in urine volume with no increase in urine osmolality >600mOsmol/L and without a fall in serum Na$^+$ suggests partial nephrogenic diabetes insipidus. Limited reduction in urine volume, with some increase in urine osmolarity but a fall in serum Na$^+$ suggests primary polydipsia.

Low dose dexamethasone suppression test

Indication: to distinguish hypercortisolism from normality. The dexamethasone suppressed CRH test is believed to have less false positives in cases of alcholic or depressive pseudo-Cushing's syndrome.

Patient preparation: patients should not be on oral steroids or drugs that increase steroid metabolism.

Overnight dexamethasone suppression test: 1mg dexamethasone is taken PO at midnight. Serum sample for cortisol is taken the following morning between 0800 and 0900h.

Interpretation: serum cortisol should suppress to <140nmol/L (usually <50nmol/L). Values 140–175nmol/L are equivocal and suggest a 2-day test should be performed. 10–15% false +ve rate.

161

2-day low dose dexamethasone suppression test (preferred): dexamethasone 0.5mg is given PO every 6h for 8 doses (2 days) starting in the early morning. Ideally tablets are taken strictly at 6-hourly intervals (0600, 1200, 1800, 0000h) which may necessitate an inpatient stay. A 24h collection for urine free cortisol is taken on the second day of the test and serum cortisol is measured at 0600h on the 3rd day, 6h after the last dose. IV administration of dexamethasone can be used if there are concerns over absorption or compliance.

Interpretation: serum cortisol 6h after the last dose should be <140nmol/L, usually <50nmol/L. Urinary free cortisol on the second day should be <70nmol/L, normally <30nmol/L. The 2-day test strictly performed has less false +ves than the overnight test.

Dexamethasone suppressed CRH test: dexamethasone 0.5mg is given PO every 6h for 8 doses (2 days) but starting at midnight and ending at 0600h. Tablets are taken strictly at 6-hourly intervals (0000, 0600, 1200, 1800h) which may necessitate an inpatient stay. Last dose is taken at 0600h and an injection of CRH (100μg IV or 1μg/kg) is given at 0800h. A blood sample for cortisol is taken at 0815h (i.e. 15min later).

Interpretation: serum cortisol level should be <38nmol/L (normal).

Yanovski JA, Cutler GB, Chrousos G *et al.* (1993. Corticotrophin-releasing hormone stimulation following low-dose dexamethasone administration: a new test to distinguish Cushing's syndrome from pseudo-Cushing's states. *JAMA* **269**, 2232–2238.

High dose dexamethasone suppression test

Indication: to distinguish between patients with Cushing's disease (ACTH-secreting pituitary tumour) and ectopic ACTH production in patients with established hypercortisolism.

Patient preparation: as low dose test except that the test can be performed immediately following the 2-day low dose test.

Procedure:
1. 2 × 24h urine free cortisol collections are made to calculate the mean basal 24h urine free cortisol.
2. Baseline serum cortisol measurement is also taken before the first dexamethasone dose, ideally at 0600h. If the low dose test is performed first, the baseline values (urine and blood) must be taken prior to the low dose test (i.e. any doses of dexamethasone).
3. Dexamethasone 2mg is given PO every 6h for 8 doses (2 days) starting in the early morning. Ideally tablets are taken strictly at 6-hourly intervals (0600, 1200, 1800, 0000h) which may necessitate an inpatient stay.
4. A 24h urine collection for urinary free cortisol (final) is taken on day 2 and a blood sample is taken for (final) cortisol 6h after the last dexamethasone dose (0600h on day 3). Creatinine excretion should be measured and compared between urine samples to confirm true 24h collections.

Interpretation: % suppression of basal cortisol is calculated as:

(basal cortisol–final cortisol)/basal cortisol × 100.

The same calculation is made for basal and day 2 urine free cortisol. 50% suppression is suggestive of pituitary-dependent disease. 90% suppression increases the likelihood (strict criteria). Thymic carcinoids and phaechromocytomas releasing ACTH are source of false positives.

Short synacthen test

Indication: suspected adrenal insufficiency. Will not detect recent-onset secondary adrenal insufficiency.

Contraindication: asthma/allergy to ACTH—risk of allergic reaction (can be performed with careful medication supervision of patient).

Preparation: patient must not take hydrocortisone on the morning of the test as this will be detected in the cortisol assay. The test can be performed on low dose dexamethasone but the morning dose should be omitted until after the test. May have some value in patients on higher dose steroid therapy to indicate the degree of suppression of adrenocortical function.

Procedure: 250µg of synthetic ACTH (synacthen) given IM or IV. Blood taken at times 0, 30 and 60min for serum cortisol. A value at any time >550nmol/L makes the diagnosis very unlikely.

Low dose test: the test can be performed with a very low dose of ACTH (e.g. 1μg). This may detect more subtle degrees of hypoadrenalism but the clinical significance of these findings remains uncertain.

Long (depot) ACTH test

Indication: distinguishing 1° and 2° adrenal failure.

Patient preparation: a short synacthen test should be performed prior to the test to diagnose adrenal failure. If patient is on steroid replacement, change to dexamethasone 0.5mg/day.

Procedure: blood is taken at 0900h for basal cortisol. 1mg of depot synthetic ACTH (synacthen) is then given IM on 2 consecutive days and blood collected 5h after each dose (1400h). A final cortisol sample is taken at 0900h on the 3rd day.

Interpretation: serum cortisol should rise to >1000nmol/L on the last day and, if adrenal failure previously indicated by a short synacthen test, such a rise indicates secondary adrenal failure (pituitary/hypothalamic cause inc. suppressive drugs).

Full blood count (FBC)

Called *complete blood count* (CBC) in the USA.

Before the advent of modern haematology blood analysers the blood count consisted of a Hb concentration (estimated using a manual colorimetric technique), a white cell count and manual platelet count. Other parameters such as MCV had to be mathematically calculated (*derived*) using the measured variables Hb, RCC and PCV.

Modern analysers use a variety of methods to provide a huge range of FBC variables including electronic impedance, laser light scatter, light absorbance and staining characteristics. The resultant FBC provides measured variables such as Hb, PCV and RCC along with derived (mathematically) MCV, MCH and MCHC. These machines also provide automated platelet counts and a 5-part differential WBC.

Sample: peripheral blood EDTA; the sample should be analysed in the laboratory within 4h, if possible.

Main parameters measured
1. Hb concentration.
2. Red cell count (RCC).
3. MCV.
4. MCH.
5. MCHC.
6. Haematocrit (Hct) or PCV.
7. Red cell distribution width (RDW).
8. White cell count.
9. WBC differential.
10. Platelet count.

Some machines are even more sophisticated and will measure *reticulocyte counts* in addition to determination of reticulocyte Hb and MCV.

Role of the FBC
Why ask for a FBC? How will this aid the diagnosis or management of the patient? The FBC assesses several different parameters and can provide a great deal of information. The red cell variables will determine whether or not the patient is anaemic. If anaemia is present the MCV is likely to provide clues as to the cause of the anaemia. The white cells are often raised in infection—neutrophilia in bacterial infections and lymphocytosis in viral (but not always so). Platelets (size or number) may be abnormal either as a direct effect of underlying blood disease or may simply reflect the presence of some other underlying pathology. Most of us take a somewhat cursory glance at the FBC when the report arrives on the ward or in clinic, but a more detailed look may reveal a great deal more!

FBC parameters

Haemoglobin concentration (Hb)

Units: g/dL or g/L (Europe uses SI units; the USA still uses g/dL or grams%).

Defines *anaemia* (Hb <lower limit of normal adjusted for age and sex). Values differ between ♂ and ♀ since androgens drive RBC production and hence adult ♂ has higher Hb, PCV and RCC than adult ♀.

Red cell count (RCC)

Unit: $\times 10^{12}$/L.

Most clinicians pay little attention to the red cell count but this parameter is useful in the diagnosis of polycythaemic disorders and thalassaemias (the latter results in the increased production of red cells that are smaller than usual and contain low quantities of haemoglobin, i.e. are microcytic and hypochromic).

Causes of a low red cell count include
- Hypoproliferative anaemias, e.g. iron, vitamin B_{12} and folate deficiencies.
- Aplasias e.g. idiopathic or drug-induced (don't forget chemotherapy).
- Parvovirus B19 infection-induced red cell aplasia resulting in transient marked anaemia.

Causes of high red cell count
- PRV.
- Thalassaemia.

Mean cell volume (MCV)

Unit: femtolitre (fL), 10^{-15}L.

Provided as part of the derived variables or can be calculated if you know the PCV and RCC (PCV $\div$ RCC, e.g. if PCV 0.45 and RCC 5×10^{12}/L then MCV is 90fL).

Irrespective of the method used to determine the MCV, this index provides a useful starting point for the evaluation of anaemia (*see table below*).

The MCV may suggest the cause of anaemia

MCV ↓	MCV normal	MCV ↑
Iron deficiency	Blood loss	B_{12} or folate deficiency
β thalassaemia trait	Myelodysplasia	Myelodysplasia
Sideroblastic anaemia	Anaemia of chronic disease	

Mean cell haemoglobin (MCH)

Unit: pg.

High
- Macrocytosis.

Low
- Microcytosis, e.g. iron deficiency anaemia.

Mean cell haemoglobin concentration (MCHC)

Unit: g/dL or g/L.

Of value in evaluation of microcytic anaemias.

High
- Severe prolonged dehydration.
- Hereditary spherocytosis.
- Cold agglutinin disease.

Low
- Iron deficiency anaemia.
- Thalassaemia.

Haematocrit or PCV

These are not entirely synonymous terms (but they are, more-or-less). If blood is placed in a microcapillary tube and centrifuged the red cells are spun down to the bottom, leaving the plasma above. The RBCs will occupy about 40% of the blood in the tube—the blood will have a PCV of 0.4 (or 40%). The Hct is similar, but derived, using automated blood counters.

PCV unit: litres/litre (although the units are seldom cited on reports).

High PCV
- Polycythaemia (any cause).

Low PCV
- Anaemia (any cause).

Red cell distribution width (RDW)

Measures the *range* of red cell size in a sample of blood, providing information about the degree of red cell anisocytosis, i.e. how much variation there is between the size of the red cells. Of value in some anaemias:

e.g. $\downarrow$ MCV with normal RDW suggests β thalassaemia trait.
$\downarrow$ MCV with high RDW suggests iron deficiency.

(Probably noticed more by haematology staff than those in general medicine!)

White cells

The automated differential white cell count is provided as part of the FBC. The red cells in the sample are lysed before the white cells are counted. A typical FBC will show the *total* white cell count and the *5-part differential white cell count*, broken down into the 5 main white cell subtypes in peripheral blood which include:
- Neutrophils.
- Lymphocytes.
- Monocytes.
- Eosinophils.
- Basophils.

Normal ranges are provided inside front cover.

The printed FBC usually shows the % of each type of white cell but unless the absolute WBC (as $\times 10^9$/L) is known this % count is of little value.

▶As a general rule ignore the % count—you cannot detect abnormalities such as neutropenia unless you have the *absolute* values.

Abnormalities of the WBC, e.g. neutrophilia, neutropenia, etc. are discussed in 📖OHCM p632.

Platelet count

Unit: $\times 10^9$/L.

Normal: 150–400 $\times 10^9$/L.

Platelets (*thrombocytes* in the USA) are the smallest cells in the peripheral blood. Traditional counting methods using a microscope and counting chamber have been replaced by automated counting on most standard haematology analysers.

Platelet distribution width (PDW)

This is analogous to the red cell distribution width (RDW) and provides information about the *range* of platelet size in a blood sample.

169

- The PDW will be *high* if there are giant platelets in the presence of normal sized platelets, e.g. essential thrombocythaemia (one of the myeloproliferative disorders).
- The PDW will be *normal* in a reactive thrombocytosis (where the platelet count is increased but they are all of normal size).

Platelet clumping

This is seen as an *in vitro* artefact in some individuals. Platelets clump in EDTA and the blood analyser will report spurious thrombocytopenia. The actual *in vivo* count is entirely normal, and the platelets function perfectly normally. Taking the blood into a citrate or heparin tube will usually show the patient's platelet count to be normal. The presence of even a small blood clot in an EDTA sample may also reduce the platelet count (the haematology technical staff will usually check to see whether the sample contains a small clot before sending out the report).

Peripheral blood film

Examining a stained peripheral blood smear under the microscope allows the examination of red cells, white cells, and platelets. In addition the blood film will help detect parasites (e.g. malaria, trypanosomes) or abnormal cells in the blood.

When to request a blood film examination

The Haematology lab will usually examine a peripheral blood film if the patient's indices are abnormal (unless there has been no major change from previous FBCs). If you suspect an underlying blood disorder you should request a film. *Note*: The lab staff may not make a film if the indices are completely normal.

Method

A fingerprick blood sample may be spread onto a glass slide (the phlebotomists may do this for you), air-dried, fixed and stained. Alternatively, a drop of EDTA blood may be treated in the same manner (the haematology lab staff will make the film). *Beware*: old EDTA samples produce strange artefacts such as extreme red cell crenation—for this reason, if a film is required it should be made from a fresh blood sample.

Sample: EDTA (as fresh as possible).

Information from the blood film

Red cells
- Size.
- Shape.
- Membrane changes (e.g. oxidative membrane damage).
- Colour.
- Basophilic stippling.
- Inclusions, e.g. Howell-Jolly bodies, malarial parasites, HbC crystals, etc.

White cells
- Number.
- Morphology.
- Abnormalities such as toxic granulation, dysplastic changes.
- Presence of abnormal cells, e.g. leukaemic blasts or lymphoma cells.

Platelets
- Number.
- Size.
- Shape.

Other features on the film
- Parasites.
- Red cell rouleaux (stacking effect, seen e.g. when ESR is ↑).
- Nucleated red cells.
- Plasma cells.
- Occasionally see circulating carcinoma cells.

📖 OHCM p630.

Red cell morphology

In health the normal RBC is a pink biconcave disc-shaped cell, and most red cells are roughly the same size, shape and colour in health. They

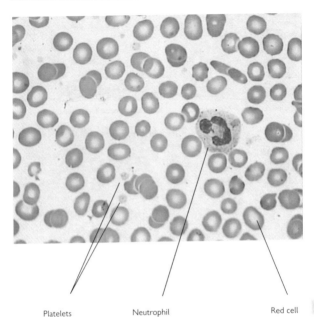

Platelets   Neutrophil   Red cell

Fig. 3.1

should be roughly the size of a small lymphocyte nucleus. Many disease and deficiency disorders alter the RBC appearance by either reducing its haemoglobin content, or altering the membrane such that characteristic morphological abnormalities are produced. Examples include target cells, sickle cells, bite cells, burr cells and many others (*see table opposite*). Most of the morphological features are *not* absolutely specific for one particular disorder, but rather they suggest a range of conditions which may be associated with the RBC feature. This should prompt you to look for conditions which might account for the abnormality.

▶Pay attention to the peripheral blood film comment (inserted on the report by the haematology lab staff, or automated blood counter)—it should help you decide which tests to carry out next. Conversely, cryptic lab comments like 'anisopoikilocytosis noted' do not help the clinician much. (Note: *aniso* = unequal, *poikilo* = varied.)

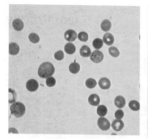

Stippled red cells in haemolysis

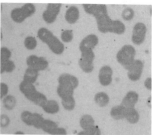

Marked rouleaux in myeloma

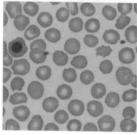

Single nucleated red cell (on left)
Fig. 3.2

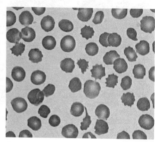

Crenated red cells

Parasites on the blood film

Although there are now highly sensitive monoclonal antibody kits for the diagnosis of diseases such as malaria, a well-stained blood film can often make the diagnosis more easily. Blood films are useful for confirming a diagnosis of:
- Malaria.
- Trypanosomiasis.
- Microfilaria.

Parasites in bone marrow

Some diseases such as Leishmaniasis require bone marrow aspiration and staining (in fact there are many infections that can be diagnosed using a bone marrow):
- *Leishmania donovani.*
- Tuberculosis.
- *Tropheryma whippelii* (Whipple's disease).
- *Cryptococcus neoformans.*

Microcytic RBCs	Fe deficiency, thalassaemia trait & syndromes, congenital sideroblastic anaemia, anaemia of chronic disorders (if longstanding).
Macrocytic RBCs	Alcohol/liver disease (*round macrocytes*), MDS, pregnancy and newborn, compensated haemolysis, B_{12} or folate deficiency, hydroxyurea and antimetabolites (*oval macrocytes*), acquired sideroblastic anaemia, hypothyroidism, chronic respiratory failure, aplastic anaemia.
Dimorphic RBCs	Two populations, e.g. Fe deficiency responding to iron, mixed Fe and B_{12}/folate deficiency, sideroblastic anaemia, post red cell transfusion.
Hypochromic RBCs	Reduced Hb synthesis, e.g. iron deficiency, thalassaemia, sideroblastic anaemia.
Polychromatic RBCs	Blood loss or haematinic treatment, haemolysis, marrow infiltration.
Spherocytes	Hereditary spherocytosis, haemolysis, e.g. warm AIHA, delayed transfusion reaction, ABO HDN, DIC and MAHA, post-splenectomy.
Pencil/rod cells	Fe deficiency anaemia, thalassaemia trait & syndromes, PK deficiency.
Elliptocytes	Hereditary elliptocytosis, MPD and MDS.
Fragmented RBCs	MAHA, DIC, renal failure, HUS, TTP.
Teardrop RBCs	Myelofibrosis, metastatic marrow infiltration, MDS.
Sickle cells	Sickle cell anaemia, other sickle syndromes but *not* sickle trait.
Target cells	Liver disease, Fe deficiency, thalassaemia, HbC syndromes.
Crenated RBCs	Usually storage or EDTA artefact. Genuine RBC crenation may be seen post-splenectomy and in renal failure ($\rightarrow$burr cells).
Burr cells	Renal failure.
Acanthocytes	Hereditary acanthocytosis, a-β-lipoproteinaemia, McLeod red cell phenotype, PK deficiency, chronic liver disease (esp. Zieve's syndrome).
Bite cells	G6PD deficiency, oxidative haemolysis.
Basophilic stippling	Megaloblastic anaemia, lead poisoning, MDS, liver disease, haemoglobinopathies, e.g. thalassaemia.
Rouleaux	Chronic inflammation, paraproteinaemia, myeloma.
↑ reticulocytes	Bleeding, haemolysis, marrow infiltration, severe hypoxia, response to haematinic therapy.
Heinz bodies	Not seen in normals (removed by spleen), small numbers seen post-splenectomy, oxidant drugs, G6PD deficiency, sulphonamides, unstable Hb (Hb Zurich, Köln).
Howell-Jolly bodies	Composed of DNA, removed by the spleen, seen in dyserythropoietic states, e.g. B_{12} deficiency, MDS, post-splenectomy, hyposplenism.
H bodies	HbH inclusions, denatured HbH (β_4 tetramer), stain with methylene blue, seen in HbH disease (−−/−α), less prominent in α thalassaemia trait, not present in normal subjects.
Hyposplenic blood film	Howell-Jolly bodies, target cells, occasional nucleated RBCs, lymphocytosis, macrocytosis, acanthocytes. Infectious mononucleosis, any viral infection, toxoplasmosis, drug reactions.

- *Penicillium.*
- *Histoplasma capsulatum.*
- *Candida albicans.*
- *Toxoplasma gondii.*

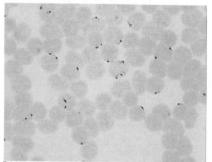

Falciparum malaria (blood film)

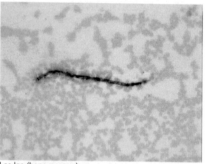

Loa loa (bone marrow)

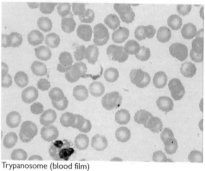

Trypanosome (blood film)

Fig. 3.3

White blood cell morphology

In much the same was as RBC morphology provides clues about underlying disease, so too does microscopical examination of stained peripheral blood WBCs. Modern counters enumerate WBCs and our greater reliance on modern technology means that visual inspection of blood films is becoming a dying art. A well-stained blood film may provide the diagnosis much more cheaply.

Blood film when WBC is ↓
- Sometimes difficult to determine diagnosis since so few WBCs.
- May suggest B_{12} or folate deficiency (are the RBCs normal or large?).
- Aplastic anaemia—are the platelets and Hb normal?
- Underlying leukaemia—are there any leukaemic blasts* present?
- Overwhelming infection—may see toxic granulation (large dark granules in the cytoplasm—not diagnostic but suggestive).
- May be immune or post-viral—atypical lymphocytes may be seen; other indices usually normal.

Blood film when WBC is ↑
What cell predominates?
- Lymphocytes? suggests viral, CLL, acute leukaemia (lymphoblastic).
- Granulocytic? (neutrophils, eosinophils, basophils)—may be reactive or CML.
- Abnormal looking WBC? Look for Auer rods (≡ AML), smear cells (CLL), bilobed neutrophils (pseudo-Pelger cells seen in MDS).

Diagnosis must be made in context
How old is the patient?
- Viral illnesses often produce bizarre films in children but beware of complacency (acute leukaemia may be the cause).
- MDS and malignancies like CLL and CML are diseases of older individuals.

Is the patient well?
- May be worth repeating FBC and film to see if abnormalities have resolved.
- If patient unwell or has lymphadenopathy or hepatosplenomegaly then underlying disease must be excluded.

175

---

*A blast is a primitive cell seen in the marrow in large numbers in leukaemia. We all have some blasts in our marrows but these should be <5% of the total nucleated bone marrow cells in health.

Some WBC abnormalities seen on FBC reports

Atypical lymphocytes	Infectious mononucleosis, any viral infection, toxoplasmosis, drug reactions.
Auer rods	Seen in myeloblasts; pathognomonic of AML. Prominent in AML M3 subtype (acute promyelocytic leukaemia).
Pelger-Huët anomaly	Bilobed neutrophils. May be hereditary (neutrophils are functionally normal) or acquired, e.g. MDS (pseudo-Pelger cells).
Left shifted	Immature WBCs seen in peripheral blood. Seen in severe infections, inflammatory disorders, DKA, marrow 'stress', MPD, CML.
Right shifted	Hypermature WBCs seen in e.g. megaloblastic anaemia and iron deficiency.
Toxic granulation	Coarse granules in neutrophils. Seen in severe infection, post-operatively and inflammatory disorders.
Smear cells	Lymphocytes in which the cell membrane has ruptured when making the blood film—there are no smear cells *in vivo*! Seen in CLL.

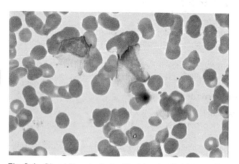

Fig. 3.4 Blood film: atypical white blood cells (this was from a patient with glandular fever, but these cells may be seen in any viral illness).

📖 OHCM p632.

Assessment of iron status

Introduction
The anaemia of iron deficiency is caused by defective synthesis of haemoglobin resulting in red cells that are smaller than normal (*microcytic*) and contain reduced amounts of haemoglobin (*hypochromic*). The diagnosis of iron deficiency anaemia is generally straightforward but it may be confused with that due to the anaemia of chronic disease (ACD) or other hypochromic anaemias (*see table*, p179).

Iron plays a pivotal role in many metabolic processes and the average adult contains between 3 and 5g of iron of which two-thirds are present in the O_2-carrying molecule, haemoglobin. Somewhat surprisingly, there is no specific excretion mechanism in humans. Iron balance is controlled at the level of gut absorption, and relies on two iron-sequestering proteins, *transferrin* (iron transport and recycling of iron) and *ferritin* (safeguards iron entry into the body, and maintains surplus iron in a safe and readily accessible form).

Ferritin

This is the primary iron-storage protein consisting of 24 apoferritin subunits forming a hollow sphere (each can hold up to 4500 Fe atoms).

Haemosiderin

Haemosiderin, located predominantly in macrophages, is a water-soluble protein–iron complex with an amorphous structure.

Transferrin and its receptor

Transferrin contains only 4mg iron and is the principal iron transport protein with more than 30mg iron transported round the body daily. Synthesis of transferrin is inversely proportional to the body iron stores, with increased transferrin concentration when iron stores are reduced.

The transferrin receptor (TfR) is a disulphide-linked dimer composed of two identical 85kDa subunits. The serum TFR concentration is elevated in iron deficiency. However, sTfR may also increase in any condition in which there is increased erythropoiesis, e.g. haemolytic anaemias, thalassaemia, polycythaemia vera and other myeloproliferative disorders.

Assessment of iron status

Several parameters are available
- Haemoglobin concentration.
- Serum ferritin.
- Serum iron and transferrin (as total iron binding capacity, TIBC).
- % hypochromic cells in peripheral blood.
- Red cell protoporphyrin assay (not widely available).
- Bone marrow aspirate (stained for iron)—the 'gold standard'.
- Soluble transferrin receptor assay (sTfR).

Remember, iron deficiency is not an 'all-or-nothing' phenomenon. In progressive deficiency there is a gradual loss of iron with subtle alterations of iron-related parameters during which the red cells may look entirely normal. In the initial stages of developing iron deficiency macrophages become depleted of iron and the serum ferritin ↓ to the lower end of the normal range; during this 'latency' period the Hb is normal. As the deficiency progresses plasma iron levels ↓ and TIBC ↑. Free RBC protoporphyrin levels ↑ as it accumulates, and eventually hypochromic RBCs appear in the peripheral blood. At this stage a full blood count will usually show ↓ Hb, MCV, MCH and MCHC, and the peripheral blood film will show microcytic hypochromic red cells.

Confirmation of simple iron deficiency anaemia
- Hb ↓.
- Serum ferritin will be ↓.

> **Beware**: serum ferritin is an acute phase protein and may be normal or even ↑ in inflammatory, malignant or liver disease. During the inflammatory response the iron/TIBC are unlikely to be of any value (iron ↓ and TIBC will be ↓). If an inflammatory process is suspected, an alternative test is required, e.g. sTfR, which is not affected by inflammatory disorders.

- Serum iron and TIBC (but little used today).
- sTfR ↑.
- MCV ↓.
- MCH & MCHC ↓.
- Microcytic & hypochromic RBCs on blood film.
- Absent marrow iron.

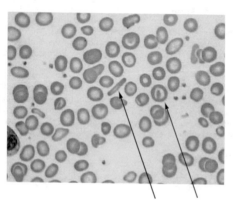

Pencil cell   Target cell

Fig. 3.5 Blood film of iron deficiency anaemia. Note the variation in cell size and shape.

📖OHCM p628.

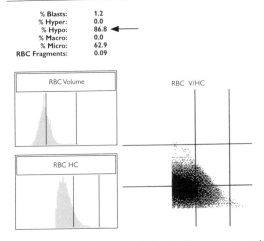

Additional Routine Parameters

% Blasts:	1.2
% Hyper:	0.0
% Hypo:	86.8
% Macro:	0.0
% Micro:	62.9
RBC Fragments:	0.09

Fig. 3.6 The % hypochromic red cells (provided by some automated counters) helps in the diagnosis of iron deficiency. Notice that the RBC volume and haemoglobin content (HC) are both shifted to the LEFT (=small pale red cells).

Hypochromic anaemias—may be confused with iron deficiency	
Disorder	Example
Disorders of Fe metabolism	Iron deficiency anaemia — Blood loss — Reduced iron intake — Impaired iron transport
Anaemia of chronic disorders	Chronic inflammatory diseases Malignant disease
Disorders of haem synthesis	Sideroblastic anaemias Hereditary Idiopathic Secondary — drugs — alcohol — lead poisoning
Globin synthesis disorders	Thalassaemias — β thalassaemia — α thalassaemia

Provan D, Weatherall D. (2000) Acquired anaemias and polycythaemia, *Lancet* **355**, 1260–1268.

Assessment of B$_{12}$ & folate status

Measurement of the serum B$_{12}$ and red cell folate levels is necessary in the investigation of macrocytic anaemia and certain other situations (see below). Serum folate levels are an unreliable measurement of body stores of folate—the red cell folate level is probably more meaningful.

B$_{12}$ unit: ng/L.

Serum & red cell folate units: μg/L.

Sample: clotted blood sample (serum B$_{12}$ and folate) and peripheral blood EDTA (red cell folate).

Deficiency of either vitamin leads to megaloblastic anaemia where there is disruption of cell division in all actively dividing cells (includes the bone marrow and gut). In the marrow there is nuclear:cytoplasmic asynchrony where the nuclei are immature despite a mature well-haemoglobinised cytoplasm. In the peripheral blood there may be anaemia, often with pancytopenia; the red cells show oval macrocytic changes with basophilic stippling and occasionally nucleated red cells. Neutrophils typically become hypersegmented (they have >5 lobes).

Until recently, B$_{12}$ and folate assays were tedious microbiological assays but these have now been replaced by automated techniques using radioisotopic methods which allow large numbers of samples to be batched and tested fairly cheaply.

Deficiency of B$_{12}$ or folate do not always cause macrocytic anaemia

In the past, deficiency of B$_{12}$ or folate were synonymous with macrocytic anaemia but deficiency of either vitamin may present without anaemia or macrocytosis—remember, these are *late* features of the disease. However, in most cases of deficiency the marrow will show characteristic megaloblastic change (nuclear asynchrony with giant metamyelocytes). ▶*Deficiency of B$_{12}$ may cause neurological problems in the absence of anaemia.*

Whom should you test?

- Patients with GIT disease, glossitis, abnormalities of taste, previous surgery or radiotherapy to stomach or small bowel.
- Neurological disease, e.g. peripheral neuropathy, demyelination.
- Psychiatric disturbance, e.g. confusion, dementia.
- Malnutrition, e.g. growth impairment in children; vegans.
- Alcohol abuse.
- Autoimmune disease of thyroid, parathyroid or adrenals.
- Patients with family history of pernicious anaemia.
- Others, e.g. drugs that interfere with vitamin absorption or metabolism such as nitrous oxide, phenytoin, etc.

Look for blood film abnormalities

▶B$_{12}$ & folate deficiencies produce similar clinical and laboratory features.
- Oval macrocytes.
- Hypersegmented neutrophils (also seen in renal failure, iron deficiency and MDS).

Which test next?

Make sure you have the following:
- FBC.

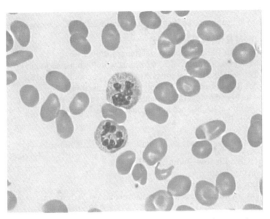

Fig. 3.7 Blood film of megaloblastic anaemia. There are large oval macrocytes and two hypersegmented (>5 lobes) neutrophils.

- Blood film.
- Serum B_{12} level.
- Serum and red cell folate level.
- Intrinsic factor antibodies (IFA), +ve in 50–75% patients with PA.
- Consider bone marrow (helps exclude MDS, myeloma and other pathologies that give rise to macrocytic anaemia, but seldom performed today since it is easy to get a B_{12} and folate result back quickly).

Interpretation of results: vitamin B_{12}
Normal ranges are based on 2 standard deviations either side of the mean, so there will be 'normal' people who have 'abnormal' B_{12} (or folate) levels.

B_{12} <normal   – deficiency
– altered metabolism
– 'normal'

The lowest levels are seen in those most deficient. What matters is whether there is *tissue deficiency* (leads to marrow and neurological changes).

Mild ↓ in B_{12} level?
Difficult, but common! Probably worth repeating the test and reviewing the patient and other results. If no evidence of tissue deficiency, can probably observe the patient. If there is evidence of tissue deficiency then the patient will require treatment.

Detecting tissue deficiency
The most reliable method is probably the measurement of serum homocysteine (accumulates in vitamin B_{12} and folate deficiency).

Beware ↓ B_{12} not associated with tissue deficiency
- Folate deficiency.

- Pregnancy.
- Myeloma.
- Transcobalamin I deficiency.

Folate

↓ level seen in hospitalised patients due to negative folate balance.

The B₁₂ level is low—what next?

Available tests for the cause of B_{12} deficiency include:

- Parietal cell (+ve in serum of 90% patients with PA but also found in other disorders and 15% of the normal elderly) and intrinsic factor antibodies (IFA better—if +ve confirms diagnosis of PA).
- Schilling test (urinary excretion method where addition of IF restores B_{12} absorption in PA but not in intestinal, e.g. ileal, disease) *or*
- Whole body B_{12} counting.
- Endoscopy with duodenal biopsy.
- Other gastroenterology tests for malabsorption (📖Ch7).

The folate level is low—what next?

- Check dietary history.
- Endoscopy with duodenal biopsy.
- Other gastroenterology tests for malabsorption (📖Ch7).

📖OHCM p634.

Erythrocyte sedimentation rate (ESR)

This simple but very useful qualitative test measures how fast a patient's red cells fall through a column of blood. It is a sensitive but non-specific index of plasma protein changes which result from inflammation or tissue damage. The ESR is affected by haematocrit variations, red cell abnormalities (e.g. poikilocytosis, sickle cells) and delay in analysis, and is therefore less reliable than measurement of the plasma viscosity. The ESR is affected by age, sex, menstrual cycle, pregnancy and drugs (e.g. OCP, steroids).

The ESR is widely used in clinical medicine and despite attempts (by haematology departments) to replace the ESR with the plasma viscosity the ESR has remained in use and appears to retain a valuable place in the armoury of disease diagnosis and monitoring.

Sample: peripheral blood EDTA; the sample should be analysed in the laboratory within 4h.

Normal ranges (upper limits)

Age	Men	Women
17–50 years	10mm/h	12mm/h
51–60	12	19
>60	14	20

There are many factors which influence the ESR causing a high or low result:

Provan D, Weatherall D. (2000) Acquired anaemias and polycythaemia, *Lancet* **355**, 1260–1268.

High ESR (significant*—look for a cause)
- Any inflammatory disorder, e.g. infection, rheumatoid.
- TB.
- Myocardial infarction (the ESR ↑ as an early response).
- Anaemia.

*Depends exactly *how high*. An ESR of 30 probably means little but if >100 is *highly significant* and indicates something seriously wrong.

Low ESR (rarely important, but useful for exams)
- Polycythaemia.
- Hypofibrinogenaemia.
- CCF.
- Poikilocytosis.
- Spherocytosis.
- Sickled cells.

▶ A normal ESR does *not* exclude organic disease.

📖OHCM p672.

Harris GJ. (1972) Plasma viscometry and ESR in the elderly. *Med Lab Technol* **29**, 405–410; Lewis SM. (1980) Erythrocyte sedimentation rate and plasma viscosity. *Ass Clin Pathol Broadsheet* **94**, 1–6.

Plasma viscosity

This test is a sensitive but non-specific index of plasma protein changes which result from inflammation or tissue damage. Provides much the same information as the ESR. The ESR and PV tend to rise in parallel but the PV is *unaffected* by haematocrit variations (e.g. severe anaemia or poly-cythaemia) and delay in analysis up to 24h, and is therefore more reliable than the ESR. It is not affected by sex but is affected by age, exercise and pregnancy. It is constant in health and shows no diurnal variation. There is a suggestion that the PV may be a more sensitive indicator of disease severity than the ESR.

Sample: peripheral blood EDTA. The sample is centrifuged and the plasma removed.

Normal range: 1.50–1.72CP (or MPA/s at 25°C).

High and low plasma viscosity
High PV generally signifies some underlying pathology; low PV can be ignored.

Note: Despite the advantages outlined the PV has not been adopted by all medical staff (who still prefer the ESR as a measure of inflammation). The PV is better for monitoring hyperviscosity syndromes, e.g. Waldenström's macroglobulinaemia.

📖OHCM p672.

Cooke BM, Stuart J. (1988) Automated measurement of plasma viscosity by capillary viscometer. *J Clin Pathol* **41**, 1213–1216.

Tests for glandular fever

This infection is caused by Epstein-Barr virus (EBV). Infected cells produce so-called heterophile antibodies (these are IgM molecules that agglutinate horse and sheep RBCs but do not agglutinate ox RBCs and do not react at all with guinea-pig RBCs).

There are various kits available that can detect the presence of heterophile antibodies and in the right clinical context will confirm a diagnosis of EBV infection. The Monospot test is probably the commonest in current use. The Paul-Bunnell test was the first to demonstrate the presence of heterophile antibodies in patients with EBV infection.

Clinical features

Glandular fever often affects young adults (12–25 years) and results in malaise, fever, tonsillitis, petechial haemorrhages on palate and lymphadenopathy. Splenomegaly is fairly common. A similar clinical picture is seen in CMV, *Toxoplasma* and early HIV infections.

Sample: EDTA.

Positive Monospot
- EBV infection.

False positives
- Toxoplasmosis.
- CMV infection.
- Rheumatoid.
- Malaria.

Hoff G, Bauer S. (1965) A new rapid slide test for infectious mononucleosis. *JAMA* **194**, 351–353.

Investigation of haemolytic anaemia

The normal red cell has a lifespan of ~120 days. Anaemia resulting from ↓ RBC lifespan is termed *haemolytic*. May be inherited or acquired and the basic underlying mechanisms may involve abnormalities of the RBC *membrane*, RBC *enzymes* or *haemoglobin*.

Extravascular vs. intravascular

Extravascular haemolysis implies RBC breakdown by the RES (e.g. liver, spleen, and macrophages at other sites) while intravascular haemolysis describes RBC breakdown in the circulation itself. There are many investigations available which will help determine the predominant site of destruction, which in turn will help define the underlying cause of haemolysis, which is why we do the tests in the first place.

Detection of haemolysis itself

The main question is whether the patient's anaemia is due to haemolysis or some other underlying mechanism such as blood loss, marrow infiltration, etc.

📖OHCM p638.

General tests of haemolysis

Is haemolysis actually occurring? Suggestive features are
- Evidence of ↑ red cell destruction.
- Evidence of ↑ red cell production (to compensate for red cell loss).
- Evidence of autoantibody in the patient's serum.

Evidence of RBC destruction
- ↑ serum bilirubin.
- ↑ serum LDH (reflecting ↑ RBC turnover).
- Spherocytes or other abnormal RBCS, e.g. fragments on blood film.
- Plasma haptoglobins may be ↓ or absent.
- ↑ Faecal & urinary urobilinogen (faecal not measured).
- ↓ RBC lifespan (seldom measured nowadays).

Evidence of ↑ RBC production
- ↑ Reticulocytes (on film, manual or automated count). Not absolutely specific, will ↑ in brisk acute bleed, e.g. GIT.
- ↑ MCV (reticulocytes are larger than mature RBCs, and don't forget folate deficiency which occurs in haemolytic disorders).

Is it mainly intravascular?
- ↑ Plasma Hb.
- Methaemalbuminaemia.
- Haemoglobinuria.

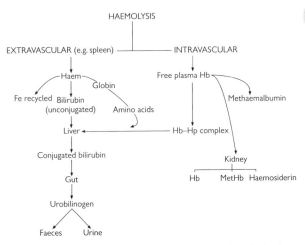

Fig. 3.8 Increased red cell breakdown may be extravascular (outside the circulation, predominantly spleen, liver and marrow) or intravascular (within the vessels).

Modified from Dacie JV, Lewis SM, eds. (1995) *Practical Haematology*, 8th edition, Churchill Livingstone, Edinburgh.

- Haemosiderinuria.

What is the cause?

Genetic
- RBC morphology (e.g. spherocytes, elliptocytes).
- Hb analysis.
- RBC enzyme assays.

Acquired
- Immune—check DAT.
- Non-immune: check RBC morphology (e.g. TTP/HUS).
- Is there some other underlying disease?
- Consider PNH (rare).

Reticulocytes

These are immature RBCS formed in the marrow and found in small numbers in normal peripheral blood. They represent an intermediate maturation stage in marrow between the nucleated RBC and the mature RBC (the reticulocyte lacks a nucleus but retains some nucleic acid). Measuring the number of reticulocytes in the blood may help determine whether the anaemia is due to ↓ RBC production. The reticulocyte count is also a useful measure of response to haematinic (iron, B_{12} or folate) replacement therapy.

Detection and measurement
- Demonstrated by staining with supravital dye for the nucleic acid.
- Appear on blood film as larger than mature RBCs with fine lacy blue staining strands or dots.
- Some modern automated blood counters using laser technology can measure levels of retics directly.
- Usually expressed as a % of total red cells, e.g. 5%, though absolute numbers can be derived from this and total red cell count.

Sample: EDTA.

Normal range: 0.5–2.5% (50–100 × 10^9/L).

Causes of ↑ reticulocyte counts

Marrow stimulation due to
- Bleeding.
- Haemolysis.
- Response to oral Fe therapy.
- Infection.
- Inflammation.
- Polycythaemia (any cause).
- Myeloproliferative disorders.
- Marrow recovery following chemotherapy or radiotherapy.
- Erythropoietin administration.

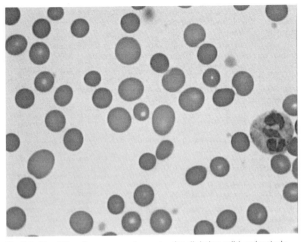

Fig. 3.9 Blood film of numerous spherocytes (small darker cells) and reticulocytes (larger red cells) in autoimmune haemolytic anaemia.

Causes of ↓ reticulocyte counts

Marrow infiltration due to
- Leukaemia.
- Myeloma.
- Lymphoma.
- Other malignancy.

Marrow underactivity (hypoplasia) due to
- Fe, folate or B$_{12}$ deficiency. *Note*: Return of retics is earliest sign of response to replacement therapy.
- Immediately post-chemotherapy or radiotherapy.
- Autoimmune disease especially RA.
- Malnutrition.
- Uraemia.
- Drugs.
- Aplastic anaemia.
- Red cell aplasia.

Howells MR *et al.* (1986) Erythropoiesis in pregnancy. *Br J Haematol* **64**, 595–599.

Serum haptoglobins

Haptoglobins (H$_P$) are plasma proteins synthesised by the liver, whose function is the removal of free plasma haemoglobin. Hp molecules bind free Hb and are taken up by the reticuloendothelial system for degradation. Hp–Hb complexes do not appear in the urine because their large size prevents them passing through the renal tubules.

The Hp–Hb complex is cleared by the reticuloendothelial system at a rate of 15mg/100mL/h which means that even very mild haemolysis will cause the disappearance of Hp from the circulation. The serum haptoglobin should be measured in patients with suspected intravascular haemolysis. However, the Hp level is frequently reduced in patients with extravascular haemolysis, and the Hp level cannot be used to determine whether the basic haemolytic process is intra- or extravascular. It should generally be accompanied by estimation of the serum methaemalbumin, free plasma haemoglobin and urinary haemosiderin.

Sample: clotted blood.

Normal range: (expressed as Hb binding capacity in mg/dL): 30–250mg/dL.

Conditions with ↓ haptoglobins

Haemolysis including
- Incompatible blood transfusion.
- Autoimmune haemolytic anaemia.
- Sickle cell disease.
- Thalassaemia major.
- PNH.

Others
- 1% population have genetic lack of haptoglobin.
- Lower levels in infancy.

188

Note: It takes about 1 week after haemolysis has stopped for haptoglobin levels to return to normal.

Conditions with ↑ haptoglobins (acute phase protein, like ferritin)
- Any disorder with ↑ ESR.
- Carcinoma especially if bony secondaries.
- Any inflammatory disorder.
- Trauma.
- Surgery.
- Steroid therapy.
- Androgen therapy.
- Diabetes mellitus.

Rougemont A et al. (1988) Hypohaptoglobinaemia as an epidemiological and clinical indicator for malaria. Results of two studies in a hyperendemic region in West Africa. *Lancet* **2**, 709–712.

Serum bilirubin

Two forms are found: prehepatic bilirubin (unconjugated) and bilirubin conjugated to glucuronic acid (conjugated). Generally serum bilirubin levels are 17–50μmol/L in haemolysis (mainly unconjugated). *Beware*: serum bilirubin levels may be normal even if haemolysis is present; a level >85μmol/L suggests liver disease.

The serum bilirubin may be modestly ↑ (e.g. 20–30μmol/L) in dyserythro-poietic disorders such as vitamin B_{12} or folate deficiency or myelodys-plasia, due to ineffective erythropoiesis where the RBCs are destroyed in the marrow before ever being released into the circulation.

Urobilin & urobilinogen

Urobilinogen is the reduced form of urobilin, formed by bacterial action on bile pigments in the GI tract. Faecal and urinary urobilinogen ↑ in haemolytic anaemias.

Urinary haemosiderin

Usage
The most widely used and reliable test for detection of chronic intravas-cular haemolysis. Results from the presence of Hb in the glomerular fil-trate.

Principle
Free Hb is released into the plasma during intravascular haemolysis. The haemoglobin binding proteins become saturated resulting in passage of haem-containing compounds into the urinary tract of which haemosiderin is the most readily detectable.

Method
1. A clean catch sample of urine is obtained from the patient.
2. Sample is spun down in a cytocentrifuge to obtain a cytospin prepara-tion of urothelial cells.
3. Staining and rinsing with Perl's reagent (Prussian blue) is performed on the glass slides.
4. Examine under oil-immersion lens of microscope.
5. Haemosiderin stains as blue dots within urothelial cells.
6. Ignore all excess stain, staining outside cells or in debris, all of which are common.
7. True +ve only when clear detection within urothelial squames is seen.

Cautions
An iron-staining +ve control sample should be run alongside test case to ensure stain has worked satisfactorily. Haemosiderinuria may not be detected for up to 72h after the initial onset of intravascular haemolysis so the test may miss haemolysis of very recent onset—repeat test in 3–7 days if −ve. Conversely, haemosiderinuria may persist for some time after a haemolytic process has stopped. Repeat in 7 days should confirm.

Causes of haemosiderinuria

Common causes	Red cell enzymopathies, e.g. G6PD and PK deficiency but only during haemolytic episodes
	Mycoplasma pneumonia with anti-I cold haemagglutinin
	Sepsis
	Malaria
	Cold haemagglutinin disease
	TTP/HUS
	Severe extravascular haemolysis (may cause intravascular haemolysis)
Rarer causes	PNH
	Prosthetic heart valves
	Red cell incompatible transfusion reactions
	Unstable haemoglobins
	March haemoglobinuria

Plasma haemoglobin

In health, haemoglobin is contained within RBCs but during intravascular haemolysis excessive quantities of Hb may be released from ruptured RBCs. Normally haptoglobins mop up free Hb. If there are insufficient haptoglobins to cope with the free Hb, the kidneys clear the Hb leading to haemoglobinuria. Some Hb may be broken down in the circulation to haem and globin; haem can bind to albumin producing methaemalbumin ($\longrightarrow$ methaemalbuminaemia).

▶The finding of free Hb in plasma is *highly suggestive* of intravascular haemolysis.

Sample: sodium citrate (but discuss with haematology laboratory before sending sample).

Causes of ↑ plasma haemoglobin

Mild ↑ (50–100mg/L)	Moderate ↑ (100–250mg/L)	Severe ↑ (>250mg/L)
Sickle/thalassaemia	AIHA	Incompatible blood transfusion
HbC disease	Sickle cell disease	PNH
	Thalassaemia major	PCH
	HbSC	Blackwater fever
	Prosthetic heart valve	
	March haemoglobinuria	

Normal range: 10–40mg/L (up to 6mg/L).

Pitfalls: any RBC damage occurring during blood sampling may result in an erroneously high reading. Great care must be taken during venepuncture.

Crosby WH, Dameshek W. (1951) The significance of hemoglobinemia and associated hemosiderinuria, with particular reference to various types of hemolytic anemia. *J Clin Lab Med* **38**, 829.

Schumm's test

Use: detection of methaemalbumin (seen after all haptoglobins used up in a haemolytic process, usually implies the haemolysis is predominantly intravascular).

This spectrophotometric test for methaemalbumin (which has a distinctive absorption band at 558nm) should be requested in patients with suspected intravascular haemolysis and may be abnormal in patients with significant extravascular (generally splenic) haemolysis. It should be accompanied by estimation of the serum haptoglobin level, free plasma haemoglobin and urinary haemosiderin.

Sample: heparinised or clotted blood.

Positive result in
- Intravascular haemolysis.
- Mismatched blood transfusion.
- RBC fragmentation syndromes.
- G6PD deficiency with oxidative haemolysis.
- PNH.
- March haemoglobinuria.
- Unstable Hbs.

Winstone NE. (1965) Methemalbumin in acute pancreatitis. *Br J Surg* **52**, 804–808; Hoffbrand AV, Lewis SM, Tuddenham EGD, eds. (2000) *Postgraduate Haematology*, 4th edition, Butterworth-Heinemann, Oxford.

Hereditary haemolytic anaemias

There are many inherited causes for haemolytic anaemia which fall into 3 major groups shown in the table below.

Mechanism	Example
Red cell membrane disorders	Hereditary spherocytosis
	Hereditary elliptocytosis
Red cell enzyme disorders	G6PD deficiency
	Pyruvate kinase deficiency
Haemoglobin disorders	Sickle cell anaemia
	Thalassaemia

Red cell membrane disorders

Hereditary spherocytosis
This is the best known inherited membrane abnormality leading to a reduced red cell lifespan and sometimes severe anaemia. Inheritance is usually autosomal dominant, and there is often a positive family history.

Osmotic fragility test
Principle of the test
The test measures the ability of red cells to take up water before rupturing (lysing). This is determined by the volume : surface area ratio. Normal red cells can ↑ their volume by up to 70% before lysing (because they are disc shaped, and have the capacity to take in extra water easily). Spherocytic red cells have an ↑ volume : surface area ratio and are able to take up less water than normal red cells before lysing (they are spheres and as such they are 'full' already).

Sample: EDTA (need normal control sample sent at the same time).

Method
- RBCs are incubated in saline at various concentrations. This results in cell expansion and eventually rupture.
- Normal RBCs can withstand greater volume increases than spherocytic RBCs.
- A positive result (confirming HS) seen when RBCs lyse in saline at near to isotonic concentration, i.e. 0.6–0.8g/dL (normal RBCs will simply show swelling with little lysis).
- Osmotic fragility is more marked in patients who have not undergone splenectomy, and if the RBCs are incubated at 37°C for 24h before performing the test.

Other supportive tests
- There will be a positive family history of HS in many cases.
- The blood film shows ↑↑ spherocytic RBCs.
- Anaemia, ↑ reticulocytes, ↑ LDH, unconjugated bilirubin, urinary urobilinogen with ↓ haptoglobins.
- DAT –ve.

Beware: this test is not diagnostic of HS, but will be +ve in any condition in which there are increased numbers of spherocytic red cells. Use this

Parpart AK et al. (1947) The osmotic resistance (fragility) of human red cells. *J Clin Invest* **26**, 636; Weatherall DJ, Provan AB. (2000) Red cells I: inherited anaemias. *Lancet* **355**, 1169–1175.

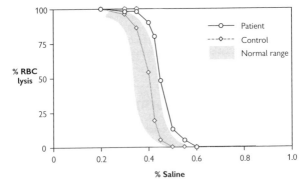

Fig. 3.10 Test and control samples subjected to varying concentrations of saline. The broad grey band represents the normal range. The red cells in the test sample (from a patient with hereditary spherocytosis) lyse at higher concentrations of saline than that seen in the normal control which suggests that HS is a likely diagnosis.

test in conjunction with a history, blood film and family studies (HS is inherited as an autosomal dominant, so one of the parents and some siblings should be affected).

Red cell enzyme assays

Numerous red cell enzymes are responsible for maintaining the integrity of the RBC in order to allow it to function efficiently in O_2 delivery and CO_2 removal. RBC enzyme defects lead to shortened RBC survival (i.e. haemolysis) and anaemia. Although there are numerous enzymopathies that may cause haemolysis, the most useful starting assays are for G6PD and pyruvate kinase.

Of course, one should start by taking a detailed history from the patient, asking about previous haemolytic episodes, family history, ethnic origin and possible drug toxicities.

Sample: fresh EDTA or heparin. The enzymes are stable for 6 days at 4°C and 24h at 25°C.

Methods: these are too numerous and complex to list here.

Essentially there are 3 methods for analysis of G6PD
- Brilliant cresyl blue decolorisation test.
- Methaemoglobin reduction test.
- UV spot test.

Normal range: varies between laboratories (check with your local lab).

Pitfalls: during a haemolytic episode in patients with G6PD deficiency the oldest RBCs are destroyed first. Younger RBCs (and especially reticulocytes) have higher levels of the enzyme than older cells. It follows therefore that if the enzyme level is assayed during an acute episode the G6PD level obtained may be falsely normal. This will rise further as reticulocytes pour into the peripheral blood, as happens during recovery from the acute attack. It is better to wait until the acute attack is over and the patient is in steady-state.

Haemoglobin abnormalities

There are 2 main classes of haemoglobin abnormalities.

Abnormality	Example
Structural Hb variants	Sickle haemoglobin, HbD, HbE
Imbalanced globin production	Thalassaemias (α, β, etc.)

Structural haemoglobin variants
If the amino acid change results in an electrical charge difference, this may be detected by protein electrophoresis (separates proteins on the basis of charge). Investigation requires full clinical history, FBC, blood film and Hb electrophoresis.

Thalassaemias
β thalassaemia is diagnosed from the blood indices, blood film, HbA_2 and HbF levels. For α thalassaemia the investigation is more complex requiring DNA analysis to detect α globin deletions. Globin chain synthesis, which examines the ratio of $\alpha : \beta$ globin production, is performed less with the advent of DNA-based methods.

Haemoglobin analysis

Haemoglobin electrophoresis
Electrophoresis is an electrical method for separating molecules on the basis of size (for DNA fragments) or overall electrical charge (for proteins). Hb electrophoresis allows the separation of different Hbs *providing* they have differing charges (Hb molecules with the same charge will move together on the gel and cannot be distinguished). The methods used take advantage of the fact that amino acid side chains on the globin molecules can be ionised. The net overall charge of a protein depends on the *pH* of

Arya R et al. (1995) Hereditary red cell enzymopathies. *Blood Rev* **9**, 165–175; Beutler E. (1992) The molecular biology of G6PD variants and other red cell enzyme defects. *Annu Rev Med* **43**, 47–59; World Health Organization Scientific Group. (1967) *Standardization of Procedures for the Study of Glucose-6-phosphate Dehydrogenase.* Technical Report Series, No. 366, WHO, Geneva.

Weatherall DJ, Provan AB. (2000) Red cells I: inherited anaemias. *Lancet* **355**, 1169–1175.

the solution it is in and the pKs of the amino acids (the pK is the pH at which half the side chains are ionised).

Electrophoretic methods used
- Cellulose acetate (at pH 8.6).
- Citrate agar (at pH 6.0).
- Isoelectric focusing (IEF).
- High-performance liquid chromatography (HPLC).

Due to space limitations each of these methods will be discussed only briefly. Other texts deal with this topic in considerable detail.

Sample: peripheral blood EDTA.

Cellulose acetate
This test is commonly performed in the diagnosis of abnormal haemoglobin production (haemoglobinopathies or thalassaemia). Because some Hbs have the same net charge they will run together, e.g. HbS will run in the same band as HbD and HbG, and HbC will run with HbE. To resolve these bands electrophoresis is next carried out at acid pH.

Citrate agar
This is similar to cellulose acetate where Hbs are separated at an acid pH (pH 6.0) to separate out Hbs that run together at alkaline pH.

Isoelectric focusing
This is a high resolution method for separating different Hb molecules. The basic principle of the test relies on the fact that all proteins and amino acids have a pH at which their net charge is zero. This is termed the isoelectric point. At this pH there is no net movement in the presence of an externally applied electric field. The Hb molecules are subjected to a pH gradient. This method has the advantage of high resolution but is more expensive than standard electrophoresis.

High-performance liquid chromatography
This chromatographic technique has been around for 20 years or more, and is being increasingly used for analysis of haemoglobin molecules. Haemoglobins are passed through a matrix column and eluted from the column at varying times, during which their absorbance is measured. Detection of standard haemoglobin variants is simple; the advantage of HPLC is that novel haemoglobin variants can also be detected, and HPLC can separate proteins that cannot be resolved using other means. HPLC is more expensive than all the techniques mentioned above.

When should you request these tests?
Haemoglobin analysis is usually carried out:
- When the MCV is ⬇⬇ but Hb normal or slightly ⬇.
- In patients from ethnic groups known to be associated with high levels of haemoglobin disorder, e.g. sickle or thalassaemia.

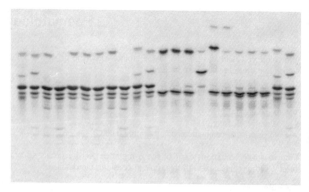

Fig. 3.11 Isoelectric focusing.

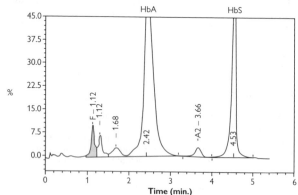

Fig. 3.12 HPLC analysis showing sickle trait (HbA + HbS).

Investigation of possible thalassaemia

1. Check FBC and look at MCV.
2. Is the MCV normal (>76fL)? If so, thalassaemia is unlikely.
3. Does the FBC show anything else? ↑ RCC with ↓ MCV and MCH are likely in thalassaemia.
4. Measure the HbA$_2$: this is generally ↑ in β thalassaemia trait (carrier).
5. Carry out HPLC.
6. Measure HbF level.
7. Look at distribution of HbF in RBCs (HbF is present in *all* RBCs in African HPFH(hereditary persistence of fetal haemoglobin), but not present in all cells in carrier for δβ thalassaemia.

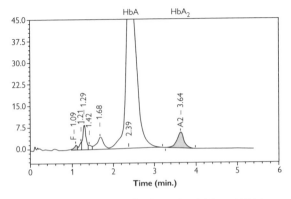

Fig. 3.13 HPLC analysis showing β thalassaemia trait (elevated HbA$_2$).

8. Assess iron status (common cause of ↓ MCV—don't miss this!).
9. Look for RBC inclusions (e.g. H bodies in α thalassaemia or Heinz bodies in unstable haemoglobin disorders).
10. Carry out DNA analysis, examining both α and β globin genes.

197

Sickle solubility test

Sickle Hb is the result of a point mutation in the β globin gene resulting in a glu→val switch at position 6 of the β globin protein. Sickle haemoglobin (HbS) forms long filaments (tactoids) reducing its solubility when O$_2$ tension is reduced. This forms the basis of the sickle solubility test.

Sample: any anticoagulant.

The patient's blood is mixed with sodium dithionite solution and left to stand. A positive sickle sample should be used as a control. When the tubes are examined a clear solution implies that there is no sickle Hb; a turbid solution confirms the presence of sickle Hb in the patient's sample.

▶ A positive result will be obtained for sickle carriers (HbAS) and sickle cell homozygotes (HbSS). If a positive result is obtained Hb electrophoresis must be carried out to determine whether the patient is a carrier or has homozygous sickle cell anaemia.

Steinberg MH et al., eds. (2001) *Disorders of Hemoglobin. Genetics, Pathophysiology, and Clinical Management*, Cambridge University Press, Cambridge.

Molecular diagnosis of sickle cell disease

This is useful for prenatal diagnosis. The β globin genes of the fetus are amplified using PCR (cells are obtained by amniocentesis or CVS) and digested with a bacterial restriction enzyme, e.g. Mst II. If the sickle mutation is present no digestion will occur (the mutation removes the restriction site).

Neonatal haemoglobin screening

- Obtain blood from neonate (e.g. heel prick) in babies at risk of sickle or β thalassaemia major (e.g. mother has gene for HbS, C, D^{Punjab}, E, O^{Arab}, β or δβ thalassaemia).
- Universal neonatal screening is generally used in areas where there is a high incidence of haemoglobinopathy.

📖OHCM p642.

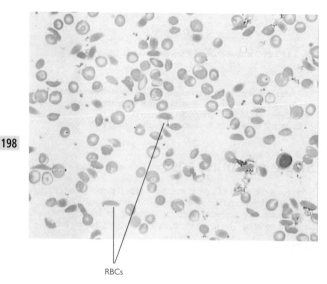

RBCs

Fig. 3.14 Blood film of homozygous sickle cell anaemia (HbSS). The lines show two sickled RBCs.

Estimation of haemoglobin A$_2$ ($\alpha_2\delta_2$)

Normal adults have 3 types of haemoglobin: HbA, HbA$_2$ and HbF. HbA ($\alpha_2\beta_2$) is the major Hb and HbA$_2$ is a minor adult haemoglobin, which is very useful for the diagnosis of β thalassaemia trait. HbA$_2$ levels are ↑ in the heterozygote (carrier state) and is a specific test for this genotype. The test is carried out using a column chromatography method.

Sample: EDTA.

Normal range: 2.0–3.2%.

Causes of ↑ HbA$_2$
- β thalassaemia trait (HbA$_2$ level is ~3.9–6.5%).

Causes of ↓ HbA$_2$
- Iron deficiency.
- δ thalassaemia.

Normal adult haemoglobins:

HbA	97% total
HbA$_2$	2.0–3.2%
HbF	0.5%

Estimation of fetal haemoglobin (HbF)

HbF makes up >50% of the total Hb at birth but decreases to ~5% by 5 months of age (as γ chain production is replaced by β chains). HbF levels may be raised in some haemoglobinopathies.

Sample: EDTA.

↑ HbF found in
- β thalassaemia trait.
- β thalassaemia major.
- Hereditary persistence of fetal haemoglobin.
- Homozygous sickle cell disease (HbSS).
- Sickle/β$^+$ thalassaemia (some cases).
- Sickle/β^0 thalassaemia (some cases).
- Juvenile chronic myeloid leukaemia.
- Multiple myeloma (uncommon and never measured).
- Acquired aplastic anaemia.

Haemoglobin H bodies (β$_4$)

HbH, consisting of a tetramer of β globins (β$_4$), is found in α thalassaemia. The β chains form tetramers due to the relative lack of α globins with which to pair. The demonstration of HbH allows the detection of α thalassaemia trait (either $-\alpha/-\alpha$ or $--/\alpha\alpha$) and HbH disease ($--/-\alpha$).

Method
The HbH body test involves staining RBCs with brilliant cresyl blue; HbH bodies are seen as large dark inclusions in the red cells.

Sample: fresh EDTA.

▶ *Note:* The presence of HbH confirms α thalassaemia but the absence of HbH bodies does *not* exclude the diagnosis.

Heinz bodies

These are red cell inclusions made up of insoluble denatured globin protein. Heinz bodies are seen when the RBCs are stained with methyl violet stain.

Sample: fresh EDTA.

Interpretation: Heinz bodies are seen close to the RBC membrane. These are normally removed by the spleen and are therefore more frequent following splenectomy.

Causes of Heinz bodies
- Oxidative haemolysis:
  - Chlorates, phenacetin, other drugs.
  - G6PD, PK deficiencies and other enzymopathies.
- Unstable haemoglobins.

Sevitt S *et al.* (1973) Acute Heinz-body anaemia in burned patients. *Lancet* **2**, 471–475.

Testing for unstable haemoglobins

Globin gene mutations may lead to amino acid substitutions that render the haemoglobin molecule unstable, leading to haemolysis. Most mutations causing unstable Hb are autosomal dominant and >80% affect the β chain. Affected individuals are heterozygotes. Heinz bodies in RBCs are intracellular Hb precipitates. Unstable Hbs can be detected electrophoretically or using the heat precipitation test, in which lysed RBCs are heated to 50°C for 1h.

Sample: fresh EDTA.

Interpretation: normal fresh haemolysates should be stable for 1h at 50°C. If there is an unstable Hb a precipitate will be seen in the tube.

Examples
- Hb Köln.
- Hb Gun Hill.

Molecular tests for diagnosis of thalassaemia

Although most haematology labs can diagnose β thalassaemia trait and β thalassaemia major, there are occasions when molecular tests are required, e.g. antenatal diagnosis where a couple are at risk of having a child with β thalassaemia major or hydrops fetalis (absence of α globin, usually lethal). In addition, the diagnosis of α thalassaemia is difficult and requires DNA analysis either using Southern blotting or PCR amplification of globin genes.

β thalassaemia

There are >100 β globin mutations now known but fortunately each population tends to have its own group of mutations (this avoids having to test for all known mutations). It is important that you include the ethnic group on the request form since this will assist the lab who will then screen for mutations commonly found in the ethnic group of the patient. Details of these mutations can be found in the *beta and delta thalassemia repository*.

Methods used for molecular diagnosis of β thalassaemia

The methods used are complex and outwith the scope of this small book (*see references below*).

How the ARMS PCR technique works

- This is amplification refractory mutation system PCR.
- Specific point mutations are known for the β globin mutations.
- PCR primers are designed to bind with the mutated sequence.
- If the patient has the mutation there will be PCR amplification.
- If the patient lacks the mutation there is no binding of the primers to the patient's DNA, and no amplification.
- So, a band on the gel means the mutation is present (and the reverse is true—if the band is absent then that particular mutation is absent).

201

Other techniques including reverse dot blots and DNA sequencing are sometimes needed if ARMS PCR fails.

Methods used for molecular diagnosis of α thalassaemia

Whereas β thalassaemia is usually the result of point mutations (single base changes), the α thalassaemias are usually the result of deletions of chunks of DNA in the region of the α globin genes. Southern blotting is useful in detecting deletions since the DNA band sizes after digestion with restriction enzymes will differ to the wild type (i.e. normal).

UK Haemoglobinopathy Reference Laboratory

This is based at the John Radcliffe Hospital in Oxford (UK). Difficult cases (e.g. α thalassaemia) can be sent to this lab (after discussing the case first); they will perform α globin gene analysis and send a detailed report containing the genotype of the patient. See end of chapter for contact details (📖p238).

Bowden DK *et al.* (1992) A PCR-based strategy to detect the common severe determinants of a thalassaemia. *Br J Haem* **81**, 104–108; Dacie JV, Lewis SM, eds (1995) *Practical Haematology*, 8th edition, Churchill Livingstone, Edinburgh; Huisman TH, Carver MF. (1988) The beta- and delta-thalassemia repository (9th edition, Part 1). *Hemoglobin* **22**, 169–195.

Acquired haemolytic anaemias

Determining the cause of haemolytic anaemia can be a complex process. Having excluded inherited disorders of haemoglobin, RBC membrane or enzymes we are left with a diverse group of disorders with a common phenotype of increased RBC destruction (and ↓ RBC lifespan).

Immune
- Autoimmune (primary, or 2° to SLE or CLL).
- Alloimmune (e.g. transfusion reactions, haemolytic disease of the newborn).
- Antibody can be warm (IgG) or cold (IgM usually).

RBC damage
- Drugs.
- Poisons.
- Burns.

RBC fragmentation syndromes
- DIC.
- TTP/HUS.
- March haemoglobinuria.

Investigations
There is little point investigating the cause of haemolytic anaemia until you have shown that haemolysis is *actually* occurring.

Look for the acquired cause
- FBC and peripheral film:
    - Spherocytes (suggests warm antibody; also present in HS).
    - ↑ WBC, e.g. might suggest underlying lymphoproliferative disorder such as CLL.
    - RBC fragments (suggests physical damage to the RBC, e.g. MAHA, TTP/HUS, burns, March haemoglobinuria, mechanical heart valves).
    - Parasites, e.g. malaria.
    - Infections, e.g. *Clostridium, Bartonella, Babesia*.
- Antiglobulin test (DAT):
    - IgG or IgG + complement (C3d) on RBC.
    - DAT is usually +ve in immune-mediated haemolysis.
- Renal function (abnormal in TTP/HUS).
- Coagulation screen (DIC with RBC fragmentation).
- LFTs (abnormal in Zieve's syndrome).
- USS for splenomegaly.
- Cold agglutinins:
    - IgM, usually against I or i proteins, RBC membrane proteins.
- Ham's test or immunophenotype if suspect PNH.

Ham's acid lysis test

This is a test for the rare acquired red cell membrane disorder called paroxysmal nocturnal haemoglobinuria (PNH) which relies on the exquisite sensitivity of red cells to lysis by normal plasma constituents. Its pathophysiology is complex and involves an abnormality of the red cell

Causes of acquired haemolytic anaemia

Mechanism	Examples
Autoimmune	**Warm antibody (IgG mainly)** Idiopathic haemolytic anaemia Secondary to other autoimmune diseases (e.g. SLE), lymphoid malignancies (e.g. CLL), infections, drugs (e.g. penicillins, methyldopa) **Cold antibodies (IgM mainly)** Cold agglutinin syndromes, cold haemagglutinin disease (CHAD), 2° to infection
Alloimmune	Haemolytic transfusion reactions, haemolytic disease of the newborn (HDN)
Infections	Many, including malaria, meningococcal, pneumococcal, viral
Chemical or physical	Drugs, burns, drowning
RBC fragmentation syndromes	Mechanical heart valves, microangiopathic haemolytic anaemia (MAHA, seen in DIC, HUS, TTP, pre-eclampsia, SLE, carcinoma)
Membrane disorders	Liver disease, PNH

membrane in PNH making it prone to complement-mediated lysis and episodes of marked intravascular haemolysis leading to free haemoglobin in the urine (haemoglobinuria).

Principle
- Abnormal sensitivity of RBCs from patients with PNH to the haemolytic action of complement.
- Complement is activated by acidification of the patient's serum to pH of 6.2 which induces lysis of PNH red cells but not normal controls.

Sample: EDTA, heparin, citrate, oxalate.

Result: +ve result indicates PNH.

Specificity: high—similar reaction is produced only in the rare syndrome HEMPAS (a form of congenital dyserythropoietic anaemia type II) which should be easily distinguished morphologically.

Sensitivity: low—as the reaction is crucially dependent on the concentration of magnesium in the serum.

Beware: may be +ve in the rare congenital dyserythropoietic anaemia (CDA) type II also called HEMPAS (hereditary erythroblast multinuclearity with positive acidified serum).

Alternative tests

- Sucrose lysis—an alternative method of complement activation is by mixing serum with a low ionic strength solution such as sucrose. Sensitivity of this test is high but specificity is low—i.e. the opposite of the Ham's test.
- Immunophenotypic detection of the deficiency of the PIG transmembrane protein anchors in PNH cells is becoming a more widely used alternative. Monoclonal antibodies to CD59 or CD55 (DAF) are used in flow cytometric analysis. The major advantage is that the test can be performed on peripheral blood neutrophils and platelets which are more numerous than the PNH red cells.

Bleeding time

This is a test of primary haemostasis, and mainly of platelet function *in vivo*, rather than a laboratory test. You will generally need to arrange this test through the haematology department who will carry out the test for you.

Procedure

A disposable spring-loaded blade is used to make 2 incisions of fixed depth into the skin of the forearm whilst a sphygmomanometer is inflated to 40mmHg. Blood from the incisions is mopped up using circular filter paper (care needs to be taken to avoid disturbing the clot which forms on the cut surface).

Normal range: up to 7min (varies depending on method used; >9min is abnormal). Longer in ♀.

Uses: best screen for acquired or congenital functional or structural platelet disorders. If bleeding time normal and history is negative (i.e. no major bleeding problems in past) this excludes an underlying platelet disorder.

Precautions

▶Don't carry out bleeding time if platelet count is $<100 \times 10^9$/L (will be prolonged). Aspirin will interfere with test—ask patients to stop aspirin 7 days before test carried out.

Causes of prolonged bleeding time

- Low platelet count.
- Platelet function defect (acquired, e.g. aspirin, paraprotein, MDS).
- von Willebrand's disease.
- Vascular abnormalities, e.g. Ehlers-Danlos.
- Occasionally low factor V or XI.
- Afibrinogenaemia.

📖OHCM p646.

Mielke CH Jr. (1982) Aspirin prolongation of the template bleeding time: influence of venostasis and direction of incision. *Blood* **60**, 1139–1142; Parkin JD, Smith IL. (1985) Sex and bleeding time. *Thromb Haemost* **54**, 731.

Prothrombin time (PT)

This tests the extrinsic coagulation pathway and is useful for detecting coagulation deficiencies, liver disease and DIC. The PT is also the main monitor for coumarin therapy (e.g. warfarin), expressed as a ratio—the *international normalized ratio* (INR). The test measures the clotting time of plasma in the presence of a tissue extract, e.g. brain (thromboplastin). The test measures prothrombin but also factors V, VII and X.

Sample: citrate.

↑ **PT**

- Oral anticoagulation therapy (vitamin K antagonists).
- Fibrinogen deficiency (factor I).
- Prothrombin deficiency (factor II).
- Deficiency of factors V, VII or X (in V or X deficiency the APTT will be ↑).
- Liver disease especially obstructive.

205

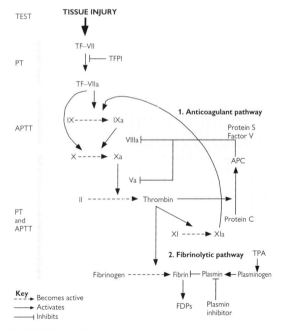

Fig. 3.15 Coagulation cascade showing the factors assayed using the various clotting tests. Modified from Provan D et al. (1998) *Oxford Handbook of Clinical Haematology*, OUP, Oxford.

- Vitamin K deficiency.
- DIC.

Activated partial thromboplastin time (APTT)

Other terms: kaolin cephalin clotting time (KCCT), partial thromboplastin time with kaolin (PTTK).

This is a test of the intrinsic coagulation system, and depends on contact factors + factors VIII, IX and reactions with factors X, V, II and I. The APTT is sensitive to circulating anticoagulants (e.g. lupus anticoagulant) and heparin.

Sample: citrate.

Uses
- Heparin monitoring.
- Screening for haemophilia A and B (VIII and IX deficiency, respectively).
- Screening for coagulation inhibitors.

Normal range: 26.0–33.5s (often expressed as ratio, APTR).

↑ APTT
- DIC.
- Liver disease.
- Massive blood transfusion.
- Heparin treatment.
- Circulating anticoagulant.
- Modest ↑ in patients taking oral anticoagulants.
- Haemophilia.

Is there an inhibitor present?
The APTT will be long if there is an inhibitor such as the lupus anticoagulant present This can be determined by mixing the patient's plasma with an equal volume of normal control plasma and repeating the APTT. If the APTT is long because of an inhibitor it will not fully correct when normal plasma is added. However, if the APTT is long because of a deficiency it will correct with the normal plasma.

Denson KW. (1988) Thromboplastin—sensitivity, precision and other characteristics. *Clin Lab Haematol* **10**, 315–328.

Turi DC, Peerschke EI. (1986) Sensitivity of three activated partial thromboplastin time reagents to coagulation factor deficiencies. *Am J Clin Pathol* **85**, 43–49; van den Besselaar AM et al. (1987) Monitoring heparin therapy by the activated partial thromboplastin time—the effect of pre-analytical conditions. *Thromb Haemost* **57**, 226–231.

Thrombin clotting time (TCT)

This is affected by the concentration of factor I (fibrinogen) and the presence of fibrin/-ogen degradation products and heparin.

Sample: citrate.

↑ **TCT**
- Low fibrinogen, e.g. DIC.
- ↑ FDPs/XDPs/D-dimers.
- Heparin*.
- Dysfibrinogenaemia (inherited, mutation in fibrinogen gene leads to amino acid change and non-functional fibrinogen).

*If suspected, check reptilase time, similar to TCT but not affected by heparin.

D-dimers

D-dimers are produced during polymerisation of fibrinogen as it forms fibrin. Measurement of D-dimer levels is more specific for this process than the older FDP (fibrinogen/fibrin degradation products) test and is now being used to detect the presence of DIC and other coagulation disorders. The test measures fibrin lysis by plasmin and is a sensitive indicator of coagulation activation (e.g. such as that seen in DIC). The assay uses a monoclonal antibody specific for D-dimers; it will not cross-react with fibrinogen or fibrin.

207

Sample: citrate (clotting screen bottle).

↑ **D-dimers seen in**
- DIC.
- DVT.
- PE.

▶▶Disseminated intravascular coagulation (DIC)

We have devoted a section to this disorder since it is a medical and haematological emergency. DIC may be seen in a variety of situations and

Modified from Dacie JV, Lewis SM. (1995) *Practical Haematology*, 8th edition, Churchill Livingstone, Edinburgh.

Summary of tests in bleeding disorders

PT	APTT	TCT	Platlets	Diagnosis
N	N	N	N	Platelet function defect., XII def. normal
↑	N	N	N	VII def., early oral anticoagulation
N	↑	N	N	VIIIC/IX/XI/XII def., vWD, circulating anticoagulant, e.g. lupus
↑	↑	N	N	Vitamin K def., oral anticoagulant V/VII/X/II def.
↑	↑	↑	N	Heparin, liver disease, fibrinogen def.
N	N	N	↓	Thrombocytopenia (any cause)
↑	↑	N	low	Massive transfusion, liver disease
↑	↑	↑	low	DIC, acute liver disease

def., deficiency; N, normal; ↑, increased; ↓, decreased.

Conditions associated with DIC

Disorder	Example
Infectious disease	Septicaemia
	Viraemia
Obstetric emergency	Placental abruption
	Eclampsia
	Amniotic fluid embolism
	Placenta praevia
	Septic abortion
Surgical	Cardiac bypass
Malignant disease	Metastatic cancer
	Acute leukaemia (esp. AML M3, i.e. acute promyelocytic leukaemia)
Shock	Trauma
	Severe burns
Transfusion	ABO mismatched transfusion
Miscellaneous	Snake bites (some)
	Liver cirrhosis

is characterised by generalised bruising and bleeding, usually from venepuncture sites, post-operatively and spontaneously. Diagnosis requires FBC, clotting screen and evidence of rapid consumption of fibrinogen. *Classic* (acute) DIC, where the test results fit the bill, is easy to spot. The situation may be more subtle and you are strongly advised to discuss the case with a haematology registrar or consultant if you are in any doubt about the diagnosis of DIC.

▶▶**Laboratory diagnosis**

FBC	↓ platelets may show RBC fragments
PT	↑ in moderately severe DIC
APTT	usually ↑
Fibrinogen	↓ (falling levels significant—but remember this is an acute phase protein so level may be normal even in florid DIC)
D-dimers	↑

209

Platelet function tests

These are specialised tests carried out by the coagulation laboratory for the investigation of patients with suspected platelet dysfunction. Because of their complexity, the platelet function tests will not be described in detail here.

Patients generally present with bleeding or bruising problems and have had normal coagulation results. Because of the labour-intensive nature and cost of these assays you will need to arrange these tests after discussion with your local haematology medical staff.

Sample: blood collection needs to be optimal with non-traumatic venepuncture, rapid transport to the lab with storage at room temperature and testing within a maximum of 2–3h.

Current tests
- Platelet count.
- Morphology.
- Adhesion.
- Aggregation.
- Platelet release.
- Bleeding time.

Platelet count

Normal range 150–400 $\times$ 10^9/L. Adequate function is maintained even when the count is <0.5 normal level, but progressively deteriorates as it drops. With platelet counts <20 $\times$ 10^9/L there is usually easy bruising and petechial haemorrhages (although more serious bleeding can occur).

Morphology

Large platelets are biochemically more active; ↑ mean platelet volume (MPV >6.5) is associated with less bleeding in patients with severe thrombocytopenia. Altered platelet size is seen in inherited platelet disorders.

Platelet adhesion

Adhesion to glass beads now rarely performed in routine lab practice, but potentially useful in vWD diagnosis.

Platelet aggregation

Most useful of the special tests is performed on fresh sample using aggregometer.

Aggregants used

- Adenosine 5-diphosphate (ADP) at low and high concentrations. Induces 2 aggregation waves: primary wave may disaggregate at low concentrations of ADP; the second is irreversible.
- Collagen has a short lag phase followed by a single wave and is particularly affected by aspirin.
- Ristocetin-induced platelet aggregation (RIPA) is carried out at a high (1.2mg/mL) and lower concentrations and is mainly used to diagnose vWD.
- Arachidonic acid.
- Adrenaline (epinephrine), not uncommonly reduced in normal people.

Platelet release

ELISA or RIA are used to measure the granule proteins β-thromboglobulin (β-TG) and heparin neutralising activity (HNA). These are sensitive markers of platelet hyper-reactivity and beyond the scope of the routine laboratory.

Practical application of tests

Their main role is in diagnosis of inherited platelet functional defects. In acquired platelet dysfunction secondary to causes such as renal and hepatic disease, DIC and macroglobulinaemia, platelet function is rarely tested.

Yardumian A et al. (1986) Laboratory investigation of platelet function: a review of methodology. J Clin Path **39**, 701–712.

Thrombophilia screening

Thrombophilia describes acquired or inherited disorders that predispose to arterial or venous thromboembolism (VTE). Thrombophilia should be suspected when the blood clot affects an unusual site, the patient is young, has recurrent thrombotic episodes, or has a strong family history of VTE.

Causes: 📖 *Symptoms & Signs*, (p74).

Which patients should be screened for possible thrombophilia?
- Arterial thrombosis, e.g. patients <30 years, without obvious arterial disease.
- Venous thrombosis:
  - Patients <40 years with no obvious risk factors.
  - Unexplained recurrent thrombosis.
  - VTE and family history of thrombosis in first degree relatives.
  - Unusual site, e.g. mesenteric, portal vein thrombosis.
  - Unexplained neonatal thrombosis.
  - Recurrent miscarriage (≥3).
  - VTE in pregnancy and the OCP.

Screen
- Exclude medical causes (check ESR, LFTs, AIP, fasting lipids).
- FBC (exclude thrombocytosis).
- Clotting screen for acquired defects (PT, APTT, LA/ACL, ↑ fibrinogen).
- Screen for inherited thrombophilia:
  - First line PC, PS, AT, APCR.
  - Check for presence of the factor V Leiden mutation in APCR +ve patients (DNA analysis).
  - Consider testing plasminogen, factor XII, homocysteine levels, prothrombin variant.
- DNA analysis for prothrombin gene mutation.

Thrombophilia investigations are time-consuming and expensive and you should discuss with the local haematology medical or lab staff before sending samples. *Note*: Some thrombophilia tests cannot be carried out in the 'acute' phase of a VTE event or while the patient is taking warfarin.

Cattaneo M et al. (1998) Interrelation of hyperhomocyst(e)inemia, factor V Leiden, and risk of future venous thromboembolism. *Circulation* **97**, 295–296; Dahlback B. (1997) Resistance to activated protein C as risk factor for thrombosis: molecular mechanisms, laboratory investigation, and clinical management. *Semin Hematol* **34**, 217–234; Lane DA et al. (1996) Inherited thrombophilia: Part 1. *Thromb Haemost* **76**, 651–662. Lane DA et al. (1996) Inherited thrombophilia: Part 2. *Thromb Haemost* **76**, 824–834.

Antithrombin, proteins C & S

These proteins are the body's *natural anticoagulants*, hence deficiencies may lead to thromboembolic disease.

Antithrombin (AT)
Used to be called AT III but no I or II so now abbreviated to AT. A useful measure in thrombophilia screening since low levels of AT are found in 4.5% patients with unexplained VTE.

↓ AT levels
- Hereditary (40–60% normal level), autosomal dominant.
- Chronic liver disease.

- Protein wasting disorders.
- Heparin therapy.
- 3rd trimester of pregnancy.
- Acute leukaemia.
- Burns.
- Renal disease.
- Gram −ve sepsis.

Protein S
- Reduced levels predispose to VTE. Individuals with 30–60% normal level may suffer recurrent thrombosis.

↓ Protein S
- Inherited (autosomal dominant).
- Pregnancy.
- Oral anticoagulants, e.g. warfarin.
- Nephrotic syndrome.
- Liver disease.

Protein C
- Similar to protein S; autosomal dominant inheritance in genetic cases.

↓ Protein C
- Hereditary.
- Liver disease.
- Malignancy.
- Warfarin therapy.
- Pregnancy.

Bone marrow examination

This is a key investigation in haematology. It may be *diagnostic* in the follow-up of abnormal peripheral blood findings, and is an important *staging* procedure in defining the extent of disease, e.g. lymphomas. It is a helpful investigative procedure in unexplained anaemia, splenomegaly or selected cases of pyrexia of unknown origin (PUO).

Preferred sites: posterior iliac crest is the usual site (allows aspirate and biopsy to be obtained). The sternum is suitable **only** for marrow aspiration.

The marrow aspirate provides
- Cytology of nucleated cells.
- Qualitative and semiqualitative analysis of haematopoiesis.
- Assessment of iron stores (if Perls' iron stain used).
- Smears for cytochemistry (helps in the diagnosis of leukaemias).

Marrow cells can also be used for
- Chromosomal (cytogenetic) analysis.
- Immunophenotype studies using monoclonal antibodies.

Marrow trephine biopsy provides information about
- Marrow cellularity.
- Identification and classification of abnormal cells.
- Immunohistochemistry on infiltrates.

Contraindications

None, other than physical limitations, e.g. pain or restricted mobility. Avoid sites of previous radiotherapy (inevitably grossly hypocellular and not representative).

Procedure

1. BM aspiration may be performed under LA alone, but short acting IV sedative (e.g. midazolam) is preferred when trephine biopsy is performed. GA used in children.
2. Place patient in (L) lateral position, or use right if he cannot lie on left side.
3. Infiltrate skin and periosteum over the posterior iliac spine with local anaesthetic.
4. Make a small cutaneous incision before introducing the aspirating needle, which should penetrate the marrow cortex 3–10mm before removal of the trocar.
5. Aspirate no more than 0.5–1mL marrow initially (to avoid dilution of sample with blood).
6. Make smears promptly (it will clot rapidly!).
7. If further samples are needed, e.g. for immunophenotyping, cytogenetics, etc. these can be aspirated after making initial slides.
8. For trephine biopsy use Islam or Jamshidi needle.
9. Advance the needle through the same puncture site to penetrate the cortex.
10. Remove the trocar and, using firm hand pressure, rotate the needle clockwise and advance as far as possible.
11. Remove the needle by gentle anticlockwise rotation.
12. Following the procedure apply simple pressure dressings.
13. Minor discomfort at the location may be dealt with by simple analgesia such as paracetamol.

213

Tests carried out on bone marrow	
Chromosomes	Standard cytogenetic analysis, looking for rearrangements suggestive of acute or chronic leukaemias and myelodysplasia
	Fluorescence *in situ* hybridisation (FISH) looking for additions or losses of chromosomes, as well as more subtle changes seen in leukaemias and lymphomas
DNA or RNA analysis	Using PCR to look for mutations or translocations which help classify leukaemias and lymphomas; also useful for monitoring disease levels in some disorders
Immunophenotype	Cell surface marker profile helps in the diagnosis of most leukaemias and lymphomas; may also be used to monitor disease levels post-treatment
Microbiology	e.g. TB culture (not routine, but occasionally useful in cases of PUO)
Cytochemical stains	To help define type of leukaemia

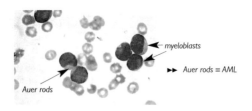

Fig. 3.16 AML marrow.

Cytochemistry tests (leukaemias)

These staining methods have been around for many years (for decades they were *all* that was available), but remain extremely useful in the diagnosis and classification of leukaemias. Modern technologies such as flow cytometry and nucleic acid analysis have refined leukaemia and lymphoma diagnosis but the examination of well-stained cytochemistry bone marrow smears remain the cornerstone of good haematology practice.

After performing a bone marrow aspirate and spreading the material onto glass slides, the air-dried unfixed microscope slides are passed to the cytochemistry lab who will fix and stain the slides according to the likely diagnosis (stains for AML differ to those for ALL, for example). Positive results with particular stains will point to a specific diagnosis. This will then be augmented by flow cytometric or molecular assays.

Cytochemical stains and their specificities

Cytochemical stain	Substrate/cell
Myeloperoxidase (MPO)	Lysosomal enzyme found in neutrophils and monocytes
Sudan black (SB)	Phospholipids in neutrophil granules
Chloroacetate esterase	Stains specific esterase in granulocytes and mast cells. Makes it easier to diagnose AML M4 subtype
α-naphtholacetate esterase (ANAE)	Esterase stain, useful for diagnosis of AML subtypes
Acid phosphatase	Enzyme found in many different WBCs. Useful for T cell malignancies
Periodic acid–Schiff (PAS)	Detects glycogen in cells. Granulocytes have diffuse staining whereas lymphocyte staining is much coarser

	Acute lymphoblastic leukaemia		Acute myeloid leukaemia		
	B lineage	T lineage	M1–3	M4–5	M6–7
Myeloperoxidase	—	—	+/++	+	—
Sudan black	—	—	+/++	+	—
Chloroacetate esterase	—	—	−/++	—	—
α-naphthol acetate esterase	—	—	—	++	—
Acid phosphatase	—	+ (focal)	—	+ (diffuse)	+ (focal)
Periodic acid–Schiff	+ (blocks)	—	—	+ (fine granular)	+

+, positive; ++, strongly positive; —, negative.

From Hoffbrand AV, Lewis SM, Tuddenham EGD (2000) Postgraduate Haematology, 4th edition, Butterworth-Heinemann, Oxford.

215

Neutrophil alkaline phosphatase

Uses

This is a cytochemical stain used to demonstrate the presence and quantity of the neutrophil enzyme alkaline phosphatase. Historically the NAP score was of value in differentiating 'reactive' states from myeloproliferative disorders, such as CML, polycythaemia rubra vera, etc.—now more often features in examination MCQs! (*Note: sometimes termed leucocyte alkaline phosphatase, LAP.*)

Procedure

Best performed on fresh blood films, made without the use of anticoagulant. EDTA samples may be used but are less satisfactory. The film should be made, air dried, fixed and then stained—all within 30min. Positive NAP activity is indicated by the presence of bright blue granules in the neutrophil cytoplasm (the nucleus is stained red).

Scoring: films are scored from 0 to 4 on the basis of stain intensity:

0	negative, no granules seen
1	weak positive, few granules
2	positive, few–moderate numbers of granules
3	strongly positive
4	very strong

Interpretation & significance

High NAP score	Low NAP score
Polycythaemia rubra vera (PRV)	Chronic myeloid leukaemia
Leukaemoid reaction	Paroxysmal nocturnal haemoglobinuria
Neutrophilia—any cause	Acute myeloid leukaemia
Myelofibrosis	
Essential thrombocythaemia	
Hepatic cirrhosis	
Hodgkin's disease	
Aplastic anaemia	
Down's syndrome	
Cushing's disease	

The NAP score is affected by corticosteroids, oestrogens and pregnancy (↑ NAP). In Hodgkin's disease the NAP score offers no advantage over simpler tests such as ESR for assessment of disease activity. Occasionally of value in a patient with aplastic anaemia who is developing PNH—the NAP score is seen to fall (both of these are very rare disorders). NAP score has been replaced in most hospitals by flow cytometry and other methods.

Dacie JV, Lewis SM. (1995) *Practical Haematology*, 8th edition, Churchill Livingstone, Edinburgh.

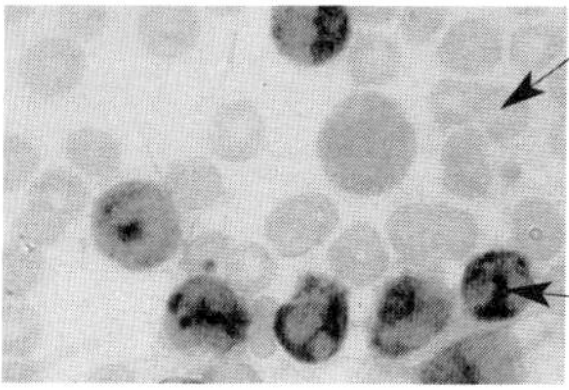

Fig. 3.17 NAP stained blood film: shows positively stained neutrophils.

Blood transfusion

Due to space limitations it is inappropriate to go into major details about the investigations used in transfusion medicine. However, we have provided the more important tests in current use which include:

- Blood group & antibody screen.
- Cross-match (compatibility test).
- Direct antiglobulin test (DAT).
- Antiplatelet and antineutrophil antibody testing.

Safe transfusion practice

217

Each year patients are transfused with the wrong blood. The commonest error is clerical and generally involves the cross-match sample being taken from the wrong patient and so the compatibility test is performed on the wrong sample. Occasionally the staff carrying out the transfusion connect the blood up to the wrong patient. In any event, the result varies from no symptoms to shock and possible death.

How to minimise errors

- First, ask yourself: *does this patient really need to be transfused* with blood or blood products (e.g. FFP, platelets, etc.)? For example, a post-operative patient who is asymptomatic with a Hb of 9g/dL probably does not require red cell transfusion. Use clinical judgement in helping decide whether or not to proceed with transfusion.
- Before taking the blood sample check that you are taking blood from the correct patient—ask for his/her name and check the identity bracelet.
- Label the patient's blood bottle at the bedside (i.e. no prelabelling of bottles:
  - Many transfusion labs insist on 1, 2, 5, 6 & 7 and either 3 or 4 from:

1. **Surname & forename (correctly spelt)**
2. **DOB**
3. **Hospital/A&E/new NHS number**
4. **First line of address**
5. **Sex**
6. **Time and date blood taken**
7. **Signature of person taking blood**

- Ensure details on form match those on the bottle.
- Complete the request form properly:
  - State what is required (e.g. 2 units of packed cells, etc.).
  - Detail any previous transfusions, reactions, antibodies (if known).
  - Let the lab know when you want the blood or blood product.

▶▶ Sticky patient labels are fine for forms but are not suitable for specimen bottles, and are usually not accepted by transfusion labs. Transfusion specimens should be labelled by hand—at the bedside.

If this sounds cumbersome and bureaucratic:

Remember many people die annually because they are transfused with the *wrong blood*. In most cases clerical error is to blame—people have filled out bottles in advance and failed to check patient identity.

Transfusion reactions

Rapid temperature spike (>40°C) at start of transfusion indicates transfusion should be stopped (suggests acute intravascular haemolysis).

If slow rising temperature (<40°C), providing patient not acutely unwell, slow IVI. Fever often due to antibodies against WBCs (or to cytokines in platelet packs).

▶▶ Immediate transfusion reaction

Intravascular haemolysis (→haemoglobinaemia & haemoglobinuria). Usually due to anti-A or anti-B antibodies (in ABO mismatched transfusion). Symptoms occur in minutes/hours. **May be fatal.**

Immediate transfusion reaction or bacterial contamination of blood

Symptoms	Signs
Patient restless/agitated	Fever
Flushing	Hypotension
Anxiety	Oozing from wounds or venepuncture sites
Chills	Haemoglobinaemia
Nausea & vomiting	Haemoglobinuria
Pain at venepuncture site	
Abdominal, flank or chest pain	
Diarrhoea	

If predominantly extravascular may only suffer chills/fever 1h after starting transfusion—commonly due to anti-D. Acute renal failure is not a feature.

Mechanism
Complement (C3a, C4a, C5a) release into recipient plasma→smooth muscle contraction. May develop DIC or oliguria (10% cases) due to profound hypotension.

Initial steps in management of acute transfusion reaction
- Stop blood transfusion immediately.
- Replace giving set, keep IV open with 0.9% saline.
- Check patient identity against donor unit.
- Insert urinary catheter and monitor urine output.
- Give fluids (IV colloids) to maintain urine output >1.5mL/kg/h.
- If urine output <1.5mL/kg/h insert CVP line and give fluid challenge.
- If urine output <1.5mL/kg/h and CVP adequate give frusemide 80–120mg.
- If urine output still <1.5 mL/kg/h consult senior medical staff for advice.
- Contact blood transfusion lab before sending back blood pack and for advice on blood samples required for further investigation (see below).

219

Complications
Overall mortality ~10%.

Urgent investigations

Your local blood transfusion department will have specific guidelines to help you with the management of an acute reaction. The following guide lists the samples commonly required to establish the cause and severity of a transfusion reaction. *If you are uncertain about the laboratory procedure or management of a patient who appears to have suffered a severe reaction you must notify your hospital's haematology medical staff* who will provide advice. ▶▶▶Delays may threaten the patient's life.

---

1. Check compatibility label of blood unit matches with patient's ID band, forms and casenotes.
2. *If mistake found tell the blood bank urgently*—the unit of blood intended for your patient may be transfused to another patient.
3. Take blood for:

   — **haematology**   FBC
                                   DAT
                                   plasma haemoglobin
                                   repeat cross-match sample
                                   coagulation screen

   — **chemistry**   U&E

   — **microbiology**   blood cultures

4. Check urinalysis and monitor urine output.
5. Do ECG and check for evidence of ↑$[K^+]$.
6. Arrange repeat coagulation screens & biochemistry 2–4 hourly.

Febrile transfusion reactions

Seen in 0.5–1.0% of blood transfusions. Mainly due to anti-HLA antibodies in recipient serum or granulocyte-specific antibodies (e.g. sensitisation during pregnancy or previous blood transfusion).

Delayed transfusion reaction

Occurs in patients immunised through previous pregnancies or transfusions. Antibody weak (so not detected at pre-transfusion stage). 2° immune response occurs—antibody titre ↑.

Symptoms and signs
- Occur 7–10 days after blood transfusion.
- Fever, anaemia and jaundice.
- ± Haemoglobinuria.

Management
- Discuss with transfusion lab staff.
- Check DAT and repeat compatibility tests.
- Transfuse patient with freshly cross-matched blood.

McClelland B (2001) *Handbook of Transfusion Medicine*, 2nd edition, HMSO, London.

Bacterial contamination of blood products

Uncommon but **potentially fatal** adverse effect of blood transfusion (affects red cells and blood products, e.g. platelet concentrates). Implicated organisms include gram −ve bacteria, including *Pseudomonas*, *Yersinia* and *Flavobacterium*.

Features
Include fever, skin flushing, rigors, abdominal pain, DIC, ARF, shock and possible cardiac arrest.

Management—as per *Immediate transfusion reaction*
- Stop transfusion
- Urgent resuscitation.
- IV broad-spectrum antibiotics if bacterial contamination suspected.

Antiglobulin test

The old term is Coombs' test. Direct antiglobulin test (DAT) detects antibodies or complement or both on the RBC surface and the indirect antiglobulin test (IAT) detects presence of antibodies in serum. A useful investigation when investigating haemolytic anaemia.

Sample: EDTA.

221

Interpretation
- Positive DAT in most AIHA.
- Lymphoproliferative disorders, e.g. CLL.
- Drug-induced haemolysis (e.g. α-methyl dopa, L-dopa).
- Haemolytic disease of the newborn, e.g. Rhesus HDN.

Note: As with many tests in medicine, things are never entirely black or white—a +ve DAT does not necessarily imply that haemolysis is actively occurring and a −ve DAT does not exclude haemolysis.

Coombs RRA. (1945) A new test for the detection of weak and 'incomplete' Rh agglutinins. *Br J Exp Path* **26**, 255; Kelton JG. (1985) Impaired reticuloendothelial function in patients treated with methyldopa. *NEJM* **313**, 596–600.

Kleihauer test

Uses
To determine (1) whether fetal red cells have entered the maternal circulation, and if so (2) determine the volume of such fetal cells.

Background

If a Rhesus (D)-negative mother has a baby that is Rh (D) +ve she may develop antibodies (maternal anti-D) against fetal red cells. This may result in fetal red cell destruction termed *Rhesus haemolytic disease of the newborn*, a serious haemolytic disorder which is seen less today due to greater understanding of the underlying mechanism and our ability to prevent it. Sensitisation to the fetal red cells occurs when fetal RBCs enter the maternal circulation, e.g. at birth or through obstetric manipulations, e.g. amniocentesis, previous pregnancies, etc.

Fetal RBCs in the mother's circulation can be detected and quantified (in mL) using the Kleihauer test, which exploits the resistance of fetal red cells to acid elution (acid washes adult Hb out of the mother's red cells but the fetal RBCs contain HbF which is not washed out). The Kleihauer test should be performed on all RH (D) −ve women who deliver a RH (D) +ve infant.

Fetal cells appear as darkly staining cells against a background of ghosts (these are the maternal red cells). An estimate of the required dose of anti-D can be made from the number of fetal cells in a low power field.

Sample: maternal peripheral blood EDTA.

Calculating the volume of fetal RBCs in the maternal circulation

Basically, a calculation is made by the laboratory staff based on the number of fetal RBCs seen in the Kleihauer film. The actual calculation is:

1800^* × ratio of $^{fetal}/_{adult}$ RBCs × $\frac{2}{3}$ (correction factor)

for example, if there are 1% fetal RBCs in maternal circulation

$1800 \times \frac{1}{100} \times \frac{2}{3} = 24mL$

*1800 is the maternal red cell volume

A 4mL bleed (i.e. 4mL fetal RBCs) requires 500IU anti-D given IM to the mother with a further 250IU anti-D for each additional mL of fetal RBCs.

Don't panic!

The lab carrying out the Kleihauer test will tell you the volume of fetal RBCs detected since they will count the cells and do the calculation for you. After this you will need to calculate the dose of anti-D to give the mother but *if you are unsure either discuss with the haematology medical staff or contact your local transfusion centre* and they will help you with the dosing. Most obstetric units will have anti-D protocols which should be available on the ward.

Chanarin I, ed. (1989) *Laboratory Haematology: an Account of Laboratory Techniques*, Churchill Livingstone, Edinburgh.

Erythropoietin assay

Erythropoietin (Epo) is the hormone produced largely by the kidney that drives red cell production. The typical anaemia found in renal disease is a result of failure of Epo production. Epo assays are of value in renal medicine and haematology. For example, in the assessment of polycythaemic states an ↑ Epo level may be appropriate (e.g. in hypoxia where the body is attempting to increase O_2 availability to tissues) or inappropriate (e.g. some tumours). The Epo assay is carried out using a radioimmunoassay method and is not available in all haematology laboratories (may need to be sent to another hospital or lab).

Normal range: 35–25mu/mL, steady state level, no anaemia. May rise to 10,000mu/mL in hypoxia or anaemia.

Causes of ↑ Epo (appropriate)
- Anaemias.
- High altitude.
- Hypoxia:
  - Lung disease.
  - Sleep apnoea syndromes.
- Cyanotic heart disease (e.g. R⟶L shunts).
- High affinity haemoglobins.
- Cigarette smoking.
- Methaemoglobinaemia.

Causes of ↑ Epo (inappropriate)

- Renal disease:
  - Hypernephroma.
  - Nephroblastoma.
  - Post-renal transplant.
  - Renal cysts.
  - Renal artery stenosis.
- Hepatoma.
- Uterine fibroids.
- Cerebellar haemangioblastoma.
- Phaeochromocytoma.

Other causes of ↑ Epo
- Androgen therapy.
- Cushing's disease.
- Hypertransfusion.
- Neonatal polycythaemia.

Causes of ↓ Epo
- Renal failure.
- Polycythaemia vera.
- Rheumatoid arthritis, and other chronic inflammatory diseases.
- Myeloma and other cancers.

Cotes PM *et al.* (1986) The use of immunoreactive erythropoietin in the elucidation of polycythemia. *NEJM* **315**, 283–287.

Immunohaematology

Immunohaematology is the study of the effects of the immune system on the blood and its components. This includes red cells, white cells, platelets and coagulation proteins.

Tests for antiplatelet and antineutrophil antibodies

These tests are usually requested by the haematology department for patients with either thrombocytopenia or neutropenia, respectively. These assays are used to detect the presence of specific antibodies against platelet or neutrophil antigens on the cell surface.

Antibodies may be alloantibodies (e.g. antibody produced by the mother against fetal antigens) or autoantibodies, which are antibodies produced by the patient against his/her own antigens.

Antiplatelet antibody tests

Generally platelet immunofluorescence tests (PIFT) or monoclonal antibody immobilisation of platelet antigens (MAIPA) are used. These are useful for detecting even weak antibodies or where there are only a few antigenic sites per cell.

Disorders with neutrophil-specific alloantibodies

- Neonatal alloimmune neutropenia.
- Febrile transfusion reactions (HLA antibodies).
- Transfusion-associated lung injury (TRALI).

Disorders with neutrophil-specific autoantibodies

- Primary autoimmune neutropenia.
- Secondary:
  - SLE.
  - Evans' syndrome (AIHA + ↓platelets).
  - Lymphoproliferative disorders (e.g. CLL).
  - Immune dysfunction (e.g. HIV, GvHD).

Elegant though these tests are, they are actually not useful in clinical practice for the diagnosis of neutropenia or thrombocytopenia where the cause is autoimmune since these are largely clinical diagnoses (platelet-associated IgG or IgM may be high in autoimmune thrombocytopenia. However, it may also be high in non-immune causes of thrombocytopenia). Where these tests are of value is in the neonatal setting where the neonate has low platelets or neutrophils.

Roitt I. (1997) *Essential Immunology*, 9th edition, Blackwell Science, Oxford.

Immunophenotyping

This describes the identification and counting of cell types using powerful monoclonal antibodies specific for cell surface proteins.

3 Haematology

Uses
- Diagnosis and classification of leukaemias and lymphomas.
- Assessment of cellular DNA content and synthetic activity.
- Determination of lymphocyte subsets, e.g. CD4+ T cells in HIV infection.
- Assessment of clonality.
- Allows identification of prognostic groups.
- Monitoring of minimal residual disease (MRD, the lowest level of malignancy that can be detected using standard techniques).

Terminology and methodology
Cell surface proteins are denoted according to their cluster differentiation (CD) number. Most cells will express many different proteins and the pattern of expression allows cellular characterisation. Monoclonal antibodies recognise specific target antigens on cells. Using a panel of different antibodies an immunophenotypic *profile* of a sample is determined. Immunophenotyping is used in conjunction with standard morphological analysis of blood and marrow cells. The antibodies are labelled with fluorescent markers and binding to cell proteins is detected by laser. For each analysis thousands of cells are assessed individually and rapidly. Some antibodies can detect antigens inside cells.

Sample: heparin

Monoclonal antibodies (MoAbs)
These are so-called because they are derived from single B lymphocyte cell lines and have identical antigen binding domains (idiotypes). It is easy to generate large quantities of MoAbs for diagnostic use.

225

- Cell populations from e.g. PB or BM samples are incubated with a panel of MoAbs, e.g. anti-CD4, anti-CD34 which are directly or indirectly bound to a fluorescent marker antibody.
- Sample is passed through a fluorescence-activated cell sorter (FACS) machine.
- FACS instruments assign cells to a graphical plot by virtue of cell size and granularity detected as forward and side light scatter by the laser.
- Allows subpopulations of cells, e.g. mononuclear cells, in blood sample to be selected.
- The reactivity of this cell subpopulation to the MoAb panel can then be determined by fluorescence for each MoAb.
- A typical result for a CD4 T lymphocyte population is shown:
  CD3, CD4 +ve; CD8, CD13, CD34, CD19 −ve.

Leukaemia diagnosis: common patterns (profiles)

AML	CD13+, CD33+, ± CD34, ± CD14 +ve.
cALL	CD10 and TdT +ve.
T-ALL	cCD3, CD7, TdT +ve.
B-ALL	CD10, CD19, surface Ig +ve.
CLL	CD5, CD19, CD23, weak surface Ig +ve.

Applications

Surface immunophenotyping	Leukaemias
	Lymphomas
	CD4:CD8 ratios in HIV infection
DNA content of tumours	Ploidy
	S phase analysis
	Proliferation markers
TdT measurement	In leukaemias & lymphomas
BMT/stem cell transplantation	
Antiplatelet antibody detection	
Reticulocyte counts & maturation	
Apoptosis	
Detection of small numbers of cells	E.g. fetal cells in mother's circulation, microorganisms in blood

Clonality assessment
Particularly useful in determining whether there is a monoclonal B cell or plasma cell population.
▶ Monoclonal B cells from e.g. NHL will have surface expression of κ or λ light chains **but not both**.
▶ Polyclonal B cells from e.g. patient with infectious mononucleosis will have both κ **and** λ expression.

Adapted from Provan D et al. (1998) *Oxford Handbook of Clinical Haematology*, Oxford University Press, Oxford.

Cytogenetics

Uses
- The study of chromosomes.
- Looks at the number of chromosomes in each cell.
- Detects structural abnormalities between chromosome pairs.

Chromosome abnormalities may be constitutional (inherited) or acquired later in life. Cytogenetic analysis of chromosome structure and number has been used for many years for the study of disorders such as Down's syndrome. Acquired chromosomal abnormalities are found in malignancies, especially haematological tumours. The analysis and detection of cytogenetic abnormalities is known as **karyotyping**. Because of the complexity of this subject area we will concentrate on two main areas where chromosome analysis is of value.

- Prenatal diagnosis of inherited disorders:
  - Detection of common aneuploidies (gain or loss of chromosomes).
  - Detection/exclusion of known familial chromosome abnormalities.

- Detecting acquired chromosome abnormalities for:
  - Diagnosis of leukaemia subtypes, e.g. t(15;17) characteristic of AML M3 subtype.
  - Markers of prognostic information in a variety of diseases such as leukaemias, e.g. t(9;22), in acute leukaemias, N-myc amplification in neuroblastoma.
  - Monitoring response to treatment (in CML the Philadelphia chromosome, t(9;22), should disappear if the malignant cells are killed).

Principal indications for cytogenetic analysis are therefore
- Haematological malignancies at diagnosis (assuming the bone marrow is infiltrated).
- Infiltrated solid tumour tissue at diagnosis.
- Patients with equivocal morphology (e.g. type of leukaemia not clear using microscopy and other markers).
- FISH analysis when required in certain treatment protocols, e.g. MRC.
- Confirmation of disease relapse.
- Accelerated phase or blast crisis in CML.

Cytogenetic assays are expensive (around £250 for a leukaemia or lymphoma karyotype) and if there is any doubt as to whether the test is indicated we would suggest you discuss the case with one of your seniors or the cytogenetics staff. Arranging karyotyping before or during pregnancy is generally carried out by the obstetrician in charge of the woman's care.

Cytogenetic terminology

227

Constitutional	Present at conception or arising during embryonic life
Acquired	Arise later in fetal life or after birth
Translocation	Exchange of material between chromosomes
Deletion	Loss of part of a chromosome
Duplication	Part of a chromosome is gained
Inversion	Part of a chromosome is rotated through 180°
Diploid	46 chromosomes (somatic cell)
Haploid	23 chromosomes (germinal cell, e.g. egg or sperm)
Trisomy	Extra copy of a chromosome
Monosomy	Loss of a chromosome
Aneuploidy	Loss or gain of certain chromosomes, e.g. monosomy or trisomy

Rooney DE. (2001) *Human Cytogenetics*, Vol 2, 2nd edition, Oxford University Press, Oxford.

Chromosome anatomy

Two chromosomes are shown. Note the banding pattern which helps identify individual chromosomes, along with position of the centromeres (mitotic spindle attaches to these during cell division), short (*p*) and long (*q*) arms, and telomeres (chromosome ends).

Cytogenetics: prenatal diagnosis

This allows both the detection of genetic diseases associated with specific chromosomal abnormalities, thereby offering the possible prevention of an affected child. With the advent of chorionic villus sampling (CVS) in the first trimester, karyotyping can be done at an early stage of development. Pre-implantation genetic diagnosis allows abnormalities to be detected even before implantation has occurred.

Sample: amniotic fluid (15–16 weeks' gestation).

Tests available
- α-fetoprotein level.
- Chromosome analysis.
- Biochemical tests, e.g. acetylcholinesterase.

Sample: CVS (9–12 weeks' gestation).

Tests available
- DNA analysis.
- Chromosome analysis.
- Biochemistry tests.

Procedure (brief)

1. Cells are obtained using amniocentesis, CVS or fetal blood sampling.
2. Cells are cultured in medium.
3. Cell division is arrested at metaphase using e.g. colchicine.
4. Chromosomes are spread onto slides and stained.
5. Chromosomes are examined directly using light microscopy or with the aid of a computerised image analysis system.

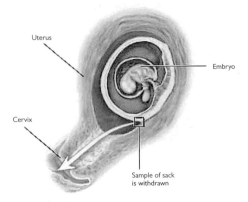

Fig. 3.18 Diagram showing method of chorionic villus sampling.

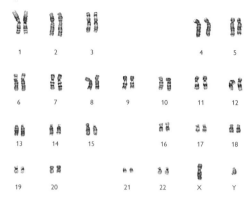

Fig. 3.19 Normal karyotype showing metaphase chromosomes (22 auto-somes, 1–22, and 2 sex chromosomes, XX or XY depending on sex of patient).

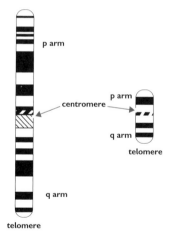

229

Fig. 3.20 Chromosome anatomy: note short (p) arms and long (q) arms.

Cytogenetics: haematological malignancies

Uses
- Aids the diagnosis and classification of haematological malignancy.
- Assessment of clonality.

- Identification of prognostic groups.
- Monitoring response to therapy.
- Determining engraftment and chimerism post-allogeneic transplant.

Terminology
- Normal somatic cell has 46 chromosomes; 22 pairs and XX or XY.
- Numbered 1–22 in decreasing size order.
- 2 arms meet at centromere—short arm denoted **p**, long arm is **q**.
- Usually only visible during condensation at metaphase.
- Stimulants and cell culture used—colchicine disrupts the spindle apparatus thereby arresting cells in metaphase.
- Chromosomes are G-banded using Giemsa or Leishman's stain to create characteristic banding patterns along the chromosome. The regions and bands are numbered, e.g. p1, q3, etc.

Common abnormalities
- Whole chromosome gain, e.g. trisomy 8 (+8).
- Whole chromosome loss, e.g. monosomy 7 (–7).
- Partial gain, e.g. add9q+, or partial loss, e.g. del5q– .
- Translocation—material exchanged with another chromosome; usually reciprocal, e.g. t(9;22)—the Philadelphia translocation.
- Inversion—part of chromosome runs in opposite direction, e.g. inv(16) in M4Eo.
- Many translocations involve breakpoints around known oncogenes, e.g. bcr, ras, myc, bcl-2.

Molecular cytogenetics
- Molecular revolution is further refining the specific abnormalities in the genesis of haematological malignancies.
- Techniques such as FISH (fluorescence *in situ* hybridisation) and PCR (polymerase chain reaction) can detect cryptic abnormalities.
- Bcr-abl probes are now used in diagnosis and monitoring of treatment response in CML.
- IgH and T cell receptor (TCR) genes are useful in determining clonality of suspected B and T cell tumours, respectively.

2 Specific probes may be used in diagnosis and monitoring of subtypes of acute leukaemia, e.g. AML, e.g. PML-RARA in AML M3, t(9;22), t(12;21), and 11q23 rearrangements in paediatric acute lymphoblastic leukaemias.

Heim S, Mitelman F. (1995) *Cancer Cytogenetics*, 2nd edition, Wisley-Liss, New York; Kingston HM. (1994) *ABC of Clinical Genetics*, 2nd edition, BMJ Books, London; Sandberg AA. (1990) *The Chromosomes in Human Cancer and Leukemia*, 2nd edition, Elsevier Science, New York.

HLA (tissue) typing

THE HLA (human leucocyte antigen) system or MHC (major histocompatibility complex) is the name given to the highly polymorphic gene cluster region on chromosome 6 which codes for cell surface proteins involved in immune recognition.

3 Haematology

Karyotypic abnormalities in leukaemia and lymphoma

CML
t(9;22)	Philadelphia chromosome translocation creates bcr-abl chimeric gene.

AML
t(8;21)	AML M2, involves AML-ETO gene—has better prognosis.
t(15;17)	AML M3 involves PML-RARA gene—has better prognosis.
inv(16)	AML M4Eo—has better prognosis.
−5, −7	Complex abnormalities have poor prognosis.

MDS
−7, +8, +11	Poor prognosis.
5q− syndrome	Associated with refractory anaemia and better prognosis.

MPD
20q− and +8	Common associations.

ALL
t(9;22)	Philadelphia translocation, poor prognosis.
t(4;11)	Poor prognosis.
Hyperdiploidy	Increase in total chromosome number—good prognosis.
Hypodiploidy	Decrease in total chromosome number—bad prognosis.

T-ALL
t(1;14)	Involves tal-1 oncogene.

B-ALL and Burkitt's lymphoma
t(8;14)	Involves myc and IgH genes, poor prognosis.

CLL
+12, t(11;14)	

ATLL
14q11	

NHL
t(14;18)	Follicular lymphoma, involves bcl-2 oncogene.
t(11;14)	Small cell lymphocytic lymphoma, involves bcl-1 oncogene.
t(8;14)	Burkitt's lymphoma, involves myc and IgH genes.

Uses

Tissue typing patients (to ensure compatibility between donor and recipient) who are undergoing transplantation to reduce the likelihood of rejection or graft-versus-host disease in the following types of transplant:

- Heart.
- Lung.
- Liver.
- Kidney.
- Bone marrow.
- Stem cells.

The gene complex is subdivided into 2 regions

Class 1   The A, B and C loci.

These proteins are found on most nucleated cells and interact with CD8+ T lymphocytes.

Class 2   Comprised of DR, DP, DQ loci present only on B lymphocytes, monocytes, macrophages and activated T lymphocytes.

Interact with CD4+ T lymphocytes.

- Class 1 and 2 genes are closely linked so one set of gene loci is usually inherited from each parent though there is a small amount of cross-over.
- There is ~25% chance of 2 siblings being HLA identical.
- There are other histocompatibility loci apart from the HLA system but these appear less important generally except during HLA matched stem cell transplantation when even differences in these minor systems may cause GvHD.

Typing methods

Class 1 and 2 antigens were originally defined by serological reactivity with maternal antisera containing pregnancy-induced HLA antibodies. There are many problems with the technique and it is too insensitive to detect many polymorphisms. Molecular techniques are increasingly employed such as SSP. Molecular characterisation is detecting vast class 2 polymorphism.

Importance of HLA typing

- Matching donor/recipient pairs for renal, cardiac and marrow stem cell transplantation.
- Degree of matching more critical for stem cell than solid organ transplants.
- Sibling HLA-matched stem cell transplantation is now treatment of choice for many malignancies.
- Unrelated donor stem cell transplants are increasingly performed but outcome is poorer due to HLA disparity. As molecular matching advances, improved accuracy will enable closer matches to be found and results should improve.

Functional tests of donor/recipient compatibility

- MLC (mixed lymphocyte culture)—now rarely used.
- CTLp (cytotoxic T lymphocyte precursor assays)—determine the frequency of cytotoxic T lymphocytes in the donor directed against the recipient. Provides an assessment of GvHD occurring.

HLA-related transfusion issues

- HLA on WBC and platelets may cause immunisation in recipients of blood and platelet transfusions.
- May cause refractoriness and/or febrile reactions to platelet transfusions.
- Leucodepletion of products by filtration prevents this (the National Blood Service removes the WBCs at source routinely nowadays).
- Diagnosis of refractoriness confirmed by detection of HLA or platelet-specific antibodies in patient's serum.

Text adapted from Provan D et al. (1998) Oxford Handbook of Clinical Haematology, Oxford University Press, Oxford; Gruen JR, Weissman SM. (1997) Evolving views of the major histocompatibility complex. Blood **90**, 4252–4265.

- Platelet transfusions matched to recipient HLA type may improve increments.

Southern blotting

This technique has been around since the mid-1970s. It explained much about the physical structure of genes and was a major advance in the diagnosis of many single gene disorders. The method is simple and elegant, but time-consuming. Not used as much today with the advent of PCR technology. Southern blotting relies on the physical nature of DNA whereby single strands are able to recognise and bind to their complementary sequences (Fig. 3.21).

Sample: EDTA sample (heparin can be used but beware inhibitory effect on PCR amplification; if any chance PCR required, send EDTA).

Procedure
1. Genomic (i.e. total) DNA is extracted from WBC in EDTA blood sample.
2. DNA is digested with bacterial restriction endonucleases (enzymes cleave DNA at specific sequences—each enzyme recognizes a different DNA sequence).
3. After digestion of the DNA, the fragments are separated on the basis of size using agarose gel electrophoresis (smallest fragments travel the farthest).
4. The fragments are transferred to a nylon membrane and fixed permanently to the membrane using UV light.
5. Membranes are 'probed' using specific (known) gene probes that are radioactively labelled using ^{32}P.
6. The location of specific binding is detected by placing the membrane next to radiographic film (standard x-ray film).
7. The film is developed using standard techniques and the autoradiograph generated will show bands corresponding to the position of binding of the labelled probe.
8. Fragment sizes are calculated and the presence or absence of mutations are worked out by determining whether enzyme cutting sites have been lost through mutation.

Applications
- Historically many diseases caused by single base changes (loss of restriction enzyme cutting site) have been diagnosed using Southern blotting.
- Globin gene disorders:
  - Sickle cell anaemia (mutation in β globin gene).
  - Thalassaemia (mutations or deletions in α or β globin genes).

233

Southern EM. (1975) Detection of specific sequences among DNA fragments separated by gel electrophoresis. *J Mol Biol* **98**, 503–517 (Southern's classic paper and probably *the* most cited molecular biology paper ever).

- Clotting disorders:
  - Haemophilia.
- Analysis of immunoglobulin or T cell receptor genes to detect clones of cells in suspected leukaemia or lymphoma.
- Detection of chromosomal translocations in leukaemia and lymphoma (e.g. t(9;22) in CML, t(14;18) in follicular lymphoma).

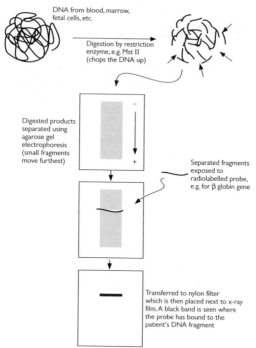

DNA from blood, marrow, fetal cells, etc.

Digestion by restriction enzyme, e.g. Mst II (chops the DNA up)

Digested products separated using agarose gel electrophoresis (small fragments move furthest)

Separated fragments exposed to radiolabelled probe, e.g. for β globin gene

Transferred to nylon filter which is then placed next to x-ray film. A black band is seen where the probe has bound to the patient's DNA fragment

Fig. 3.21

PCR amplification of DNA

The ability to use an enzyme to amplify specific DNA sequences has revolutionised modern diagnostic pathology. Whereas Southern blotting might take up to 1 week to produce a result, PCR can do the same thing in 2–3h! PCR is now in routine use in the analysis of oncogenes, haematological malignancies, general medicine, infectious disease and many other specialties. Because the system amplifies the starting DNA up to a million-fold there need only be one cell as starting material; in practice much more DNA is required but because of the extreme sensitivity of the technique PCR has been used in forensic medicine where there may be only a few cells available for analysis (e.g. blood or semen stain).

Advantages
- Requires very little DNA.
- DNA quality does not matter (can be highly degraded, e.g. with age and still be amplified—DNA from Egyptian mummies has been amplified).
- Rapid results.

Disadvantages
- Expensive, but less so than it used to be.
- DNA sequence of the gene of interest must be known in order to design the short PCR primers (oligos). With the near completion of the Human Genome Project this is less of a problem now.
- Highly sensitive, and contamination of samples may occur (DNA fragments float through the air constantly; if these drop into the reaction tube a false +ve result may be obtained).

Procedure (in brief)
- Two short DNA primers on either side of the gene of interest bind to the fragment of interest.
- The region between the primers is filled in using a heat-stable DNA polymerase (Taq polymerase).
- After a single round of amplification has been performed the whole process is repeated.
- This takes place 30 times (i.e. through 30 cycles of amplification) leading to a million-fold increase in the amount of specific sequence.
- After the 30 cycles are complete a sample of the PCR reaction is run on agarose gel and bands are visualised.
- Information about the presence or absence of the region or mutation of interest is obtained by assessing the size and number of different PCR products obtained after 30 cycles of amplification.

235

Applications
- PCR is currently used to amplify immunoglobulin genes, HIV loci, tuberculosis genes and many other targets that are of use in molecular medicine (cystic fibrosis, haemophilia, thalassaemia, sickle cell disease and many others).
- PCR can be used to quantitate mRNA species in blood samples and tissue samples. Allows gene 'activity' to be measured.

Saiki RK. (1988) Primer-directed enzymatic amplification of DNA with a thermostable DNA polymerase. *Science* **239**, 487–491.

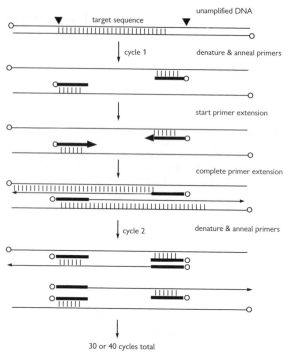

unamplified DNA

target sequence

cycle 1   denature & anneal primers

start primer extension

complete primer extension

cycle 2   denature & anneal primers

30 or 40 cycles total

236   Fig. 3.22

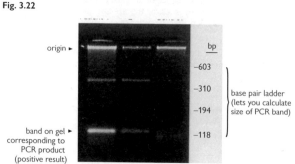

origin ▶

bp

−603

−310

−194

−118

base pair ladder
(lets you calculate
size of PCR band)

band on gel ▶
corresponding to
PCR product
(positive result)

Fig. 3.23

In situ hybridisation & FISH

Like PCR and other techniques, *in situ* hybridisation and FISH are concep-
tually simple techniques that rely on the ability of a DNA probe to 'find'
its counterpart on a chromosome, bind, and if a fluorescent tag is present

it will light up the region of binding (this modification is termed fluorescence *in situ* hybridisation, or FISH). These techniques have evolved from standard cytogenetic analysis of metaphase chromosomes in which metaphase chromosomes were prepared on glass slides to which specific labelled probes were applied.

Sample: discuss with your local cytogenetics or haematology lab (they will have specialised medium for maintaining cells from blood or marrow so that they will divide and be suitable for hybridisation studies).

In situ hybridisation
The location of binding of the probe is detected by visualising the signal produced after coating microscope slides with photographic emulsion, which generate a black area around the probe which is labelled with ^{32}P.

FISH
A further modification based on the original principles, whereby specific gene probes are hybridised to chromosomes without the need for metaphase preparations (interphase cells can be used). Instead of ^{32}P the probes are labelled with fluorescent dye and hybridisation may be detected as red, blue or other coloured dots over the cells.

Applications of FISH
- Used in the analysis of trisomies (chromosome gains) and monosomies (chromosome losses) associated with leukaemias and lymphomas. The presence of trisomy is detected as three fluorescent dots within the cell whilst monosomy is seen as a single fluorescent dot within the cell.
- FISH has been used widely within paediatric leukaemias, such as ALL, where abnormalities of chromosome number are common.

237

Sinclair PB et al. (1997) Improved sensitivity of BCR-ABL detection: a triple-probe three-color fluorescence in situ hybridization system. *Blood* **90**, 1395–1402; Vaandrager JW. (1996) Direct visualization of dispersed 11q13 chromosomal translocations in mantle cell lymphoma by multicolor DNA fiber fluorescence in situ hybridization. *Blood* **88**, 1177–1182; Mathew P et al. (1997) Detection of the t(2;5)(p23;q35) and NPM-ALK fusion in non-Hodgkin's lymphoma by two-color fluorescence in situ hybridization. *Blood* **89**, 1678–1685.

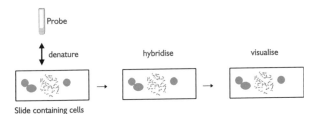

Fig. 3.24 FISH.

Specialised haematology assays

The following laboratories provide specialised molecular, biochemical and cellular investigations for rare haematological disorders. Please contact the laboratory before tests are requested to confirm the specimen(s) required.

Thalassaemia disorders

Dr John Old
National Haemoglobinopathy Reference Laboratory, Institute of Molecular Medicine, John Radcliffe Hospital, Headington, Oxford OX3 8DU
Tel: 01865-222449; Fax: 01865-222500
E-mail: jold@hammer.imm.ox.ac.uk

Professor Swee Lay Thein
Haematological Medicine, King's College Hospital, Denmark Hill, London SES 9RS
Tel: 020-7346-1682; Fax: 020-7346-6168
E-mail: sl.thein@kcl.ac.uk

Dr Mary Petrou
Perinatal Centre, University College Hospital, 84–86 Chenies Mews, London WC1E 6HX
Tel: 020-7388-9246; Fax: 020-7380-9864
E-mail: m.petrou@ucl.ac.uk

Dr Tom Vulliamy
Haematology, ICSTM, Hammersmith Hospital, London W12 0HS
Tel: 020-8383-1136; Fax: 020-8742-9335
E-mail: t.vulliamy@ic.ac.uk

Haemoglobin variants, unstable and altered affinity haemoglobins

Dr John Old
National Haemoglobinopathy Reference Laboratory, Institute of Molecular Medicine, John Radcliffe Hospital, Headington, Oxford OX3 8DU
Tel: 01865-222449; Fax: 01865-222500
E-mail: jold@hammer.imm.ox.ac.uk

Professor Sally Davies[1] & Joan Henthorn[2]
Department of Haematology, Central Middlesex Hospital, Acton Lane, London NW10 7NS
1 Tel: 020-8453-2112; Fax: 020-8965-1115
E-mail: sally.davies@dol.gso.gov.uk
2 Tel: 020-8453-2323

Dr Barbara Wild
Haematological Medicine, King's College Hospital, Denmark Hill, London
SE5 9RS
Tel: 020-7737-4000 Ext 2283; Fax: 020-7346-3514
E-mail: barbara.wild@kcl.ac.uk

Glycolytic defects, G6PD deficiency other erythroenzymopathies

Dr Mark Layton
Haematology, ICSTM, Hammersmith Hospital, London W12 0HS
Tel: 020-8383-2173; Fax: 020-8742-9335
E-mail: m.layton@ic.ac.uk

Dr Barbara Wild
Haematological Medicine, King's College Hospital, Denmark Hill, London
SE5 9RS
Tel: 020-7737-4000 Extn 2283; Fax: 020-7346-3514
E-mail: barbara.wild@kcl.ac.uk

Porphyrias

Dr Allan Deacon
Clinical Biochemistry, King's College Hospital, Denmark Hill, London SE5
9RS
Tel: 020-7346-3856; Fax: 020-737-7434

Dr Michael Badminton[1] & Ms J Woolf/Dr S Whatley[2]
Porphyria Service, Medical Biochemistry, University Hospital of Wales,
Cardiff CF14 4XW
1 Tel: 02920-748349; Fax: 02920-748383
E-mail: badminton.mn@cardiff.ac.uk
2 Tel: 02920-743565

239

Red cell membrane defects

Dr May-Jean King
International Blood Group Reference Laboratory, Southmead Road,
Bristol BS10 5ND
Tel: 0117-991-2111; Fax: 0117-959-1660
E-mail: may-jean.king@nbs.nhs.uk

Immunology

Autoimmunity and complement

Introduction
Tissue damage associated with autoimmune activation can be termed organ specific if tissue damage is confined to individual organs or non-organ specific if there is multi-organ involvement. Although associated disease mechanisms involve both the humoral and cellular immune mechanisms, humoral autoimmunity is the best characterised with regard to investigations, and laboratory tests are based upon:

- The detection or quantification of autoantibodies, typically IgG antibodies.
- The measurement of complement components.
- The detection of changes in concentration of non-specific inflammatory markers.

What the relationship is between these antibodies and the disease mechanism is usually debatable and only in a few instances, e.g. antiglomerular basement membrane antibody, is there direct pathological involvement between the antibody and the disease. In most instances, e.g. rheumatoid factors, the presence of antibodies should be seen as good diagnostic markers of the likelihood of the disease being present.

Spectrum of autoimmune disease

	Organ/tissue	Disease
Organ specific	Pituitary	Hypophysitis
	Thyroid	Thyrotoxicosis
		Hypothyroidism
	Adrenal	Addison's disease
	Pancreas	Insulin-dependent diabetes
	Gonad	Premature ovarian failure
		Male infertility
	Stomach	Atrophic gastritis
		Pernicious anaemia
	Intestine	Coeliac disease
	Liver	Primary biliary cirrhosis
		Autoimmune hepatitis
	Heart	Dressler's syndrome
	Eye	Phacogenic uveitis
		Sympathetic ophthalmia
	Skin	Pemphigus vulgaris
		Bullous pemphigoid
	Neuromuscular	Myasthenia gravis
		Lambert-Eaton syndrome
	Bone marrow	Haemolytic anaemia
		Idiopathic thrombocytopenia
	Kidney	Goodpasture's syndrome
		Crescentic glomerulonephritis
	Blood vessels	Systemic vasculitis
		Wegener's granulomatosis
		Polyarteritis nodosa
Non-organ specific	Connective tissue	Sjögren's syndrome
		Scleroderma
		Systemic lupus erythematosus
		Rheumatoid arthritis
		Antiphospholipid syndrome

243

Detection of autoantibodies

Autoantibodies are detected by immunochemical techniques. Test samples are reacted with target antigens in representative tissue or as purified or recombinant preparations. Common techniques used are immunofluorescence, particle agglutination, immunodiffusion, counterimmunoelectrophoresis, immunoprecipitation, immunoblotting, ELISA and related assays and radioimmunoassays.

Endocrine disease

Gastric parietal cell and intrinsic factor antibodies

Autoimmune gastritis (type A) and pernicious anaemia (PA) are associated with antibodies to gastric parietal cells (GPC) in intrinsic factor (specificity 90%). GPC may also be found (40%) in other organ-specific autoimmune diseases, e.g. autoimmune thyroid disease, and may also be present in elderly patients without autoimmune disease (10–15%).

Antigen on parietal cell—β subunit of H^+ and K^+-ATPase. Intrinsic factor antigen 70kDa glycoprotein secreted by parietal cells of gastric mucosa. Intrinsic factor antibodies may be type 1, a blocking antibody (in 70% with PA), or type 2, a binding antibody (in ~35% PA).

Antibodies associated with diabetes mellitus

There are many autoantibodies associated with type 1 diabetes mellitus (type 1 DM). Their clinical application is limited but they may have a use in predicting disease in relatives of patients with type 1 DM. Positive response to 2 or more of the following markers is associated with a high incidence of onset of type 1 DM within 5–7 years.

• Glutamic acid decarboxylase (GAD) antibody

GAD is the enzyme converting glutamic acid to γ-aminobutyric acid and is involved in the control of release of insulin from the secretory granules.

• Islet cell antibody

Antibodies are reactive with whole islets and with increasing β-cell destruction their levels fall such that they are not usually seen after the first year of disease. Prevalence at diagnosis is 75%, first degree relatives 2–5%, general population 0.4%.

• Insulin antibody

Prior to administration of exogenous insulin, these antibodies are present in 40% of newly diagnosed patients with type 1 DM. Titres diminish once β-cell destruction is advanced. May be seen in other autoimmune polyendocrinopathies.

Sperm antibody

Considered specific and characteristic of immunological infertility. In direct agglutination tests if greater than 40% of the sperm are coated with particles a diagnosis of immunological infertility due to antisperm antibodies is highly probable.

Steroid cell antibodies

Present in Addison's disease, autoimmune endocrinopathies, premature ovarian failure and gonadal failure.

Antigen: cytochromic P450 enzymes in the steroid biosynthetic pathways.

Thyroid antibodies

May be primary, pathogenic antibodies or secondary antibodies which may be useful as a diagnostic marker.

Primary thyroid antibodies

Thyrotropin receptor antibodies (TRAB) are useful in the diagnosis of Graves' disease. Anti-TRAB is seen in 50–80% of Graves'. Does not distinguish between stimulatory and inhibitory antibodies, which can only be achieved by a functional or bioassay.

Secondary thyroid antibodies

Major autoantibodies associated with autoimmune thyroid disease are thyroglobulin (TG) and thyroid peroxidase (TPO). The TPO antibody is the more clinically relevant and often seen at high titre in 80–95% of patients with Hashimoto's thyroiditis, but also seen in patients with Graves' disease (50–80% intermediate titre).

📖OHCM p409.

Gastrointestinal disease

245

Autoantibodies associated with coeliac disease

Coeliac disease is gluten-sensitive enteropathy. There is abnormal immunological responsiveness to wheat protein, α-gliadin. IgA-α-gliadin and IgG and IgA-endomysial antibodies are sensitive and specific markers for coeliac disease and IgA-endomysial antibodies are the antibody of choice for primary screening for coeliac disease. α-gliadin antibodies are a useful adjunct in the assessment of children with suspected coeliac disease and may be used to monitor the efficacy or compliance with a gluten-free diet. IgA deficiency must obviously be excluded in patients under investigation.

Autoantibodies associated with liver disease

Antibodies associated with autoimmune liver disease are mitochrondrial, smooth muscle (SM) and liver/kidney microsomal (LKM) antibodies. Antinuclear antibodies (ANA) may also be seen. The titre of the antibodies is of clinical significance.

Autoantibodies associated with chronic liver disease

Disease	Antibody	Frequency
Primary biliary cirrhosis (PBC)	Mitochondrial	>95%
	SM	50%
Autoimmune hepatitis I	SM	70%
	Mitochondrial	30%
Autoimmune hepatitis II	LKM	80%
Autoimmune sclerosing cholangitis	ANA	
	SM	

Neuromuscular disease

Acetylcholine receptor (ACR) antibody

ACR antibodies are pathologically associated with myasthenia gravis (MG, 80% of patients) and there are three types:
- Binding.
- Blocking.
- Modulating.

Glycolipid antibodies

These antibodies have been noted in association with peripheral neuropathy in which it is thought that they have a pathological role. Up to 50% of patients with multifocal motor neuropathy and less frequently in Guillain-Barré syndrome have antibodies to ganglioside M1 (GM1). The main clinical associations are set out below.

Syndrome	Antibody to
Chronic sensorimotor demyelinating neuropathy	SGPG and MAG
Chronic axonal sensory neuropathy	Sulphatide
Multi-focal motor sensory neuropathy	GD1b, GT1b, GQ1b
Miller-Fisher syndrome	GQ1b, GT1a
Guillain-Barré syndrome	GM1, GD1a

SGPG, sulphated glucuronic acid epitope of peripheral nerve glycolipid, sulphated glucuronyl paragloboside; MAG, myelin-associated glycoprotein; G, ganglioside M, D, T and Q subtypes.

Antibodies to myelin-associated glycoproteins have been reported in multiple sclerosis (MS), MG and SLE. Monoclonal IgM proteins may have anti-MAG activity.

Paraneoplastic antibodies

Associated with neurological manifestations in association with an underlying malignancy.

Enteric neuronal antibodies
– Small cell carcinoma of the bronchus.

Glutamic acid decarboxylase antibodies
– Stiff man syndrome.

Neuronal antibodies
– In CSF in 74% of patients with cerebral SLE.

Neuronal nuclear antibodies (ANNA)
– Small cell carcinoma of the lung, carcinoma of the breast.

Purkinje cell antibodies
– Gynaecological cancer or Hodgkin's disease.

Retinal antibodies
– Small cell carcinoma of the lung.

Voltage-gated calcium channel antibodies
– Lambert-Eaton myasthenic syndrome (associated with small cell carcinoma of the lung.

Renal disease

Glomerular basement membrane (GBM) antibodies

Antigen: non-collagenous portion of Type 4 collagen. Detected in classical untreated Goodpasture's syndrome. May also coexist with anti-neutrophil cytoplasmic antibody in patients with systemic vasculitis and rapidly progressive glomerulonephritis. The concentration of anti-GBM antibodies may be used to monitor the patient's response to therapy.

Antineutrophil cytoplasmic antibodies (ANCA)

Antigen: a variety of intracellular enzymes within the neutrophil leucocyte. Associated with necrotising vasculitis, and vasculitis associated with rheumatic and inflammatory bowel diseases. There are two major types of indirect immunofluorescence staining:
• Cytoplasmic (C-ANCA).
• Perinuclear pattern (P-ANCA).
Atypical staining patterns may also be reported.

C-ANCA with specificity for serine protease 3 (PR3)
Associated with Wegener's granulomatosis.

P-ANCA with specificity for myeloperoxidase (MPO)
Associated with microscopic polyangiitis and Churg-Strauss syndrome.

'Atypical' ANCA patterns can be seen to antigens such as BPI (bactericidal permeability increasing protein), elastase, cathepsin, lactoferrin and lysozyme.

247

Antibody and disease association

Pattern	Disease	Frequency
C-ANCA	Wegener's granulomatosis	90%
PR3-associated	Micropolyarteritis	30%
	Churg-Strauss syndrome	30%
	Polyarteritis nodosa (PAN)	11%
	RPGN	8%
P-ANCA	Churg-Strauss syndrome	60%
MPO-associated	Anti-GBM disease	30%
	Crescenteric glomerulonephritis	65%
	Microscopic polyangiitis	45%
	Wegener's granulomatosis	10%

Note: P-ANCA can be seen in association with ANA; RPGN, rapidly progressive glomerulonephritis.

Rheumatic disease

Phospholipid antibodies
A group of antibodies directed against phospholipid binding proteins or conformational epitopes involved in the binding proteins.

Cardiolipin antibody
Antigens: negatively charged phospholipids. Specifically associated with primary antiphospholipid syndrome. Specific antigen: phospholipid binding plasma proteins, e.g. β2-glycoprotein I. IgG class antibodies are the most prevalent.

Antiphospholipid antibodies include
- β2-glycoprotein 1 antibody.
- Phosphatidylserine antibody.
- Phosphatidylinositol antibody.
- Phosphatidic acid antibody.
- Calpastatin antibody.

Coagulation assays, e.g. activated partial thromboplastin time (APTT) and dilute Russell's viper venom time (DRVVT) detect the functional activity of phospholipid antibodies. They are referred to as *lupus anticoagulants*.

Both types of assays should be used in evaluating a patient for antiphospholipid syndrome (APS) to assess:
- Risk of thrombosis in patients with SLE.
- Risk for fetal loss in pregnancy.

Nuclear antibodies
Group of antibodies associated with autoimmune rheumatic diseases, identified by IIF. They can be either:
- Against structural or insoluble proteins *or*
- Against saline soluble antigens—extractable nuclear antigens.

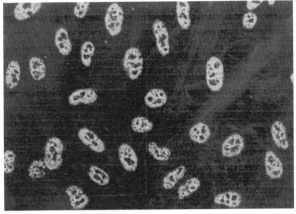

Fig. 4.1   ANA: Hep2 cells in a speckled pattern.

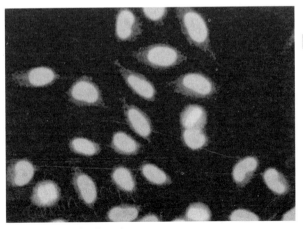

Fig. 4.2   ANA: Hep2 cells in a homogeneous pattern.

Nuclear antibody patterns (indirect immunofluorescence) and disease associations

IIF pattern	Antigen	Disease
Peripheral	DsDNA	SLE
Homogeneous	DNA–histone complex	SLE
Speckled	Sm	SLE
	RNP	Mixed connective tissue disease
	SSA/Ro	Sjögren's syndrome, SLE
	SSB/La	Sjögren's syndrome, SLE
	Centromere	Systemic sclerosis
Nucleolar	Nucleolar RNA	Systemic sclerosis
	Scl70	Systemic sclerosis
	PM/Scl	Polymyositis
Cytoplasmic	Jo-1	Dermatomyositis
	Ribosome-P	SLE

Drug association

Drug-induced ANA can occur and the half-life of the presence of the antibody is usually approximately 3 months. Drugs associated with drug-induced lupus syndrome are procainamide, isoniazid, phenytoin, hydralazine, methyldopa, chlorpromazine, penicillamine, minocycline.

Centromere antibodies

Antigen: kinetochore of the centromere. Associated with systemic sclerosis. CREST variant.

Double-stranded DNA antibody

Disease association: SLE (60%).

Single-stranded DNA antibodies

70% of patients with SLE but also in other autoimmune rheumatic diseases and inflammatory conditions. Clinically of limited value.

ENA antibodies

SSA/Ro

Disease associations: sub-acute cutaneous lupus erythematosus, neonatal lupus (90%); may be associated with partial or complete heart block; primary Sjögren's syndrome; SLE (30%) with interstitial pneumonitis; systemic sclerosis (60%).

SSB/La

Clinical associations: primary Sjögren's syndrome (65%); increased incidence of extraglandular disease; SLE (15%).

RNP
Clinical associations: overlap syndrome or mixed connective tissue disease. Specific for SLE but lacks sensitivity.

Sm
Clinical association: SLE 20–30%.

Scl70
Clinical association: diffuse cutaneous systemic sclerosis.

PM/Scl (PM-1)
Clinical associations: polymyositis and systemic sclerosis overlap syndrome (25%).

Aminoacyl-tRNA synthetase antibodies
Disease associations: polymyositis and dermatomyositis.

Clinical association: myositis (20%), Jo-1 the most common. May also be associated with interstitial lung disease and arthralgia.

Examples
Jo-1	histidyl TRNA synthetase
PL-7	threonyl tRNA synthetase
PL-12	alanyl tRNA synthetase
EJ	glycyl tRNA synthetase
OJ	isoleucyl tRNA synthetase

Histone antibodies
Clinical associations-SLE (18–50%); drug-induced SLE (95%); IgG isotype is clinically significant.

Ribosomal-P antibodies
Clinical associations: SLE (10–15%) often in absence of anti-DsDNA antibodies. Association with neuropsychiatric SLE.

Rheumatoid factor
Antibody against Fc portion of IgG. Clinical association: rheumatoid arthritis—significant serological marker. *Note*: IgM rheumatoid factor found in 2–10% of healthy adults. Poor marker for monitoring disease.

Frequency of IgM rheumatoid factors
Rheumatoid arthritis	50–90%
Systemic lupus erythematosus	15–35%
Systemic sclerosis	20–30%
Juvenile rheumatoid arthritis	7–10%
Polymyositis	5–10%
Infection	0–50%
Normal	2–10%

Other isotypes
GAD and E have been described. Their specific measurement is not yet of established clinical use.

Heart disease

Cardiac muscle antibodies are associated with myocarditis, idiopathic dilated cardiomyopathy, rheumatic carditis and Dressler's syndrome. Antigens include adenine nucleotide translocator protein, cardiac myosin and tropomyosin.

Skin disease

Skin antibodies are used in investigating bullous skin diseases. There are two types:
- Intra-epidermal/desmosome antibody (pemphigus antibody)—associated with all forms of pemphigus.
- Basement membrane zone antibody (pemphigoid antibody)—associated predominantly with bullous pemphigoid. Present in serum of 70–90% of affected individuals.

Complement

The complement system consists of three sections, the *classical pathway*, the *alternate pathway* and the *terminal lytic sequence*. The glycoprotein components are number C1 through C9 and the system is completed with a number of inhibitory and regulatory proteins. Activation of the classical or alternate pathways feeds into the central biological event which is the attachment or fixation of the third component C3. The activation of C3 activates the terminal lytic sequence causing cell damage and inflammation.

Clinical assays
The function of complement can be assayed by the lysis of red cells; individual components can be measured and evidence for activation of the complement system can be obtained by detecting breakdown products.

Complement (CH50)

Clinical uses of complement assays
- Monitor overall complement activity.
- Screen for complete defects of components other than C3 and C4.
- A variation of the assay can be used to determine the functional integrity of the alternate pathway (AP50).

Complement C3 and C4
Low concentrations indicate either increased consumption or decreased synthesis.

Increased consumption can be due to
- Antigen–antibody complex can activate the whole of the complement system. C3 and C4 will be low.
- Endotoxin or other microbial product activation of the alternate pathway. C3 low, C4 normal.

Decreased synthesis
Congenital homozygous deficiencies of C3 and C4 are rare. Heterozygous states are not uncommon. There is an increased incidence of C4 heterozygosity in association with SLE and type 1 DM.

Clinical use in which C3 and C4 concentrations may be useful
- Renal disease, joint disease and multi-system disorders with evidence of vasculitis, e.g. SLE and also severe systemic infection.
- Low complement is suggestive of active disease.
- Low C3 and normal C4 concentrations may be seen in patients with Gram −ve septicaemia, some forms of glomerulonephritis (e.g. acute nephritis) and sub-acute or chronic proliferative and mesangiocapillary nephritis.

In patients with recurrent infections, complement concentrations and CH50 should be measured as genetic and acquired defects can sometimes present as immunodeficiency. A low CH50 should be followed with specific complement component measures to identify any deficiency.

Other complement investigations
Complement allotypes: MHC markers of certain diseases, confirmation of hereditary complement deficiency status.

Complement activation products: anaphylatoxins C3a, C4a & C5a
Limited use—relatively unstable and non-specific.

Complement C3 nephritic factor (C3 NEF)
If C3 concentration is ↓ and C4 normal, the presence of C3 NEF in a patient with renal disease is suggestive of mesangiocapillary nephritis.

253

C1 esterase inhibitor (C1 INH)
Hereditary angio-oedema is due to the deficiency of C1 esterase inhibitor and is the most frequent of the inherited complement component deficiencies. Functional C1 INH may be needed in acquired angio-oedema.

Immunoglobulins

The monomeric immunoglobulin molecule is composed of two identical heavy chains (G, A, M, D and E) and two identical light chains (κ and λ). Immunoglobulins are variants of this basic structure.

Measurement of serum concentrations of IgG, A & M
These are useful in:
- Diagnosis and monitoring of primary and secondary immunodeficiency.
- Monitoring of patients receiving immunoglobulin replacement therapy.
- Diagnosis of B cell malignancy.

Immunoglobulin G (IgG) subclasses

IgG has four subclasses:

IgG$_1$	60–70%
IgG$_2$	14–20%
IgG$_3$	4–8%
IgG$_4$	2–6%

Reference ranges are age-related. Viral antibody responses are mainly IgG$_1$ and IgG$_3$, whilst antibody to parasitic antigen is usually IgG$_4$. In children polysaccharide antibody responses are mainly IgG$_1$, whereas in adults they are IgG$_2$.

Clinical uses
- IgG subclass deficiency.
- Total IgG is usually within the age-related reference range.
- Sub-class assays may be useful to define an isolated sub-class deficiency in patients with multiple recurrent infections in whom total IgG is not deficient.

IgG deficiencies
IgG$_2$	Children
IgG$_3$	Puberty
IgG$_1$	Usually in combination with defects of other immunoglobulin isotypes

Monoclonal immunoglobulins—paraproteins

Proliferation of a single clone of B cells results in single heavy chain class, light chain type and idiotype. This is called a paraprotein. Immunoglobulin fragments produced by tumour cells are more common in malignant conditions. Both serum and urine analysis is important. Most frequently seen paraprotein in urine is called the Bence Jones protein.

Clinical uses
- Paraprotein assays are necessary for identifying B-cell tumours.
- Monitoring benign and malignant paraproteins.

Immunoglobulin E

IgE exerts its activity only when bound to blood basophils or tissue mast cells. When antigens bind to membrane, specific IgE mediators are released from these cells resulting in immediate hypersensitivity reactions. An ↑ serum IgE concentration suggests atopy, atopic tendency or parasitic infestation.

Clinical conditions associated with ↑ total serum IgE
- Atopic allergic disorders.
- Bronchopulmonary aspergillosis.

- Churg-Strauss granuloma.
- Post-bone-marrow transplantation.
- Parasitic disorders:
  - Visceral larva migrans.
  - Hookworm.
  - Schistosomiasis.
  - Filariasis.
- Immunodeficiency states:
  - Wiskott-Aldrich syndrome.
  - Hyperimmunoglobulinaemia E syndrome.
- Malignancies:
  - Hodgkin's disease.
  - IgE myeloma (very rare).
  - Sézary syndrome.

Allergen-specific IgE
Assays provide a rapid and reproducible measure of the presence of specific antibodies of serum IgE.

Clinical use
- To demonstrate the presence of an antibody and antigen that may be responsible for allergic reactions.

Note: The significance of a +ve result can only be interpreted in the context of a full allergic history.

Situations in which specific IgE analysis may be considered
- History of previous anaphylaxis following antigen exposure.
- Dermatographism.
- Extensive eczema.
- Very young children.
- Suspected sensitivities to some foods.
- Bee and wasp venom sensitivity.
- Patients receiving antihistamine therapy.
- Suspected penicillin sensitivity.
- Suspected occupation allergy.

255

Studies of immune paresis

Immunodeficiency may be primary (congenital) or secondary (acquired) and may also occur transiently in infancy. It can occur at any age. Primary immunodeficiencies may occur with:
- Predominant antibody defects.
- Predominant cell mediated immunity defects.
- Deficiencies associated with other defects.

Investigations
Cellular and humoral immunity investigations may be carried out and humoral assays may include those for functional antibodies in response to

infection or challenge. Mannose binding lectin deficiencies (📖*Complement* (p252)) are generally associated with increased risk of infection in children.

Cryoproteins

Cryoproteins precipitate when serum or plasma is cooled and re-dissolved when warmed. Cryoproteins may be due to the presence of mixed cryoglobulins, polyclonal with monoclonal components, monoclonal cryoglobulins, cryofibrinogens and cold agglutinins (poly and monoclonal).

Clinical uses
Cryoprotein studies should be carried out in patients showing clinical manifestations which include cold intolerance associated with pain in exposed areas, Raynaud's phenomenon and skin abnormalities including purpura, urticaria and ulcers and renal impairment.

Chapter 5

Infectious & tropical diseases

Introduction to infectious diseases

'Everything about microscopic life is terribly upsetting... how can things so small be so important?' (Isaac Asimov—1920–92).

Throughout history, infectious diseases have had a huge impact on the human species. Although they are present in human populations at all times to some degree, and indeed modern societies sometimes almost forget that infections exist, the effects of epidemics remain noticeable and spectacular. Furthermore, almost the only new diseases that come along are infections—some of the 21st century's most pressing problems are pathogens which have only appeared in the 20 years prior to this book being written (e.g. HIV, hepatitis C, hepatitis E, *Helicobacter pylori*, new variant CJD), though 'golden oldies' such as tuberculosis, pneumococcus and malaria are still merrily 'doing the rounds'.

As we enter the 21st century several factors are serving to increase the relative importance of infection over other areas of medicine. New infections are continually emerging, antimicrobial resistance is increasing, numbers of immunosuppressed patients are increasing as a consequence of improving therapies for hitherto untreatable diseases (cancer, transplantation, etc.), international travel and migration is increasing, and there is a growing fear of bioterrorism. Accordingly, many diseases currently considered 'tropical', and hence too remote and exotic to be much of a problem in London or New York, are likely to become increasingly important in differential diagnosis lists throughout the developed world.

It is always worth bearing in mind that infectious diseases are often treatable—in a differential diagnosis it is always better to consider treatable options above non-treatable options, hence infection-related possibilities should enter a differential diagnosis wherever appropriate. Furthermore, some infectious diseases have major public health consequences—e.g. MDR-TB, MRSA, VHF, HIV, hepatitis C—and it is always worth making special consideration of them if only because of the potential for spread to other human beings.

Infection is a great mimic

Infectious diseases present a clinical challenge
The same infectious disease is often capable of causing a wide variety of clinical pictures (e.g. tuberculosis, syphilis and HIV disease have many manifestations). This is not so surprising when one considers that identical twins (etc.) apart, every human being on the planet is completely different, hence individually tailored responses to a bewildering variety of infecting agents should be expected rather than come as a surprise.

Some clinical syndromes can be caused by many quite different pathogens. Good examples might be pneumonia, cellulitis and endocarditis.

Furthermore, some infectious diseases can resemble non-infectious diseases. For example, syphilis can cause a variety of rashes (including good imitations of lichen planus and of the palmo-plantar pustulosis of Crohn's disease), amoebic colitis can resemble ulcerative colitis, a brain abscess

5 Infectious & tropical diseases

can resemble a brain tumour, and tuberculosis of the vertebral column can resemble metastatic malignancy. Getting it wrong can be catastrophic for the patient.

Other diseases can mimic infections

Non-infectious diseases can resemble infection. Examples include gout of the first metatarso-phalangeal joint rather than cellulitis, cervical lyphadenopathy due to lymphoma rather than tuberculosis, familial Mediterranean fever as a cause of PUO, SLE leading to Libman-Sachs endocarditis, and an inflammatory carcinoma of the female breast resembling a pyogenic breast abscess. Again, getting it wrong can be catastrophic for the patient.

The importance of epidemiological factors

Epidemiological infection can be crucial in determining which, if any, infectious problems are an issue in a given patient.

Geography: this is very important.

Some infections are common the world over and include

- *Salmonella* infections.
- Pneumococcal pneumonia.
- Gonorrhoea.
- Thrush (candidiasis).
- Tuberculosis.
- Influenza.
- Epstein-Barr virus.
- HIV.
- Hepatitis C.
- Herpes simplex.
- Threadworm (*Enterobius*).

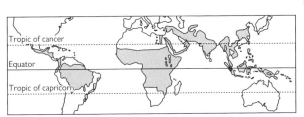

Fig. 5.1 The importance of taking a geographic history. Malaria, which can be life threatening, is a very common disease in many parts of the world (see map), but is not indiginous to most parts of the developed world. Making a diagnosis depends heavily upon the clinician eliciting the clues in the patient's history. Even if they have been taking antimalarial drugs, a patient who has been on holiday to Kenya, Thailand, or Brazil may die if the disease is not diagnosed. Clinical suspicion should lead to blood films (on 3 consecutive days) and a platelet count. Bear in mind that the patient may not have been taking adequate prophylaxis, may have been missing tablets, or may not have been absorbing them.

Some infectious diseases are only common in the developing world, e.g.
- Malaria.
- Diphtheria.
- Rheumatic fever.
- Enteric fever (typhoid and paratyphoid).
- Hepatitis E.
- Poliomyelitis.
- Rabies (although Eastern Europe has significant disease).
- Viral haemorrhagic fever (aka VHF, e.g. Lassa fever).
- Onchocerciasis (river blindness).
- Schistosomiasis.
- Leishmaniasis.
- Ascariasis.
- Cutaneous myiasis (e.g. tumbu fly).

Some infectious diseases are common in some parts of the developed world but not in other parts of the developed world, and include
- Lyme disease.
- Babesiosis.
- Histoplasmosis.
- Hydatid disease.
- Anisakiasis.

Indeed, only certain areas of the USA, for example, are endemic for
- Lyme disease.
- Coccidioidomycosis.
- Babesiosis.
- Histoplasmosis.

The 'Andromeda strain' phenomenon (with all due credit to Michael Crichton MD) should be borne in mind. The disease in front of you might be the first ever presentation! Almost the only significant new human diseases that will appear in the future will be infectious diseases, and they will keep appearing till the end of the human species.

Sexual and drug-taking activity: searching and personal questions may need to be asked. For example, HIV disease may not be suspected until a married man with three children admits to physical expression of bisexuality, or an anaesthetist with a hepatitis illness admits to injecting opiates recreationally. The patient may have a headache and photophobia because of HSV-2 infection acquired from a new regular partner. It may not be immediately obvious that the fever, rash and hypotension in a woman may be related to her tampon usage (toxic shock syndrome), yet menstruation can be a difficult subject to discuss in some cultural settings. It is not in the best interests of a patient that these sorts of issues are not broached if they are thought to be clinically relevant.

Social and professional: pets, hobbies and jobs may well be important. The patient with pneumonia and a budgie could have psittacosis. The tropical fish salesman with a chronic rash on his hand could have *Mycobacterium marinum* infection (aka 'fish tank granuloma'). The jaundiced volunteer cleaning out canals at weekends could have leptospirosis related to contact with rats.

Assessing the patient
Medicine is not easy, or everyone would be doing it! The recognition of an infectious disease in a patient (or the absence of one) goes far beyond the petri dish, the microbiology bench and PCR testing technology.

5 Infectious & tropical diseases

Assessment should include
- Detailed history.
- Full physical examination (including temperature).
- The generation of a differential diagnosis.
- Laboratory tests.
- Non-invasive procedures (including radiological tests where appropriate).
- Invasive procedures.
- The making of a definitive diagnosis (wherever possible).

When considering the possibility of an infective process, one should always consider the basic infection groups
- Bacteria (including primitive forms).
- Mycobacteria.
- Fungi.
- Viruses.
- Protozoa.
- Helminths.
- Prions.
- Myiasis.

When assessing a patient, it can be helpful to think in terms of

Syndrome—do the signs and symptoms link up into a specific picture (e.g. glandular fever, infective endocarditis, a shocked asplenic patient with possible overwhelming pneumococcal septicaemia, the unilateral discharging neck mass caused by tuberculosis)?

Pathology—e.g. is the weight loss due to specific pathologies, such as tuberculosis (curable) or HIV (treatable)?

Systematically—work through the systems and ask if an infection could be responsible for the clinical feature(s) that is (are) being observed.

261

Examples might include
- Premature dementia and CJD.
- Dyspepsia and gastric MALToma due to *Helicobacter pylori*.
- Fever in a returning traveller and malaria.
- An infective process in a site that is not immediately obvious, such as testicular infection, dental sepsis, a cervical spine abscess.

Where has the patient been? What have they been getting up to?
- The strange perianal lesion with granulomatous features may be leishmaniasis picked up sitting on the beach in Malta.
- The increasingly bizarre behaviour manifested by a 40-year-old businessman who regularly visits Eastern Europe without his wife could be meningovascular syphilis.
- Haematuria in a 22-year-old medical student may be due to the *Schistosoma haematobium* infection he acquired swimming in Lake Malawi while on an elective.
- HIV-2 may be the cause of a glandular fever-like illness in an oil company worker having recently returned from West Africa.
- A febrile illness in a holidaymaker returning from Kenya could be *Plasmodium falciparum* malaria if they had only been taking a chloroquine/proguanil combination for prophylaxis.

- Paratyphoid and typhoid fevers are suggested by a history of possibly drinking contaminated water in Morocco.
- Brucellosis must be considered after visiting a farm in Turkey and drinking unpasteurised milk.
- Massive and unremitting pruritus in a 28-year-old VSO returnee from Cameroon may be due to onchocerciasis.
- The diagnosis might be right—e.g. tuberculosis or pneumococcal meningitis—but the TB may be resistant to isoniazid/rifampicin (ask about travel history, e.g. to Pakistan) or the pneumococcus to penicillin.

Sexual history
e.g. HIV, syphilis, PID, herpes simplex, etc.

Contact with animals (job, hobbies, pets, etc.)
e.g. tuberculosis, brucella, psittacosis, leptospirosis, etc.

Drug-injecting history
e.g. HIV, HCV, HBV, endocarditis, deep sepsis

Travel history (holidays, business, military, etc.)
e.g. malaria, VHF, Legionnaire's disease, gastroenteritis, etc.

Menstrual history
Toxic shock syndrome

Fig. 5.2 Infection and history taking

Investigations available to the ID physician
(or general physician assessing a patient with a possible infectious disease)

Many tests will be performed with a view to making a diagnosis. Investigation of a patient should be rational and evidence-based wherever possible. As with any other branch of medicine, the history and examination will point the way, although the interrogative armamentarium of the infectious diseases and tropical medicine physician is enormous.

Results will emerge which, while not producing a diagnosis as such, will nevertheless require following up. For example, low C5 levels in recurrent meningococcal septicaemia may need immunological assessment. IgG deficiency leading to recurrent pneumonia may require regular infusions of γ globulins. A low CD4+ cell count, which is not due to HIV infection, could be a feature of sarcoidosis.

Making a diagnosis alone is not the only issue at stake. Some tests must be done if a patient is going to be treated safely. Examples might include: G6PD levels before administering primaquine for hypnozoite eradication;

TB cultures for antibiotic sensitivity prior to starting empirical therapy; exclusion of pregnancy before using certain antibiotics such as doxycycline and ciprofloxacin. Other tests relate to the fact that some infectious diseases are dangerous to others: a prime example of this would be multi-drug-resistant tuberculosis, which is potentially dangerous for the population at large and needs to be identified (or at least suspected wherever appropriate) and treated in an isolation unit.

Investigating the infectious diseases/tropical medicine case

Patient history and examination
- Generate a differential diagnosis.
- Consider, as appropriate, all major groups of infecting/infesting organisms (bacteria, mycobacteria, viruses, fungi, protozoa, helminths, prions, myiasis).
- Decide on and gather most appropriate specimens for the infectious agents under consideration (there are many useful books and web sites to assist here).

Available diagnostic techniques include
Serology (📖Serology (p265)).

Direct detection
- Microscopy:
  - Direct: e.g. faecal parasites (± iodine), cutaneous fungi, urinary microfilaria in onchocerciasis.
  - Special stains: these include Gram, acid/alcohol-fast, Calcofluour white, silver stain, immunofluorescence (e.g. for some viruses, and polyvalent direct fluorescence, or DF, for *Legionella*).
  - Electron microscopy: for viruses and other pathogens as appropriate (e.g. aspirate from vesicle for herpes varicella-zoster, Whipple's disease in jejunal biopsy material).
- Presence of toxin (e.g. *Clostridium difficile*—demonstration of a cytotoxin in a stool sample using a specific cytotoxic assay).
- Antigen detection (📖Serology (p265)).
- Molecular assays (📖*Molecular diagnostics* (p279)): these include gene probes, amplification assays (e.g. polymerase chain reaction, or PCR).

Culture
Possible and desirable on almost any tissue, aspirate, bodily fluid, etc. For maximum yield of useful information, expert and appropriate collection of specimens from body surfaces, of fluids normally considered sterile, and of non-sterile fluids is critical.
- Identification through special growth media (e.g. McConkey agar, thioglycolate broth).
  [⌁] http://www.bact.wisc.edu/MicrotextBook/NutritionGrowth/culturemedia.html

- Identification by biochemical reactions (often available as commercial identification panels or key tests, e.g. catalase test, coagulase test).
- Identification with specific antisera (by agglutination, Quellung reaction, or fluorescent antibody tests).
- Identification using molecular-based methods (e.g. specific probes, restriction enzyme patterns, DNA sequencing).
- Antimicrobial susceptibility testing, if indicated.

Other tests as appropriate: see appropriate sections
- Biochemistry.
- Culture and sensitivity.
- Haematology.
- Immunology.
- Molecular tests.
- Radiology.
- Serological tests.
- Stool & bowel contents.
- Tissue biopsy and deep aspiration specimens.
- Other tests.

Investigation of pyrexia of unknown origin (PUO)

This is not an uncommon problem in hospital medicine. There is a huge potential differential diagnosis.

PUO is best defined as
A body temperature ≥38.3°C centrally (rectally) for 3 weeks or longer without the cause being discovered, despite extensive investigation for at least 1 week.

Assessment should include

Observation of the fever pattern
- ►Some conditions, such as typhoid and malaria, may exhibit character-istic fever patterns.

Complete and repeated detailed history, with emphasis on the recognised differential diagnosis including
- Travel history.
- Antimalarial usage.
- Vaccination history.
- Past use of medical services in foreign parts may be especially impor-tant (e.g. blood transfusions, splenectomy post-trauma, needlestick assaults).
- Drug-using history (including illicit drugs and especially injecting).
- Exposure to certain agents and/or animals (e.g. pet ownership, occupa-tional risk of animal contact, such as veterinary medicine, nursing, farming, meat packing).
- Hobbies (e.g. cave spelunking is linked to histoplasmosis and canal fishing to leptospirosis).
- Sexual history (and risk taking).

- Menstrual history.

Complete and repeated physical examination, including re-evaluation of previous findings, e.g.
- Check the skin, eyes, nail beds, lymph nodes, heart and abdomen.
- A new sign, such as cardiac murmur, may have developed over time.

The judicious use of repeated tests is also critical, depending upon the context
- Laboratory and radiological tests, taking into account new data, e.g. blood cultures, blood films, autoantibody screen, radiological findings.
- Non-invasive procedures, taking into account new data, e.g. genito-urinary assessment, such as high vaginal swab.
- Invasive procedures, e.g. liver biopsy, bone marrow biopsy, laparoscopy, Waldeyer's ring assessment by otolaryngologist.

The common groups of causes of a PUO in an adult are
- Infections.
- Connective tissue diseases.
- Occult neoplasms (especially leukaemia and lymphoma).

A list of relevant pathologies might include
HIV, tuberculosis, endocarditis, osteomyelitis, malaria, syphilis, zoonoses (e.g. brucellosis, Lyme disease, tularaemia), viral hepatitis (especially hepatitis C and B), typhoid/paratyphoid, pelvic inflammatory disease, chronic meningococcaemia, dental sepsis, tumours such as lymphoma, renal carcinoma, liver metastases, familial Mediterranean fever, multiple pulmonary emboli, drugs, rheumatological (Still's disease, temporal arteritis, SLE, vasculitis), atrial myxoma, factitious fever, Munchausen's syndrome, Munchausen's syndrome by proxy.

With improved non-invasive and microbiological techniques, most cases of PUO are found not to be caused by infections but rather by other systemic diseases, such as sarcoidosis, SLE and temporal arteritis. However, there are also infectious diseases capable of causing prolonged fever that should always be considered and factored into the assessment because they are often treatable and/or transmissible to others and will have serious consequences if missed.

Serology

Immunological methods are in wide usage to detect pathogens present in clinical samples. Serology refers to the laboratory usage of antigen–antibody reactions for such diagnostic purposes. This testing methodology is based on the knowledge that antigen–antibody reactions are very specific. Diagnosis is arrived at by detecting antibody or antigen in blood and/or other bodily fluids, or by the identification of pathogens in culture.

Both DIRECT and INDIRECT serological tests exist.

Indirect serological techniques employ antigen–antibody reactions to detect specific antibodies manufactured in response to an antigen or antigens on an infecting pathogen's surface and circulating in the patient's blood or present in other body fluids (such as saliva). Some are non-specific (e.g. cold agglutinins, VDRL, monospot), others are specific to given pathogens.

Direct serological techniques employ antibodies to detect specific antigens. Because this technique can be used to identify and type cultured organisms (📖*Culture techniques* p270), it not only has individual clinical value but also has important epidemiological applications. Indeed, the identification and typing of organisms is extremely valuable in the public health scenario, such as with the study of outbreaks.

Hepatitis B (HBV) is a good example of an infection where both antigen and antibody profiles are diagnostically, therapeutically, prognostically and epidemiologically important:
- *Antibody detection* of specific antibody, e.g. antihepatitis Be antigen (anti-HBe antibody), antihepatitis B surface antigen (anti-HBs antibody).
- *Antigen detection*, e.g. hepatitis B e antigen (HBeAg), hepatitis B surface antigen (HBsAg).

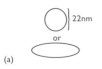

(a)

HBsAg (hepatitis B surface antigen)
Tests:
1) HBsAg can be measured in plasma
2) Generates anti-HBs antibodies, which can be measured in plasma (useful in assessing response to vaccination)

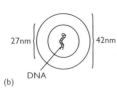

(b)

HBcAg (hepatitis B core antigen, Dane particle)
Contains viral DNA.
HBeAg (e antigen) arises out of HBcAg
Tests:
1) HBeAg can be measured in plasma
2) Generates anti-HBc antibodies and anti-Hbe antibodies
3) Plasma hepatitis B DNA levels

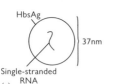

(c)

Hepatitis D (HDV, delta agent)
Can only infect when patient is already HBV-infected
Tests:
1) Antibodies to delta agent (anti-HDV)
2) Delta antigen

Antibody tests
A wide variety of methodologies for assessing antibody response are available, such as immunofluorescence, agglutination and ELISA (enzyme-linked immunosorbent assay). This is a complex subject and beyond the range of this book.

5 Infectious & tropical diseases

http://www.eawag.ch/publications_e/proceedings/oecd/proceedings/Torrance.pdf

Sub-classification of organisms, through serogrouping, is very valuable epidemiologically, e.g. while investigating an outbreak of meningococcal (*Neisseria meningitides*) disease, if the culprit is determined to be type C, vaccination can be utilised to control the outbreak (if it is a type B outbreak, there is currently no vaccine available).

In the 'direct fluorescent antibody' (DFA) technique, a fluorescent monoclonal antibody is used to react with an antigen specific for a given organism (e.g. herpes simplex virus) and a positive result will be detected microscopically. If the fluorescent antibody does not react with the antigen, the antibodies will be washed off the slide and the antigen will not fluoresce.

General principles
1. Elevated specific IgM levels indicates a 'new' infection.
2. Elevated specific IgG levels indicates a 'new' or a 'previous' infection.
3. Increasing IgG ('rising titre') when two samples ('paired sera') are taken with an appropriate intervening interval between them indicates a 'new' infection or re-infection. Diagnosis (as indicated by seroconversion) necessitates a diagnostic antibody titre or a four-fold increase in antibody titre.
4. **Seroconversion** is said to have occurred in situations 1 and 3.

267

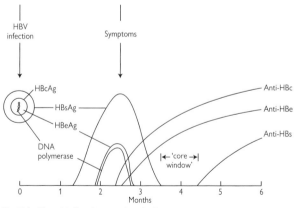

Fig. 5.4 Hepatitis B antigens and antibodies

Viral antibody tests
These can be very useful because once viral shedding has ceased, viral culture is of no further value. They include tests for HIV-1, HIV-2, HTLV-1, HTLV-2, hepatitis A, hepatitis B, hepatitis C, delta agent (hepatitis D), hepatitis E, EBV, CMV, dengue, Ebola fever, Lassa fever, RSV, mumps, measles, rubella, influenza, parainfluenza, St Louis encephalitis, yellow fever.

Bacterial antibody tests

These include ASO (for streptococcal infection), anti-DNAse B (for streptococcal infection) and anti-staphylococcal (for *Staphylococcus aureus* infections) tests.

Can also test for: cat scratch fever (*Bartonella henselae*), *Bordetella pertussis*, Lyme disease (*Borrelia burgdorferii*), *Brucella abortus*, *Burkholderia pseudomallei* (melioidosis), *Campylobacter jejuni*, *Chlamydia* spp., Q fever (*Coxiella burnetti*), *Escherichia coli* 0157, *Francisella tularensis*, *Helicobacter pylori*, *Legionella pneumophila*, *Leptospira interrogans*, *Listeria monocytogenes*, *Mycoplasma pneumoniae*, *Neisseria meningitidis*, *Neisseria gonorrhoeae*, *Rickettsia prowazekii*, *Salmonella* spp., *Treponema pallidum* (including TPHA, VDRL, FTA-ABS, IgM-FTA, IgM-ELISA), *Yersinia enterocolitica/Y. pseudotuberculosis*, Widal test.

Protozoal antibody tests

Include tests for malaria (*Plasmodium* spp.), amoebiasis, toxoplasmosis, leishmaniasis (kala azar), African trypanosomiasis (sleeping sickness), American trypanosomiasis (Chagas' disease), babesiosis, *Toxoplasma gondii*.

Helminthic antibody tests

Include tests for *Echinococcus granulosus* (hydatid disease), *Echinococcus multicularis* (alveolar echinococcosis), *Microsporidium* spp., *Pneumocystis carinii*, schistosomiasis (bilharzia), strongyloidiasis, filariasis, onchocerciasis, *Trichinella spiralis*, *Toxocara canis*, *Taenia solium* (cysticercosis, or pork tapeworm), paragonimiasis (Chinese lung fluke), gnathostomiasis.
🔗 http://www.medcor.mcgill.ca/~tropmed/td/txt/services.htm

Fungal antibody tests

Include tests for *Aspergillus fumigatus*, *Aspergillus niger*, *Aspergillus nidulans*, *Aspergillus versicolor*, *Blastomyces dermatitidis*, *Candida albicans*, *Coccidioides immitis*, *Cryptococcus neoformans*, *Histoplasma capsulatum*, Mukorazeen.
🔗 http://www.clinical-mycology.com/

Note: Some tests, such as complement fixation (CF) antibody assays for antibodies to coccidiomycosis, are specific and do not require proof of rising levels. They can accordingly provide indispensable confirmatory evidence for a diagnosis of coccidiomycosis as well as an indication of the relative risk of extrapulmonary dissemination. In chronic meningitis, a positive CF for anti-coccidioidal antibodies in the CSF often provides the only definite diagnostic indication of the need for aggressive antifungal therapy. Otherwise, most tests for antifungal antibodies, are of limited usefulness at present.

Antigen tests

Antigen measurement is achieved through techniques such as complement fixation and immunodiffusion. A variety of bodily fluids can yield diagnostically-useful antigens, including serum, urine, CSF and fresh stool—the choice depends upon the clinical context.

Viral antigen tests

Include mumps, cytomegalovirus, influenza, HIV, hepatitis B, respiratory syncytial virus, parainfluenza viruses, adenovirus and varicella-zoster virus.

5 Infectious & tropical diseases

Bacterial antigen tests

Include *Legionella pneumophila* (serotype 1) and *Borrelia burgdorferii* (in urine), β-haemolytic streptococci, pneumococcus, *Clostridium difficile*, *Haemophilus influenzae*, *Neisseria meningitidis*, *Helicobacter pylori*, *Campylobacter jejuni*.

Helminthic antigen tests

Filariasis.

⌁ http://www.tdlplc.co.uk/lab-reports/lr_spring-2000.htm

Protozoal antigen tests

Include giardiasis, *Trypanosoma cruzi* (Chagas' disease).

Fungal antigen tests

Include *Cryptococcus neoformans*, *Histoplasma capsulatum*, mannoprotein antigen in *Candida albicans*[1].

⌁ http://www.clinical-mycology.com/

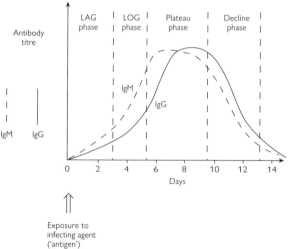

269

Fig. 5.5 Relative rate of appearance and disappearance of IgM and IgG.

1 Sendid B et al. (1999) New enzyme immunoassays for sensitive detection of circulating *Candida albicans* mannan and antimannan antibodies: useful combined test for diagnosis of systemic candidiasis. *J Clin Microbiol* **37**, 1510–1517.

Culture techniques

Microorganisms exist in nature as mixed populations. Diagnosis of an infection means identifying the relevant pathogen in the face of this plethora of 'pretenders to the crown'. Furthermore, different organisms can cause the same disease (a good example would be pneumonia) and yet require very different treatment and management and have different prognoses. While some specimens (e.g. stool, sputum) contain extremely large numbers of a variety of organisms, some specimens (e.g. blood, cerebrospinal fluid, urine) should be sterile unless infected or contaminated during their collection.

Microbial culture assists with the aetiological diagnosis of a bacterial, fungal, protozoal or viral illness by enabling identification and susceptibility testing of the isolated organism(s). Bacterial culture was the first to evolve, but useful data on other pathogenic groups can also be obtained through the use of culture-based methodologies (although options for treatment are currently more limited for viruses and fungi than for bacteria). Furthermore, culture of viruses and fungi usually takes longer than most bacterial culture, therefore the data obtained is most valuable for the late confirmation of the diagnosis or for epidemiological purposes (e.g. for predicting the appropriate constituents for a polyvalent influenza vaccine).

This account is by no means comprehensive. For greater depth, the reader is directed towards the major texts on the subject of microbiological culture.

Bacteria
Three major steps are involved in extracting pure cultures from a diverse population of microorganisms and identifying a pathogen.

1. An isolation plate is created—to do this, the mixture must be diluted until the various individual microorganisms have been dispersed far enough apart on an agar surface so that, after incubation, they will form visible colonies isolated from the colonies of their neighbours. This can be accomplished through several mechanical techniques, such as the 'streak plate method', the 'pour plate method' and the 'spin plate method'. Specialised culture media (such as selective media, differential media, enrichment media, and combination selective and differential media—a great many exist) may be used to supplement mechanical techniques of isolation. Culture can be aerobic or anaerobic (*Note*: specimens for the isolation of anaerobic pathogens require special care as anaerobic bacteria die in the presence of oxygen. Such specimens should therefore be transported in a reduced container).

2. A pure culture is created—to achieve this, an isolated colony will be selected out and aseptically 'picked off' the isolation plate for transferring to a new sterile medium. Accordingly, following incubation all the organisms in the new culture will be descendants of the same organism.

3. The organism can then be identified through various manoeuvres:
• The colony appearance.
• The microscopic appearance.
• The staining responses (e.g. Gram +ve *vs.* Gram −ve).

5 Infectious & tropical diseases

- The use of a range of biochemical tests designed to uncover characteristics typical of a particular organism, e.g. catalase reaction, sugar fermentation.
- The use of antisera (direct serology) for culture confirmation of certain organisms:
  - Agglutination and latex agglutination tests are used on colonies to identify *Escherichia coli* 0157, *Streptococcus pneumoniae*, serogroups of *Neisseria meningitidis*, *Shigella* and *Salmonella*, Lancefield groups of β-haemolytic streptococci and serotypes of *Haemophilus influenzae*.
  - Detection of specific antigens by DFA (direct fluorescent antibody) staining can be used to identify colonies of *Streptococcus pyogenes*, *Bordetella pertussis* and the species and serotypes of *Legionella*.
  - The Quellung reaction, a technique which employs specific antisera to interact with capsular polysaccharides of *Streptococcus pneumoniae*, can be used to confirm the identification of the pneumococcus as well as to determine the serotype of the cultured organism.

Bacteriological diagnosis at the bench

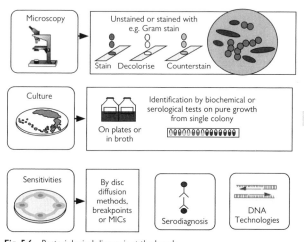

Fig. 5.6 Bacteriological diagnosis at the bench.

The process of bacterial culture and identification takes varying durations of time.

Type of organism being cultured	Approximate time needed to process
Aerobic bacterial (culture & sensitivity)	3 days
Anaerobic bacterial	7–10 days
Fungal	21 days
Mycoplasma spp.	28 days
Mycobacterium ulcerans	28 days (at 30°C, not at 37°C)
Mycobacterium paratuberculosis	13 weeks
Listeria spp.	1–2 months
Leptospira spp.	1–2 weeks

Ideally, specimens for bacterial culture should be taken BEFORE antibiotics are administered. Clearly this may not always be feasible but the information yield may well be less than ideal.

Antibiotic sensitivity
Once a bacterium is isolated, it can be cultured in the presence of an antibiotic or antibiotics to assess if it is susceptible to that agent or not (i.e. resistant). The minimum inhibitory concentration (MIC) is the lowest antibiotic concentration at which the microorganism under assessment shows no visible growth *in vitro*. The reporting of MICs can provide the clinician with precise information regarding the infecting bacterium's degree of antibiotic susceptibility and enable him/her to avoid antibiotics to which the organism shows resistance. When this data is linked up with the clinician's knowledge of the site and severity of the infection and the pharmacokinetic and pharmacodynamic properties of the various antibiotics available, a rational choice of the most appropriate antibiotic(s) can then be made that best suits the individual patient's needs.

For organisms exhibiting unusual resistance patterns, susceptibility panels using methodologies such as broth microdilution, gradient diffusion, and/or disc diffusion have been created to assist clinicians.
🔗 http://www.aruplab.com/guides/clt/tests/clt_a-62.htm#1142466

On occasions, this data will need to be linked to testing of blood levels for some antibiotics (e.g. gentamicin, vancomycin, cycloserine). Although its value is not universally accepted, the serum bactericidal test (SBT) can be utilised to determine whether concentrations of the antibiotic in a patient's serum are capable of killing the infecting microorganism in a particular clinical scenario (e.g. bacterial osteomyelitis, bacterial endocarditis, immunocompromised patients suffering from unusual infections, situations where unusual drug combinations are being used).
🔗 http://www.aruplab.com/guides/clt/tests/clt_a-79.htm#1144958

Viruses
Viral culture is very different from bacterial culture. Viruses require a very different type of medium for the organism to grow in, cell cultures, and viral growth is recognised through the cytopathic changes that appear in

cell culture. New techniques appear regularly, particularly rapid culture techniques.

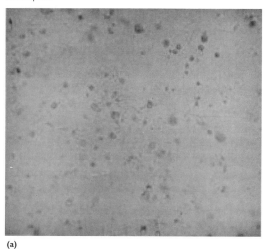

(a)

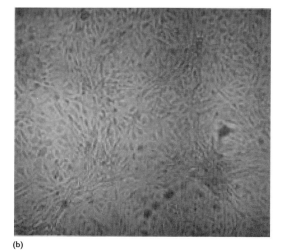

(b)

Fig. 5.7 Diagnosing viral infections using cell culture: (a) enterovirus cytopathogenic effect from a sample of stool in monkey kidney tissue culture, and (b) normal monkey kidney tissue culture. From Grist NR *et al.* (1987) *Diseases of Infection—an Illustrated Textbook*, Oxford University Press, Oxford.

273

The appropriate type of specimen to collect, the best means of transport, and the most appropriate cell culture to use will vary with the particular virus suspected, the specimen site and the time of the year.

- The choice of specimen is very important: numerous viruses enter via the mucosa of the upper respiratory tract, yet that virus may compromise multiple or distant tissues and organs.
- Swabs can be used to collect a variety of specimens from the body surfaces for viral detection, such as the nose, the throat, the eye, the skin and the rectum. Deeper specimens, such as blood and CSF, will be appropriate for some viruses. Different viruses will need different collection approaches—for example, heparin, citrate and EDTA (ethylene-diamine tetraacetic acid) are all acceptable for the detection of CMV by culture or by antigenaemia testing, but for some other viruses only citrate should be used if they are to be cultured. Issues like the temperature during transport of specimens must be taken into account.
- Unlike many bacterial or fungal pathogens, the time of year is important to keep in mind when making a diagnosis of certain viral diseases. For example, enteroviruses (such as poliomyelitis) circulate almost exclusively in the summer months and influenza likewise circulates during the winter months, so these viruses are unlikely to cause problems during other seasons of the year.
- Timing is important when collecting specimens for viral detection. They should be collected as early as possible after the onset of symptoms as once viral shedding ceases, culture will be impossible and serological and molecular techniques may be the only way of diagnosing the viral pathogen.
- Some viruses as yet cannot be cultured—e.g. viral agents of diarrhoea (caliciviruses, astroviruses and coronaviruses), hepatitis (HCV, HBV).

Swab or sample site (swabs in viral transport media)	Viruses cultured include
Eye swab	Adenoviruses, herpes simplex (HSV)
Throat swab	Adenoviruses, enteroviruses (echovirus, coxsackie, poliomyelitis), herpes varicella-zoster (HVZ), HSV, measles
Nasopharyngeal aspirate	Enteroviruses, influenza A, influenza B, RSV
Blood	CMV
CSF	Enteroviruses, HSV, HVZ
Faeces	Adenoviruses
Tissue fragments (biopsy)	CMV, HSV
Urine	Adenovirus, CMV, HSV, HVZ, measles, mumps

Cell culture techniques enable detection of a wide range of viral pathogens and can allow for dual or mixed viral infections to be diagnosed (which are common). Once specimens arrive at the laboratory, they are processed and inoculated into a variety of cell cultures that support the growth of common viral isolates, and inoculated cell cultures are then observed daily for the development of a viral cytopathic effect. Viruses vary in their cell culture requirements, and laboratories must use more than one cell line for culture. For example, when attempting to identify a respiratory viral pathogen, influenza and parainfluenza viruses favour replicating in primary cell lines such as primary Rhesus monkey kidney (RhMK) cells while respiratory syncytial virus (RSV) and adenoviruses prefer heteroploid cell lines such as human epidermoid larynx carcinoma (Hep-2) cells.

Among the newer viral culture techniques are shell vial spin amplification cultures. These offer a more rapid turnaround time than traditional viral cultures for detection of the more common respiratory viruses and some other agents. Rather than having to examine for a cytopathic effect, fluorescein-labelled monoclonal antibodies are unemployed to detect antigens of replicating viruses. This system can be utilised for detecting CMV, HSV, influenza A and B, parainfluenza 1, 2 and 3, adenovirus and RSV, and can detect, for example, HSV in as little as 1 or 2 days.

Laboratory assays for antiviral susceptibility testing include phenotypic and genotypic assays. Phenotypic assays require growth of the virus *in vitro*, and are useful for HSV and CMV for aciclovir and ganciclovir, respectively. Viruses for which *in vitro* culture systems are not available, such as HCV and HBV, cannot be tested with these types of assays, and in these circumstances genotypic assays (📖*Molecular diagnostics* (p279)) may be available and useful.

Fungi

Unlike bacterial and viral diseases, in skilled hands direct microscopy can often be used with a high degree of confidence to diagnose fungal infections (this being based on the distinctive morphological characteristics of the invading fungi (e.g. tinea) and/or the judicious use of special stains such as Calcofluor white). However, histopathological diagnoses should be confirmed by culture wherever possible. Conversely, although diagnoses are usually made by isolating the causative fungus (e.g. from sputum, urine, blood, bone marrow or biopsies from infected tissues), the presence of a fungus in a culture does not mean that it is invading the tissues (e.g. *Candida* isolation from sputum), and an aetiological role can be established with certainty only by confirmation of tissue invasion. There are also a range of serological tests available for systemic mycoses (📖*Serology* (p265)), but few provide definitive diagnoses by themselves.

Fungal culture techniques are similar to the bacterial scenario. They are most useful for detecting the dimorphic fungi, which manifest both mycelial and yeast forms. This group includes *Candida* spp., *Cryptococcus neoformans*, *Blastomyces dermatidis*, *Histoplasma capsulatum* and *Coccidioides immitis*. Rates of colony growth vary extremely widely, e.g. *Coccidioides immitis* may appear after 1 day, while *Histoplasma* may take a month or more. Special culture media, such as Niger seed agar, may be required.

Identification requires skill and experience and is based mainly upon the microscopic appearance of the hyphae and the appearance and arrangement of the spores. Definitive diagnosis of a dimorphic fungus may require inoculation into a living creature, such as a mouse, to convert the agent into the parasitic (i.e. yeast) form.

Protozoa

Protozoa of the genera *Acanthamoeba* and *Naegleria* may cause fatal CNS disease. *Acanthamoeba* spp. are free-living amoebae associated with keratitis; they may also cause a granulomatous encephalitis. Another free-living amoeba, *Naegleria fowleri*, is able to cause an acute fulminant meningoencephalitis, usually associated with a history of swimming in freshwater lakes or brackish water. In suspected cases, CSF and other suspicious clinical material may be cultured on a non-nutrient agar plate seeded with a 'lawn' of a Gram-negative bacteria (such as *E. coli*). Pathogenic amoeba can be identified microscopically.

Collection of specimens

Principles of good specimen collection
- Good-quality specimen and clinical information produces the most valuable data.
- Optimal time of collection: e.g. if at all possible, take bacterial specimens before administering antibiotics.
- Collect the optimal type of specimen wherever possible: e.g. pus is preferable to a 'pus swab'.
- Acquire expertise in specimen collection: ensure minimal contamination by normal flora (e.g. mid-stream specimen of urine (MSU), use of a tongue depressor for throat swab collection).
- Freshness of specimens: rapid transport to the laboratory is essential (especially for anaerobic organisms, and for 'hot stools' for parasite diagnosis).
- Collect the appropriate number of specimens at the appropriate intervals: e.g. paired antisera should be taken at least 1–6 weeks apart if a diagnostic rising titre is to be demonstrated.
- Be aware of biological hazards: category 3 organisms (e.g. tuberculosis, *Burkholderia pseudomallei*, hepatitis C, HIV) and category 4 organisms (e.g. viral haemorrhagic fever, possible bioterrorism cases such as smallpox).

Surface specimens include

Anal/anorectal: e.g. gonococcus (*Neisseria gonorrhoeae*).

Cervical swab: e.g. HSV, gonococcus, HPV.

Ear swab: e.g. otitis externa, otitis media, bacterial and fungal infections.

Foreign bodies: almost always infected if causing trouble! (includes iatrogenic FBs, such as arthroplasties, cardiac valves, pacemakers, ventriculo-peritoneal shunts, etc.). Foreign bodies in the ear, nose or vagina can lead to prolonged (and often unpleasant) discharges.

Genital ulcers: dark ground microscopy for syphilis organisms. Also chancroid, *Entamoeba histolytica*.

Indwelling catheters: these represent a breach of the integrity of the skin or mucosal surface. Include urinary catheters, intravenous cannulae, portacaths, etc. If a catheter is thought to be the source of an infection, cultures should be set up, and if the catheter or cannula is removed, this should be sent for culture.

Laryngeal swab: can be useful for tuberculosis.

Nasal, pharyngeal, gingival and throat: e.g. meningococcus, *Staphylococcus aureus* carriage, streptococcal infections, pertussis, adenovirus. Naso-pharyngeal aspirates are useful diagnosing for influenza and RSV (respiratory syncytial virus) through direct immunofluorescence (DIF) tests and culture. In lepromatous leprosy, a swab from the anterior nares may reveal acid-fast bacilli indicative of this infection.

Ophthalmic: e.g. bacterial conjunctivitis, adenovirus, rabies (from corneal impressions[1]. For trachoma, direct fluorescein-labelled monoclonal antibody (DFA) and enzyme immunoassay (EIA) of conjunctival smears is useful.
⌐ http://www.emedicine.com/OPH/topic118.htm

Skin: •abscess—culture for bacteria and other, unusual, organisms; •dermal scrapings, nail clippings: fungal infections (tinea—includes pedis, capitis, cruris, versicolor forms); •petechial rash scrapings: meningococcus (occasionally gonococcus).

Throat: e.g. *Candida albicans*, diphtheria, gonococcus, croup organisms.

Urethral: e.g. *Chlamydia*, gonococcus.

Vagina (high vaginal swab): e.g. *Staphylococcus aureus* in toxic shock syndrome (including toxin testing), *Gardnerella*, gonococcus.

Normally sterile fluids include

Amniotic fluid: bacterial infection can cause premature delivery, and rDNA was detected by PCR (⌐*Molecular diagnostics* (p279)) in samples from 15 (94%) of 16 patients with positive amniotic fluid cultures[2]. From the fetal point of view, hydrops fetalis can be caused by congenital infections (CMV, parvovirus B19, toxoplasmosis, syphilis and Chagas' disease), and making a diagnosis may involve analysis of amniotic fluid with cultures, PCR, etc.

Ascites: always consider tuberculosis (consider laparoscopy for biopsying peritoneal lesions for culture as well as histology, ⌐*Gastrointestinal tract investigations* (p284)). In some instances, bacterial (especially pneumococcal) infection is a possibility.

Blood: multiple samplings at separate times from separate body sites may need to be taken, such as in endocarditis. For some organisms and pathologies, an extended period of culture may be needed. Aerobic bacteria, anaerobic bacteria, mycobacteria and fungi all come into the frame.

Cerebrospinal fluid (CSF): possibilities include e.g. meningococcus, pneumococcus, *Listeria monocytogenes*, tuberculosis, fungi (e.g.

277

Cryptococcus neoformans), viruses (📖*Tissue biopsy & deep aspiration specimens* (p287)).

Ejaculate (semen): if the semen contains a high number of leucocytes, this may be an indication of either infection or inflammation. White blood cells are considered significant if more than one million are found in each millilitre of the ejaculate. STDs such as gonorrhoea or *Ureaplasma*, and prostate infections come into the differential diagnosis. *Schistosoma haematobium* (bilharzia) may cause haemospermia, and be found in ejaculate[3]. Acute mumps orchitis can be associated with loss of spermatozoa.

Ocular fluids (intra-): include aqueous humor, vitreous humor. Bacterial, fungal and parasitic problems can affect the interior of the eye.

Pericardial fluid: the most common organisms will include staphylococci, streptococci, pneumococci, *Haemophilus influenzae*, meningococci and tuberculosis.

Pleural fluid: numerous pathologies, including underlying bacterial pneumonia, tuberculous pleurisy, parasitic infections (such as strongyloidiasis) and fungal diseases (such as histoplasmosis).

Synovial fluid (joint aspirate): bacterial infections can be very destructive and the options are legion. Tuberculosis must always be borne in mind. Viral arthritides are usually self-limiting and treatment is supportive.

Urine: standard culture and sensitivity, e.g. **midstream specimen** (MSU), catheter specimen (CSU) —useful for diagnosing cystitis, pyelonephritis, prostatitis, etc. (prostatic massage may be helpful for improving diagnosis of prostatic infections); **EMU** ('early morning urines') for tuberculosis and a **terminal specimen** for *Schistosoma haematobium* (bilharzia).

Normally infected fluids include

Pus: e.g. abscess contents (such a collection can exist in almost any site in the body), wound swab/aspirates, drainage swabs. Usually bacterial (consider both aerobic and anaerobic options), but amoebic and hydatid options need to be considered when the lesion is in the liver.

Saliva: normally contains a wide range of commensal flora. Cannulation of a parotid gland duct may yield a specific pathogen that is causing a problem in that gland.

Sputum: includes tracheal aspirate, induced sputum (obtained with physiotherapy assistance) and bronchoalveolar lavage (BAL), which may be needed in sicker patients unable to produce sputum or in conditions where copious sputum production may not be a feature (such as *Pneumocystis carinii* pneumonia in HIV infection). Culture and sensitivity assists with identifying a vast range of organisms, including and especially tuberculosis (always ally sputum culture to direct microscopy).

Stool: vast range of uses (📖*Gastrointestinal tract investigations* (p284)). Includes *Salmonella*, *Campylobacter*, *Shigella*, *E. coli* 0157, typhoid and paratyphoid, *Plesiomonas shigelloides*, rotavirus, enteroviruses, etc. 'Hot stools' (from patient to the microbiology bench in less than 1h) are needed for amoebae, strongyloides larvae, etc.

1 Zaidman GW, Billingsley A. (1998) Corneal impression test for the diagnosis of acute rabies encephalitis. *Ophthalmology* **105**, 249–251; 2 Hitti J *et al.* (1997) Broad-spectrum bacterial rDNA polymerase chain reaction assay for detecting amniotic fluid infection among women in premature labor. *CID* **24**, 1228; 3 Torresi J, Yung A. (1997) Usefulness of semen microscopy in the diagnosis of a difficult case of *Schistosoma haematobium* infection in a returned traveler. *J Travel Med* **4**, 46–47.

Molecular diagnostics

Molecular diagnostics represents a growing and constantly changing area of medicine. Currently, these tests are expensive and are often only available in larger or specialist laboratories, but their potential power is considerable and simplification of the technology involved will increasingly place them within the reach of an ever-wider range of clinical laboratories.

While a full understanding of these complex technologies can present some conceptual difficulties to the average clinician, they are destined to become an increasingly important part of mainstream clinical practice. For example, in the setting of HIV/AIDS, viral load and anti-retroviral drug resistance are considered mainstream tests, while examination of the CSF for JC virus DNA by PCR is the method of choice for the diagnosis of progressive multifocal leucoencephalopathy.

The areas of greatest value include
- Detection and quantification of viruses to monitor therapy, e.g. HCV, HIV, HBV, CMV.
- Detection of slow-growing organisms, e.g. TB, atypical mycobacteria.
- Diagnosis of pathogens which are potentially too dangerous for the laboratory staff to handle, e.g. viral haemorrhagic fever, smallpox.
- Detection of organisms killed by antibiotics prior to culture samples being taken, e.g. meningococcal sepsis.
- Detection of organisms that cannot be cultured, e.g. hepatitis C virus (HCV).
- Detection of unusual diseases, e.g. helminthic diseases, fungi.
- Detection of toxins elaborated in small quantities by bacteria, e.g. toxic shock syndrome toxins.
- Where it is wished to quantify the level of an infection (e.g. viral load in HIV disease).
- Detection of mutations manifesting resistance to antimicrobial agents (genotypic resistance testing), e.g. HIV, CMV, TB. Unlike phenotypic assays, the major drawback of genotypic assays is that they can detect only resistance caused by known mutations, but unlike phenotypic assays there is no requirement for the virus to be cultured.
- Elucidation of pathogens that are as yet 'undiscovered'.

Available molecular techniques include
- PCR (polymerase chain reaction): this test uses probes to look for the presence of the genes of infecting organisms. Essentially the PCR technique is a primer extension reaction for amplifying specific nucleic

acids *in vitro*. In this way a short piece of DNA (the 'target sequence') can be amplified around one million fold, which enables its nucleotide sequence to be established and the organism it came from to be determined.

  - There are numerous PCR tests available now, and it is particularly valuable for hepatitis C (including for genotyping), HIV and TB. A universal eubacterial PCR (for genus and species identification of prokaryotes) and universal fungal PCR (genus and species identification of fungi) are available. HBV DNA quantification is accomplished through PCR.
  - Choosing the appropriate sample for the application of PCR testing is very important (e.g. biopsy of possible Kaposi's sarcoma lesion and KSHV (HHV-8); BAL fluid and PCP; small bowel biopsy and Whipple's disease; CSF and meningococcal disease or herpes simplex virus).

- LCR (ligase chain reaction): LCR works through specific probe amplification through the use of DNA-ligase. To date, this has found greatest value in *Chlamydia* infection.
- TMA (transcription mediated amplification): TMA uses an isothermal amplification system. Amplified telomerase products are RNA and these are detected using a non-isotopic hybridization protection (HPA) system. Quantitative analysis is based on the principle of differential hydrolysis of the bound and free probe. Identification of HCV, tuberculosis, gonococcus and *Chlamydia* are among its potential uses.
- Branched chain DNA (bDNA): a signal amplification methodology able to quantify HIV RNA levels.
- NASBA (nucleic acid sequence-based amplification): a quantitative test for HIV RNA. It also has value with CMV.
- Hybridisation with nucleic acid probes: this detects specific ribosomal RNA, and is most widely used for culture confirmation of an organism (e.g. fungi, mycobacteria).

280

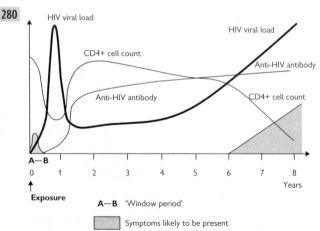

Fig. 5.8 The immunological profile of HIV disease.

- Sequencing: organisms are identified by direct sequencing of amplified gene fragments. This has been applied to tuberculosis, *Helicobacter pylori*, enteroviruses and HIV (for assessing drug resistance).
- Restriction fragment length polymorphisms (RFLP): restriction enzymes are used to cut up DNA into pieces, and the fragments are then subjected to gel electrophoresis (such as Southern blotting). The patterns produced can be used to identify organisms; this has other uses outside, but relevant to, infection medicine. For example, RFLP has been used for hepatitis C, adenovirus, tuberculosis, lymphoma and sickle cell disease.

Shanson DC. (1999) *Microbiology and Clinical Practice*, 3rd edition, Butterworth-Heinemann, Oxford

Haematology

Many infectious diseases manifest haematological changes that are diagnostically valuable.

Blood film: the blood smear examination provides general data on the size and appearance of cells as well as data on particular cell segments, while pathogens may be seen, e.g. malaria, trypanosomiasis, babesiosis, borreliosis, bartonella, filaria (time of day the blood is taken may be significant in this condition), haemolysis and evidence of hyposplenism. Thick and thin blood films should be considered, especially where malaria is concerned, and to exclude this potentially lethal condition it is recommended that at least three blood films each taken 24h apart should be performed. Blood films are also useful in assessing if a patient has developed disseminated intravascular coagulation (DIC)—*see below*.

Bone marrow examination: useful in e.g. culture (for TB, brucellosis and typhoid), microscopy (for leishmaniasis), establishing cell line integrity (e.g white cell abnormalities). An aspirate is generally very useful for culture purposes and for establishing what cells are present in the marrow, but a trephine is needed if structural information is required (e.g. to establish if granulomata suggestive of tuberculosis are present).

Coagulation studies, fibrin degradation products, D-dimers: useful where DIC is suspected. DIC is a common association of severe sepsis (especially meningococcal disease). Coagulation abnormalities are also present in conditions such as viral haemorrhagic fevers, *Plasmodium falciparum* malaria, rickettsial diseases, etc. D-dimers may assist with the diagnosis of deep venous thrombosis, although this is not universally accepted.

Cold agglutinins: a haemagglutination-based test. Can be caused by *Mycoplasma pneumoniae* (most commonly), influenza A, influenza B, parainfluenza and adenoviruses.

Differential white cell count in peripheral blood: useful associations include (1) eosinophilia and parasitoses, (2) neutrophilia and bacterial sepsis,

(3) neutropenia and atypical pneumonias, (4) atypical lymphocytes and Epstein-Barr virus (EBV), (5) neutropenia and pyrexia.

ESR: together with the C-reactive protein (📖*Biochemical tests* (p286)), the rate of erythrocyte sedimentation is sensitive to the extent of a body's response to a lesion or disease. The ESR is important for pointing to the possible existence of an organic disease, but a normal result does not exclude the presence of disease. An elevated ESR points to the need for additional investigations and, if elevated, is very useful in monitoring the course of a disease.

Ferritin levels: reduced in iron deficiency, such as that associated with hookworm infestation of the bowel (*Ancyclostoma duodenale, Necator americanus*) or *Helicobacter pylori*-associated gastritis. Serum iron and TIBC may be helpful (📖*Biochemical tests* (p286)).

Glucose 6-phosphate dehydrogenase: useful in the rational therapy of benign malarias, such as *Plasmodium vivax* and *P. ovale* (a deficiency will cause therapeutic problems with primaquine usage to kill the hypnozoite phase and prevent relapse).

Haemoglobin level and red cell parameters (especially MCV): useful in e.g. anaemia of chronic infection, haemolysis, iron deficiency (microcytosis) associated with hookworm infestation of the bowel or *Helicobacter pylori*-associated gastritis, macrocytosis due to vitamin B_{12} deficiency with *Diphyllobothrium latum* (fish tapeworm) infestation.

Haemolysis screen (including reticulocyte count): may be abnormal in e.g. DIC, EBV, viral haemorrhagic fever, *E. coli* 0157 gastroenteritis, rickettsial infections, dengue, gas gangrene. Haptoglobin levels can be useful (📖*Biochemical tests* (p286)).

Monospot test (Paul Bunnell test): diagnostic of EBV infection.

Sickling test: uncovers sickle cell disease, known to be associated with *Salmonella* osteomyelitis, chronic leg ulcers, etc.

Thrombocytopenia: characteristic in some conditions, e.g. HIV disease, *Plasmodium falciparum* malaria.

Vitamin B_{12} levels: reduced in *Diphyllobothrium latum* (fish tapeworm) infestation, tuberculosis of the terminal ileum, etc.

Radiology

Plain x-rays
- *Chest*: the potential diagnoses are legion. They include pneumonia, TB, pleural effusion/empyema, bronchiectasis, *Pneumocystis carinii* pneumonia (PCP), tropical eosinophilia and other parasite-related diseases (e.g. paragonimiasis), occupational risks for infections (e.g. silicosis and TB), post-varicella calcification.
- *Plain abdominal x-ray*: e.g. bowel dilatation, perforation, calcification of adrenal glands and lymph nodes (e.g. TB, histoplasmosis), 'babies head' sign of schistosomal bladder calcification.
- *Dental radiological studies*: occult dental sepsis.

- *Elsewhere*: e.g. limbs for osteomyelitis, skeletal muscles for calcified cysticercosis lesions, joints for Charcot changes (such as in syphilis).
- *ERCP* (endoscopic retrograde cholangiopancreatography): an upper gastrointestinal endoscopic approach, using contrast medium and radiographs to define the anatomy of the biliary tree and pancreatic duct. Useful for HIV-associated biliary tree disease (including porta hepatis nodal lymphoma), parasites (e.g. *Clonorchis sinensis*, *Ascaris lumbricoides*) and pancreatic disease such as tuberculosis.
- *IVP* (IVU, intravenous pyelography or urography): defines the renal anatomy. Renal infection such as pyelonephritis, renal calculi, malignancy or anatomical abnormalities (including congenital) leading to recurrent infections.

More sophisticated imaging

Magnetic resonance imaging (MRI) including with contrast enhancement
- Cranial: variant CJD or vCJD (exhibits bilateral pulvinar high signal), encephalitis, rabies, sagittal sinus thrombosis.
- Elsewhere in the body: defining solid lesions, fluid-filled lesions, etc.
- MRCP (MRI utilised with ERCP): further defines the hepatopancreatic-biliary tree anatomy.

Computed tomography (CT) including with contrast enhancement
- Cranial: e.g. brain abscess, paranasal sinus disease, middle ear disease, orbital sepsis, cysticercosis, mastoid air cells.
- Chest: e.g. cardiac lesions (possibly with associated endocarditis risk), mediastinum (e.g. lymphadenopathy, including retrosternal), lung lesions such as bronchiectasis, lung abscess, other non-infectious pathologies.
- Abdomen: delineates intra-abdominal abscesses and abnormalities in retroperitoneal and mesenteric lymph nodes, defects in the spleen, liver, kidneys, adrenals, pancreas and pelvis.
- Spiral CT scan: e.g. useful for defining pulmonary emboli as a cause of PUO.

283

Ultrasound
- Abdomen: evidence of pancreatic, liver, renal and biliary tree/gallbladder abnormalities (e.g. abscess, hepatic cyst, presence or absence of spleen, ascites, gallstones, etc.).
- Thoracic: pleural effusion, empyema (can assist with drainage).
- Echocardiography: to help exclude the cardiac vegetations of endocarditis, TB pericarditis (with effusion), myocarditis. Note that both transthoracic and transoesophageal (TOE) approaches are available, each yielding data of differing value in different situations.
- Doppler studies of blood vessels: to exclude deep vein thrombosis (DVT), such as in the legs.
- Biopsy: to specifically pick out an area for sampling, e.g. liver lesion, lymph node, mediastinal mass.
- Drainage: to specifically pick out an area for draining, e.g. liver abscess, pleural effusion.

Radionuclide scanning
- Indium (^{111}In)-labelled granulocyte scan: helps localise many infectious or inflammatory processes (i.e. deep sepsis).
- Technetium bone scan: bone and joint sepsis.
- Ventilation/perfusion (V/Q) lung scan: to exclude pulmonary embolus as cause of PUO, to delineate consolidation, abscess, bronchiectasis, etc.

PET (positron emission tomography)
- Has enormous potential for locating localised infective processes, especially in the brain. Limited availability at time of writing.

Gastrointestinal tract investigations

Biopsy-based

Duodenal biopsy (Crosby capsule and endoscopic methods, ± electron microscopy): e.g. Whipple's disease, giardiasis, cryptosporidium, strongyloidiasis.

Gastric biopsy: Helicobacter pylori.

Laparoscopy: useful to exclude tuberculosis and other infections in the presence of ascites (biopsies should be sent for both histology and for culture and sensitivity). (📖*Culture techniques* (p270)).

Liver biopsy: 📖*Tissue biopsy and deep aspiration specimens* (p287).

Oesophageal biopsy: e.g. candidiasis, cytomegalovirus (e.g. in advanced HIV disease).

Sigmoidoscopy and bowel biopsy: e.g. amoebiasis, pseudomembranous colitis (*Clostridium difficile* infections), exclusion of idiopathic colitis and Crohn's Disease.

GI contents-based

Baermann concentration technique: the method of choice for the detection of *Strongyloides stercoralis*.

Duodenal aspirate: e.g. giardiasis, cryptosporidium, strongyloidiasis.

Enterotest (string test): e.g. giardiasis, cryptosporidium, strongyloidiasis.

Hot stools: 📖*Culture techniques* (p270).

Salivary amylase: mumps.

Stool culture and sensitivity: 📖*Culture techniques* (p270).

Stool microscopy: for ova, cysts, parasites (e.g. for protozoa such as amoebae, helminths such as *Ascaris lumbricoides*).

Stool electron microscopy: especially good for viruses, such as rotavirus.

Stool chromatography: Clostridium difficile toxin

Sellotape® (adhesive) strip test: for the threadworm, *Enterobius vermiformis*. To perform this test, roll some clear adhesive tape around 4 fingers of a hand, sticky side out, while an assistant spreads the buttocks. In good lighting, identify the involved perianal area, and apply the with tape 1–2 times to the affected perianal area. Place the tape on a slide with the clean side downwards, trim the tape, label the slide and send to the laboratory.

284

Toxin tests: the definite diagnosis of botulism is the examination of faeces for the organism and toxin (EMG is also helpful): *Clostridium difficile*, *E. coli* 0157.

GI tract function

D-xylose absorption test: for malabsorption syndromes, such as Whipple's disease and tropical sprue.

^{13}C breath test for detection of *Helicobacter pylori:*
⊕ http://www.infai.de/scripten/iquery.cgi?res=ae19

Immunology

Immunology is a rapidly advancing field. Some immunological tests are very valuable in the assessment of patients. Cutaneous hypersensitivity tests are dealt with elsewhere (📖*Other tests* (p291)).

Complement (especially 'terminal' complements C5 to C9): deficiencies lead to a tendency to recurrent meningococcal sepsis, pneumococcal disease, etc.

Differential white cell count (📖*Haematology* (p281)): neutropenia is associated with bacterial sepsis.

Immune globulins: deficiencies lead to recurrent infections (some cases may be hereditary). Levels may also be ↑—IgM tends to be high in brucellosis, malaria, trypanosomiasis and toxoplasmosis.

Splenic dysfunction: indicated by a history of surgical removal (this may not always be clear!) or of a condition associated with hyposplenism (e.g. coeliac disease/dermatitis herpetiformis), an abnormal blood film, and an absent spleen on abdominal imaging. This state may be associated with recurrent meningococcal infection and life-threatening pneumococcal sepsis. Once diagnosed, the patient will need appropriate vaccinations and advised to always carry a warning card and/or wear a MedicAlert® bracelet or similar.

T cell subsets: the absolute CD4+ (T4) cell count and the CD4+/CD8+ (T4/T8) cell ratio is of value. HIV disease, tuberculosis and sarcoidosis are associated with reduced CD4+ cell levels, HIV with a reversed CD4+/CD8+ cell ratio. Underlying lymphoma may be hinted at by suggestive cell markers.

Cytokine studies: these are currently experimental but the field is gathering pace.

Biochemical tests

A number of biochemical tests are useful in the diagnosis and assessment of a range of infectious illnesses.

α-fetoprotein (AFP): ↑↑ in hepatocellular carcinoma (associated with HCV and HBV). *Note:* Much higher AFP than in other causes of hepatocellular damage.

Arterial blood gases: assessment of sepsis, assessment of pneumonia.

CA-125: ↑ in peritoneal tuberculosis.

C-reactive protein (CRP): together with the ESR, a valuable method for monitoring infections (although it is elevated in connective tissue conditions and neoplastic disease). CRP is an acute phase reactant, ↑ in bacterial infections and reduced in viral infections.

Creatinine phosphokinase (CPK) level: ↑ in *Legionella pneumophila* infection[1]. Also raised with zidovudine (AZT) usage in HIV disease.

Glucose metabolism: diabetes mellitus is a common association of infection. Consider performing a fasting glucose level, an oral glucose tolerance test (OGTT) or checking haemoglobin A_{1c} levels.

Haptoglobin levels: part of the haemolysis screen (📖*Haematology* (p282)). Iron levels (serum iron), total iron binding capacity (TIBC): iron ↓ (TIBC ↑) in iron deficiency, such as that associated with hookworm infestation of the bowel (*Ancyclostoma duodenale*, *Necator americanus*) or *Helicobacter pylori*-associated gastritis. Serum ferritin may be helpful.

Lactate levels: may be ↑ in the HIV-associated mitochondrial toxicity syndrome. Also high in severe sepsis syndrome.

Lipid abnormalities (cholesterol, triglycerides): HIV drug toxicity.

Liver function tests: abnormalities are present in many conditions, e.g. hepatitis, leptospirosis, yellow fever, antimicrobial drug toxicity (e.g. in tuberculosis).
- *Alkaline phosphatase (AP)*: in the serum of healthy adults, AP mostly originates from the liver (in children and adolescents, growing bone is a significant source). Biliary obstruction, which is often associated with sepsis, leads to an increase in the serum concentration of AP.
- *Bilirubin*: determination of the bilirubin levels (and the relative levels of conjugated and unconjugated bilirubin) is of great importance in the differential diagnosis of jaundice.
- *γGT*: an increase in the serum concentration of γGT is the most sensitive indicator of liver damage.

Pancreatic amylase level: ↑ with pancreatitis in e.g. mumps (consider also salivary amylase), toxicity with antiretroviral drugs (e.g. dideoxyinosine or DDI).
Pleural fluid analysis: analysis for lactate dehydrogenase (LDH) levels are useful (as well as albumin, total protein and amylase). An exudate, which implies infection in the differential diagnosis, is defined by at least one of the following criteria: pleural fluid/serum total protein ratio >0.5, pleural fluid/serum LDH ratio >0.6, or pleural fluid LDH >two-thirds of upper limits of normal of serum LDH.

Pregnancy test: some infections, such as varicella, genital herpes (simplex) and tuberculosis, are often more serious in pregnancy. The use of some antibiotics, such as ciprofloxacin and tetracyclines, is relatively contra-indicated in pregnancy.

Serum Na⁺ levels: hyponatraemia is strongly associated with Legionnaire's disease[1].

Synacthen test: tuberculosis and histoplasmosis can damage the adrenal glands, leading to an Addisonian state.

Vitamin D levels: if deficient, this may lead to difficulties with resolving tuberculosis infections (consider checking levels in patients with dark skins, especially those with a culture of wearing clothing over most of their skin).

1 Kociuba KR et al. (1994) Legionnaires' disease outbreak in south western Sydney, 1992. Clinical aspects. *Med J Aust* **160**, 274–277.

Tissue biopsy & deep aspiration specimens

Whatever part of the anatomy they are taken from, biopsy specimens should be evaluated both histopathologically (with specialised stains used wherever appropriate) and by culture for bacteria, mycobacteria, fungi, viruses and prions (utilising specialised culture techniques where appropriate).

Bone marrow biopsy

📖*Haematology* (p281). Important for tuberculosis, brucellosis, typhoid, leishmaniasis.

Cerebrospinal fluid (CSF)

While the main objective of a lumbar puncture is usually to obtain fluid for microscopy, culture and sensitivity, there are numerous other useful tests that can be performed. The opening pressure should be between 10–20cmH$_2$O—infective and other processes will alter this. While the usual approach to obtaining CSF is through a lumbar puncture, if the pressure is high a cisternal puncture can be performed instead. In neonates, foramenal puncture is a possibility.

Along with the Gram-staining process and microscopy, other tests to consider include a complete blood cell count and differential, measurement of glucose and protein levels, Ziehl-Nielsen staining for tuberculosis, and bacterial, mycobacterial, viral and fungal cultures. On occasions, other tests that might be considered include:

• A wet mount (for amoebae such as *Acathamoeba*; 📖*Culture techniques* (p270)).
• PCR for herpes simplex virus, herpes varicella-zoster and enteroviruses (📖 *Molecular diagnostics* (p234, 279)).
• Antibodies to specific pathogens (viruses such as arboviruses; 📖 *Serology* (p265)).
• An India ink capsule stain (for cryptococcosis).

- Cryptococcal antigen (📖*Serology* (p265)).
- VDRL for syphilis (📖*Serology* (p265)).
- 14-3-3 protein, a specific protein marker present in the CSF of patients with vCJD.
- Xanthochromia to help exclude subarachnoid haemorrhage.
- Cytology to help exclude carcinomatous meningitis.
- Assessing comparative CSF protein-cellular levels if Guillain-Barré syndrome (a recognised association of infections such as *Campylobacter* gastroenteritis) is being considered.

Liver biopsy

This procedure is very useful for many reasons. The indications are numerous and include assessment of viral hepatitis (especially HBV and HCV, including possible cirrhosis and/or hepatocellular carcinoma), assessment of PUO (including tuberculosis) and determining if a patient has a medication-induced liver disease. On less than 1% of occasions does the liver biopsy overestimate the amount of hepatic damage.

The biopsy is commonly preceded by an ultrasound examination of the liver to determine the best and safest biopsy site. Sometimes the biopsy is conducted under ultrasonic guidance. Coagulation status should be optimal at the time of biopsying.

Assessing Hepatitis C (HCV)

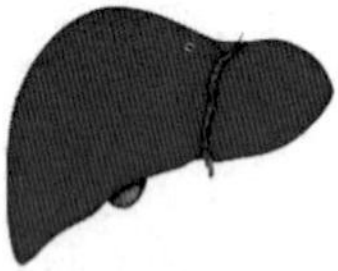

1. Counsel and test for antibodies to HCV.

2. If antibody-positive, test blood for HCV RNA (the 'hepatitis C PCR test')

3. If PCR-positive, organise liver ultrasound and biopsy, and check hepatic enzymes and coagulation profile. Histology looks at inflammation, focal necrosis, bridging necrosis and fibrosis, and the histological appearance is scored, e.g. Knodell score (X/22).

4. If score is high (e.g. Knodell score $\geq$ 6/22), consider treatment for HCV. Vaccinate against HBV & HAV.

5. If score is low (e.g. Knodell score < 6/22), observe patient regularly, watch HCV RNA levels, re-biopsy liver at ~ 2–3 years. Vaccinate against HBV & HAV. Watch α-fetoprotein levels.

Fig. 5.9

The risks of the traditional liver biopsy (not performed under ultrasound guidance) include: • pain (1 in 5 patients) • haemorrhage (1 in 500 patients) • bleeding to such an extent that a patient may require transfusions or surgery (1 in 1000 patients) • pneumothorax and/or puncture of the gallbladder, kidney or bowel (1 in 1000 patients) • death (1 in 5000 patients) (🔗 http://pages.prodigy.com/hepc/hepc6.htm). Equivalent figures are not currently available for ultrasonic-guided liver biopsy, but the technique is well established.

5 Infectious & tropical diseases

Liver biopsy material should always be subjected to microbiological culture as well as to histological assessment.

Lymph node sampling
The likely pathologies depend upon whether or not the lymphadenopathy is regional or generalised, and upon the site.

Biopsy: for histology and culture, especially for tuberculosis, for tropical infections such as chancroid, and for other relevant infections such as the cat scratch fever agent, *Bartonella henselae*. If regional, the differential diagnosis varies with the site; if intra-abdominal, for example, TB, *Yersinia enterocolitica* and adenovirus will come into the picture.

Fine needle aspirate (FNA): generally as useful as full biopsy for culture purposes, but no structural information available (similar to the aspirate *vs.* trephine issue in bone marrow sampling; 📖*Haematology* (p281)).

Respiratory samples
Sputum tests
- *Microscopy*: can perform direct microscopy (e.g. for *Aspergillus* spp., eggs of paragonimiasis), Gram stain, ZN, PCP (silver staining needed).
- *Induced sputum*: e.g. for TB, PCP.
- *Tracheal aspirate*: used in ill individuals. May produce similar material.

Bronchoscopy
- *Bronchoalveolar lavage* (BAL): useful for TB and other mycobacteria, PCP, fungi, melioidosis, resistant bacteria (e.g. *Pseudomonas*), RSV, paragonimiasis. *Lung biopsy*: useful for TB and other mycobacteria, PCP (needs silver staining), fungi, melioidosis, resistant bacteria (e.g. *Pseudomonas*), RSV paragonimiasis.

Open lung biopsy
- When it is not feasible to obtain intrathoracic tissue by less invasive means.

Pleural disease: effusion, empyema, biopsy
Consider e.g. tuberculosis, pneumococcal sepsis, underlying neoplasm (and rarer conditions, like strongyloidiasis, which will come up from time to time). Biochemical analysis of pleural fluid can help (📖*Biochemistry* (p286)). An empyema will have a high white cell count, a high protein, a low pH, LDH changes compatible with an exudate, and, possibly, organisms visible and/or culturable within the fluid. A pleural biopsy can be obtained with an Abraham's needle, but pleuroscopy may have developed into a better option in recent times.
🔗 http://blue.temple.edu/~pathphys/pulmonary/pleural_disease.html

Skin biopsy
Biopsy and hair sampling
- Useful in numerous ways, including e.g. TB, Kaposi's sarcoma (caused by HHV-8 and associated with HIV), onchocerciasis (see below), the aetiology of warts (common viral warts versus molluscum contagiosum—the distinction can be important in view of the therapeutic

options and the potential for malignant change in some sites, such as the female cervix).
- The identification of pathogenic arthropod parasites, such as myiasis (the invasion and feeding on living tissues of humans or animals by dipterous larvae, such as that of the tumbu fly), scabies, lice, ticks and chigger fleas, depends on the offending agent being seen and correctly recognised or the appropriate specimen (e.g. excision biopsy) being taken and examined histologically.

Skin snips
- Filarial infestations: examination of skin snips will identify microfilariae of *Onchocerca volvulus* and *Mansonella streptocerca*. Skin snips can be obtained using a corneal-scleral punch, or more simply a scalpel and needle. The sample must be allowed to incubate for 30min to 2h in saline or culture medium, and then examined microscopically for microfilariae that would have migrated from the tissue to the liquid phase of the specimen.
  🖑 http://www.dpd.cdc.gov/dpdx/HTML/Filariasis.asp?body=Frames/A-F/Filariasis/body_Filariasis_page2.htm

Nodulectomy is also of value, as is examination of the eye with a slit lamp.
- Leprosy: acid-fast bacilli are present in the skin.
- Ebola virus: These have diagnostic value.
  🖑 http://www.uct.ac.za/microbiology/promed21.htm

Other tissues and collections are numerous and include
- Bone infection/abscess/osteomyelitis: consider e.g. pyogenic sepsis, TB, atypical mycobacteria, sickle cell disease, ectopic ova of schistosomiasis. The history is important, e.g. with a history of fight trauma to a hand, anaerobic bony infection may be more likely.
  🖑 http://www.worldortho.com/database/etext/infection2.html
- Brain lesions and abscesses: biopsy and drainage useful for e.g. TB, herpes simplex, rabies, cysticercosis, encephalitis, vCJD, JC virus and toxoplasmosis (in HIV infection).
- Cervix: HPV.
- Joint infections: aspirate synovial fluid and consider e.g. pyogenic sepsis, TB. An acute attack of gout (diagnosed through identifying the birefringent crystals of sodium urate) can mimic an acute infective arthritis and should be excluded.
  🖑 http://www.rheumatology.org/publications/primarycare/number6/hrh0033698.html
  🖑 http://www.worldortho.com/database/etext/infection2.html
- Liver abscess: consider *Streptococcus milleri*, hydatid disease, amoebic dysentery, necrotic hepatocellular carcinoma in hepatitis C or hepatitis B, obstruction of biliary tree by *Ascaris lumbricoides* or liver flukes such as *Clonorchis sinensis*.
- Muscle biopsy:
  - Cardiac: may point towards a myocarditis or Chagas' disease.
  - Skeletal: may be used to identify parasites, including e.g. trichinosis, cysticercosis.
- Nerve biopsy: peripheral nerve biopsy (e.g. posterior auricular nerve) may reveal tuberculoid leprosy.
- Ocular:
  - Vitreous humor: e.g. intraocular infections, including fungal, HSV, HVZ, pyogenic bacterial.
  - Cornea: e.g. rabies, CJD.
  - Retina: e.g. herpes varicella-zoster, toxocariasis.

- Paranasal sinus aspirates: e.g. bacteria, fungal (such as mucomycosis).
- Pericardial biopsy: particularly important for establishing a diagnosis in a chronic pericarditis, e.g. tuberculosis, fungal.
- Peritoneal infection: via laparoscopic tissue sampling and ascites sampling (📖*Gastrointestinal tract investigations* (p284)).
- Splenic aspiration: useful in the diagnosis of visceral leishmaniasis (kala-azar) by microscopic examination and culture and demonstration of the organism.
  🖰 http://www.who.sci.eg/Publications/RegionalPublications/Specimen_Collection/
- Tonsillar biopsy: of particular value for diagnosing vCJD: also consider MRI scanning (📖*Radiology* (p282)), EEG and 14-3-3 protein in CSF.
  🖰 http://w3.aces.uiuc.edu/AnSci/BSE/Human_MAFF_vCJD_Diagnosis_and_Map.htm

Other tests

Dermatological tests

- Tuberculosis skin tests: measure delayed hypersensitivity. The Mantoux test usually involves the intradermal injection of 10 tuberculin units of purified protein derivative (PPD), and the response is quantified. The reaction is read at 48–72h. They are most useful epidemiologically, their individual clinical value being relatively limited. Multiple puncture techniques (the Heaf and Tine tests) are likely to be more convenient for large group study.
- Casoni test: an immediate hypersensitivity skin test employed to detect sensitisation to hydatid antigen (*Echinococcus granulosus*). No longer used.
- Histoplasmin test: a positive intradermal skin reaction to histoplasmin (the histoplasmin test) may be the only sign of past infection with *Histoplasma capsulatum*. The main value is epidemiological. A similar skin test exists for *Coccidioides immitis*.
- Mazzotti (DEC) test: for filariasis. This test relied on the intense pruritic response induced by microfilariae after treatment with the antifilarial agent diethylcarbamazine (DEC). Used in a minute quantity, it can nevertheless be associated with side effects, ranging from mild discomfort, fever, headaches and intolerable pruritus to tachypnoea, tachycardia, and even pulmonary oedema. Pre-treatment with antihistamines and corticosteroids may lessen the discomfort. Rarely used now.
- Schick test: for assessing susceptibility to diphtheria. A small amount of diphtheria toxin is injected into the skin; in individuals with low levels of specific antibody the injection will produce an area of redness and swelling, indicating that vaccination is needed. When the patient is immune to diphtheria, serum antibody to diphtheria toxin will neutralise the injected toxin, and no skin reaction will develop. The test is hardly used.
- Skin testing for antibiotic allergy: this can be performed in the same way as for other allergens.

Ophthalmology

- Slit lamp examination: in the hands of an expert, this technique can help with the diagnosis of infective and parasitic ocular problems, e.g. uveitis (syphilis, Reiter's syndrome), *Onchocerca volvulus* larvae, toxocariasis, toxoplasmosis, candidiasis.

Cardiac

- Electrocardiography (ECG): serial ECGs can be of value in rheumatic fever, pericarditis, myocarditis and toxic shock syndrome. The ECG is also of value in conditions where the cardiac conduction mechanism has been damaged, such as in Chagas' disease (American trypanosomiasis) and with a valve root abscess in severe infective endocarditis. In cholera and enteric fever (typhoid and paratyphoid), the cardiac rate will often be slower than one might anticipate for the degree of fever.
- Echocardiography: 📖*Radiology* (p282).

Neurological

- EEG: may help with making a diagnosis of encephalitis (e.g. in patients with HSV encephalitis, the EEG may exhibit focal unilateral or bilateral periodic discharges localised in the temporal lobes), of brain abscess or of cerebral cysticercosis. It may also be of value in vCJD.
- Lumbar puncture: material for culture and sensitivity can be obtained, but much additional information is also gathered, for example, the opening pressure is usually elevated in infections (📖*Tissue biopsy & deep aspiration specimens* (p287)).
- EMG: offers rapid bedside confirmation of the clinical diagnosis of botulism. It shows a pattern of brief, small, abundant motor unit potentials. In Guillain-Barré syndrome (a recognised association of infections such as *Campylobacter* gastroenteritis), the EMG is helpful with excluding primary muscle disease.
- Nerve conduction studies: helpful with diagnosing neuropathies (e.g. HIV, leprosy, Guillain-Barré syndrome).

Pulmonary

- Pulmonary function tests: bronchial hyperreactivity can be assessed for (often provoked by infection) and interstitial lung disease checked for (which can include, for example, tuberculosis, fungal infections, etc.).

Narcotics and anabolic steroids screen

- If positive, these may point towards occult drug use and a concomitant risk of blood-borne viruses (HIV, hepatitis C, hepatitis B). vCJD has been transmitted through anabolic steroid injecting.

Antibiotic plasma concentration monitoring

- Some drugs are toxic if the plasma levels rise too high and their use is futile if the levels are too low (indeed, this may promote the development of resistant bacteria, etc.). Monitoring serum drug levels ensures that plasma drug levels remain within the therapeutic range. Antimicrobial drugs that may require this approach include gentamicin, netilmicin, vancomycin, kanamycin, amikacin, tobramycin, chloramphenicol, streptomycin, cycloserine, amphotericin B, 5-fluorocytosine, ketoconazole, fluconazole and itraconazole.

Clinical investigation in action

Endocarditis

Endocarditis is a deep-seated infection that behaves like a deep-seated abscess—indeed, an abscess can form adjacent to an infected cardiac valve or shunt. The diagnosis of endocarditis involves thoughtful clinical assessment, including whether or not there is a history of injecting drug use, and requires multiple blood cultures and cardiac assessment. Assess clinically for likelihood, e.g. background of injecting drug use, congenital heart disease, prosthetic valves, rheumatic fever, scarlet fever. May manifest changing cardiac murmurs over a period of time, as well as a number of additional signs.

- Establish diagnosis: echocardiography (especially TOE)—to look at valves, cardiac chambers, shunts, etc.
- Establish aetiology:
  1 blood cultures (multiple)—consider culturing for unusual organisms such as fungi, HACEK organisms, *Listeria* monocytogenes, etc.,
  2 serology—Q fever (*Coxiella burnetti*) phase I and II, *Candida albicans*.
- Assess clinical status:
  1 ECG—tachycardia, conduction abnormalities,
  2 CXR—cardiac size, pulmonary emboli with right-sided endocarditis,
  3 U&E—to assess renal compromise, if any,
  4 haematology—white cell count,
  5 inflammatory markers—ESR, CRP,
  6 proteinuria—to assess renal compromise, if any,
  7 blood-borne virus status—HIV, hepatitis C, hepatitis B if there is a history of drug injecting.
- Assistance with therapy:
  1 antibiotic sensitivity testing,
  2 serum antibiotic levels (e.g. gentamicin, vancomycin).
- Prevention: dental assessment—for prevention in the future.
  Endocarditis warning card. MedicAlert® bracelet.

Tuberculosis

Consider pulmonary versus extrapulmonary disease and other epidemiological parameters, and factor into the assessment.
- Establish diagnosis/aetiology:
  1 radiological evidence (depends on what sites are, or appear to be, involved—can generate 'hard' or 'soft' data),
  2 bodily fluids (e.g. sputum, early morning urines, gastric washings) and biopsies (*see below*)—always consider performing induced sputum even with a normal CXR; histology may show caseating granulomata,
  3 PCR testing,
  4 Mantoux test,
  5 CA-125 levels—abdominal TB in women.
- Assess clinical status:
  1 inflammatory markers—ESR, CRP,
  2 T cell subsets—low CD4+ cell count characteristic,

    3 body weight,
    4 HIV testing—may be an association,
    5 glucose metabolism—may be an association (fasting glucose,
      OGTT, HbA_{1c}).
- Assistance with therapy:
    1 antibiotic sensitivity testing,
    2 serum antibiotic levels (e.g. cycloserine),
    3 liver function tests,
    4 skin testing,
    5 vitamin D levels,
    6 gene probes (for rifampicin resistance).

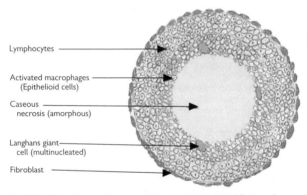

Lymphocytes

Activated macrophages
(Epithelioid cells)

Caseous
necrosis (amorphous)

Langhans giant
cell (multinucleated)

Fibroblast

Fig. 5.10 Caseating granulomata are the principle histological feature of tuberculosis together with acid-fast bacilli (detected using the Ziehl-Neelsen stain). In any tissue affected by tuberculosis, caseating garanulomata may be present and are accordingly of immense assistance diagnostically.

- Prevention: notify cases to public health authorities. Contact tracing.

▶Tuberculosis and biopsies: in any biopsy of any tissue, the possibility of extrapulmonary TB should be borne in mind. If histology is performed, caseating granulomata may be seen, and appropriate staining for acid-fast bacilli (such as the Ziehl-Neelsen stain) may reveal the presence of TB organisms. Wherever possible, appropriate cultures for TB should also be set up, both for diagnostic and for drug sensitivity purposes. Molecular techniques, including gene probes and PCR, will increasingly augment the diagnostic armoury for TB in the future.

Malaria (fever in the returning traveller)
Always consider malaria in the febrile individual returning from overseas—a detailed geographical history and malaria prophylaxis history is essential. Always consider the possibility of a coexistent second diagnosis (especially in *P. falciparum* infestation), such as *Salmonella* septicaemia (so-called 'algid malaria').

- Establish diagnosis/aetiology:
  1 thick and thin blood films × 3 (each 24h apart),
  2 molecular tests,
  3 platelet count—thrombocytopenia suggestive of *P. falciparum*,
  4 haematology—white cell count,
  5 inflammatory markers—ESR, CRP,
  6 malaria antibodies—not useful in acute situation, but useful epidemiologically.
- Assess clinical status:
  1 blood cultures—to exclude algid malaria,
  2 haemoglobinopathy—assess for sickle cell disease,
  3 assess the very ill patient thoroughly for possible cerebral malaria (includes LFTs, blood film for haemolysis, coagulation status, CXR, ECG, arterial blood gases, glucose levels, lactate levels, etc.). Note that severe falciparum malaria can present as a diarrhoeal illness.
- Assistance with therapy:
  1 G6PD levels,
  2 tests of hearing—deafness can occur with quinine.
- Prevention: avoid blood donation.

Jaundice (acute)

Jaundice can be pre-hepatic, post-hepatic or a combination of both. Epidemiological factors are important (drug injecting, travel, unsafe food, unsafe sex, job, hobbies, vaccination history, alcohol, prescribed medications, herbal remedies, etc.). The patient may have a chronic liver disease (e.g. hepatitis C) which has only just been recognised through an acute exacerbation. Always remember Courvoisier's law (*distended gall bladder in a patient with obstructive jaundice means cancer*) and Charcot's triad (the characteristic presentation of acute cholangitis, with biliary colic, jaundice and spiking fevers with rigors). Haemolysis may lead to jaundice without liver disease being present.

295

- Establish diagnosis:
  1 LFTs—conjugated and unconjugated bilirubin levels,
  2 urinalysis,
  3 stool examination—colour, flushability,
  4 haemolysis screen—blood film, coagulation studies, antiglobulin test, etc.
- Establish aetiology:
  1 serology—e.g. hepatitis A through to E, EBV, CMV, toxoplasmosis, leptospirosis, hantavirus, yellow fever,
  2 blood culture,
  3 stools for ova, cysts and parasites (e.g. *Clonorchis sinensis*, ascariasis),
  4 monospot for EBV,
  5 hepatobiliary ultrasound— obstruction by malignancy or parasites, liver parenchyma status, gallstones,
  6 ERCP/MRCP—may diagnose parasitic invasion of biliary tree, MV/crypotosporidial disease/porta hepatis lymphadenopathy associated with HIV, etc.,
  8 paracetamol levels.

- Assess clinical status:
    1 hepatobiliary ultrasound—serial scans can assess hepatobiliary status sequentially,
    2 clotting screen,
    3 α-fetoprotein levels—may suggest hepatocellular carcinoma associated with hepatitis C and hepatitis B infection.
- Assistance with therapy:
    1 HIV testing—if appropriate: co-infection with HIV, HCV and HBV an increasing problem world-wide,
    2 ethanol assessment—γGT levels, ↑ MCV,
    3 molecular tests: PCR testing for HCV, circulating DNA levels in HBV,
    4 antigens—hepatitis B.
- Prevention:
    1 notify cases to public health authorities; safe sex education; safe drug-injecting education possible once viral diagnosis of HCV, HBV and/or HIV established,
    2 assess family, sexual partners, etc. for possible infection (HIV, HBV, HCV) and/or need to vaccinate (HBV),
    3 vaccination strategies: HBV, HAV as appropriate.

Diarrhoea

Diarrhoea can be acute versus chronic, or acute on chronic. For example, a gastroenteritis illness may uncover pre-existing inflammatory bowel disease, such as Crohn's disease, or malabsorption (such as coeliac disease or pancreatic insufficiency). Drugs such as opiates can lead to 'overflow' diarrhoea. Also bear in mind that where there is one bowel pathogen, another one might be present. Antibiotic resistance is common among some bowel pathogens. Diarrhoea can appear infective, but, for example, might be endocrine in origin (e.g. carcinoid syndrome, Zollinger-Ellison syndrome, medullary carcinoma of thyroid), while the possibility of bowel cancer must always be borne in mind. Note that the presence of *Streptococcus bovis* in blood cultures is ALWAYS highly indicative of the presence of a bowel cancer until proven otherwise. Irritable bowel disease is being increasingly diagnosed. Malaria can present as diarrhoea (see earlier).

- Establish diagnosis:
    1 examine stools,
    2 keep stool chart on ward.
- Establish aetiology:
    1 stool culture and sensitivity,
    2 stool microscopy for ova, cysts and parasites,
    2 sigmoidoscopy and biopsy,
    3 *Clostridium difficile* toxin,
    4 staphylococcal enterotoxin (food poisoning),
    6 string test,
    7 malabsorption screen including antigliadin/antiendomysial antibodies,
    8 serology for *Yersinia*, amoebic, strongyloidiasis, typhoid.
- Assess clinical status:
    1 haematology: white cell count,
    2 inflammatory markers—ESR, CRP,
    3 HIV test—may be the overall underlying problem,
    4 TB assessment—may be the underlying pathology,

5 deficiencies: with problems where malabsorption is a possible problem, vitamin, iron, etc. deficiency, etc. must be investigated.

- Assistance with therapy: antibiotic sensitivity testing.
- Prevention: notify cases to public health authorities; isolate as necessary.

Pneumonic illness

Pneumonia is multi-aetiological. If recurrent, this throws up certain diagnostic possibilities that must be considered. Many epidemiological considerations are important, such as travel history, occupation, pet keeping, hobbies, sexual activity, etc. Osler's triad of rigors, pleuritis and rust-coloured sputum is said to be characteristic of pneumococcal pneumonia.

- Establish diagnosis/aetiology:
  1 CXR (or CT chest),
  2 serology: atypical pneumonia organisms (*Legionella pneumophila, Mycoplasma pneumoniae, Coxiella burnetti, Chlamydia psittaci*), hantavirus, RSV, influenza,
  3 sputum including induced sputum, bronchoscopy and BAL: microscopy and culture,
  4 blood cultures,
  5 blood cultures,
  6 serum Na$^+$ level—*Legionella*,
  7 serum creatinine phosphokinase level—*Legionella,*
  8 antigen—pneumococcal (blood), *Legionella* (urine),
  9 nasopharyngeal aspirate (NPA) for viral culture—RSV, influenza,
  10 cryoglobulins, e.g. *Mycoplasma pneumoniae,*
  11 molecular—various PCR tests.
  12 HIV test—if appropriate.
- Assess clinical status:
  1 arterial blood gases,
  2 ultrasound of chest—if effusion developing (drain if necessary),
  3 pulmonary function tests if appropriate.
- Assistance with therapy:
  1 antibiotic sensitivity testing,
  2 if recurrent: consider tuberculosis testing (*see earlier*), HIV testing, immunoglobulin levels (to check for deficiency), assessing for hyposplenism, checking terminal complement levels (C5–C9).
- Prevention:
  1 notify appropriate cases to public health authorities (e.g. *Legionella,* tuberculosis); isolate as necessary,
  2 vaccination strategies: influenza, *Pneumococcus, Haemophilus influenzae B* (HiB),
  3 cessate smoking if relevant.

297

Meningitic illness (headache and photophobia)

Meningitis can be extremely serious, particularly bacterial, mycobacterial, fungal and protozoal forms, but viral meningitis is generally less serious. Meningitic infection is often mimicked by much less serious infections, such as urinary tract infection (especially in women), throat infections (ASO, monospot), atypical pneumonias and sinusitis (especially ethmoidal, sphenoidal). A similar picture can also be generated by a subarachnoid haemorrhage. Meningococcal infection can be life-threatening without ever causing meningitis. If a bacterial meningitis is recurrent, certain diagnostic possibilities must be considered. Brain abscess (think of injecting drug use, congenital heart disease, immunodeficiency, etc.) and, under certain circumstances, encephalitis can present in a similar fashion to meningitic illnesses. Where the patient has a marked petechial rash and a history of travel to Africa, Ukraine or South America, even viral haemorrhagic fever (particularly the Congo-Crimean variety) comes into the picture.

- Establish diagnosis/aetiology:
  1. lumbar puncture (LP)/cisternal puncture/foramenal puncture (in neonates): for CSF pressure, microscopy, bacterial and mycobacterial culture (including special cultures, e.g. for *Listeria*), viral culture, biochemistry (e.g. protein, glucose), differential cell count, viral PCR, xanthochromia, India ink stain, cryptococcal antigen testing,
  2. CT scan of head: sometimes necessary to help exclude raised intracranial pressure prior to performing LP (cisternal puncture and foramenal puncture possible in skilled hands); to exclude paranasal sinusitis, mastoiditis, brain abscess,
  3. CXR and assessment for atypical pneumonia if appropriate (*see earlier*),
  4. NPA (*see earlier*),
  5. petechial rash sampling: aspirate material from a fresh purpuric lesion using a small-needle insulin syringe, and culture,
  6. molecular: meningococcal PCR (blood and CSF), pneumococcal PCR (blood and CSF),
  7. serology: urine and blood for cryptococcal antigen; blood for pneumococcal antigen; urine for mumps antigen; ASO, antibodies to EBV, *Cryptococcus*,
  8. nasopharyngeal swab for meningococcus,
  9. stool for enteroviral culture,
  10. monospot test for EBV.
- Assess clinical status:
  1. CT scan/MRI scan of head: assess for raised intracranial pressure, exclude SAH (xanthochromia), sagittal vein thrombosis; exclude skull fracture, especially of cribriform plate (this can lead to recurrent pneumococcal meningitis—if there is a nasal drip, test fluid for glucose to exclude presence of CSF as CSF contains glucose),
  2. differential white cell count in blood,
  3. inflammatory markers: ESR, CRP,
  4. coagulation screen and platelet count: for meningococcal sepsis,
  5. arterial blood gases: to assess acid-base balance in severe cases,
  6. synacthen test: adrenal failure in severe meningococcal sepsis (Waterhouse-Friederichsen syndrome),
  7. HIV test—suggested by some pathologies, and may be the overall underlying problem,
  8. TB assessment—may be the underlying pathology.
- Assistance with therapy:
  1. antibiotic sensitivity testing,
  2. serum antimicrobial levels, e.g. amphotericin, flucytosine.
- Prevention:

5 Infectious & tropical diseases

1 notify relevant cases to public health authorities; isolate as necessary,
2 vaccination strategies: meningococcus A and C, pneumococcus, influenza, HIB,
3 history of skull fracture: may need neurosurgery, etc.

Urethritis (with or without haematuria)

Pain on micturition can simply represent a urinary tract infection, or there may be a sexually transmitted disease such as gonorrhoea present. More exotic problems can be relevant to the case if the patient has been travelling. The sexual and travel history is therefore important. Renal calculi can produce clinical pictures resembling infection, as can dermatological condition such as Stevens-Johnson syndrome. Urinary tract infections are more common during pregnancy.

- Establish diagnosis/aetiology:
  1 urine collection (MSU): culture (bacterial infections), microscopy (parasites, etc. such as schistosomiasis—use terminal specimen), molecular techniques (LCR for *Chlamydia*),
  2 sexually transmitted diseases and pelvic inflammatory disease: perform HVS and urethral swabs, screen for gonococcus (includes throat and anal swabs),
  3 calcular disease: exclude with urine microscopy, radiology, etc.,
  4 prostatitis: prostatic massage, cryptococcal antigen,
  5 tuberculosis—can present like any other UTI,
  6 Reiter's syndrome: slit lamp examination of the eye, urine and stool culture/LCR for *Chlamydia*.
- Assess clinical status:
  1 biochemistry: exclude renal failure (urea, creatinine, etc.),
  2 markers of inflammation: CRP, ESR,
  3 white cell count,
  4 check all other mucosal surfaces of the body (mouth, conjunctivae, nose, etc.) to help exclude Stevens-Johnson syndrome.
- Assistance with therapy:
  1 pregnancy test,
  2 PSA to exclude prostatic carcinoma (recurrent UTIs in older men),
  3 radiology of renal tract: ultrasound, IVP (to exclude underlying renal tract anatomical problems, TB involvement, calculi, etc.).
- Prevention:
  1 history of unsafe sex, recent new sexual partner, drug injecting: consider VDRL, HIV, viral hepatitis testing,
  2 tuberculosis: notify, contact trace, etc.,
  3 calculi: exclude hypercalcaemia, hyperuricaemia, etc.

Red painful swollen lower leg

One of the most difficult things in medicine is to distinguish effectively between a distal deep venous thrombosis and cellulitis—and a combination of both! Sometimes the problem is in the tissues, and sometimes in

1. A detailed travel history and a high index of suspicion are essential in making the diagnosis of VHF. A recent travel history to an area where one of these viruses are known to be particularly prevalent is suggestive, particularly Africa (e.g. Uganda and Ebola, Nigeria and Lassa) and South America — the incubation period ranges from 3 to 21 days, depending upon the variety. Many VHF cases presenting together may suggest a bioterrorism attack.

Biohazard

5. Almost always, the true diagnosis will not be a VHF, but they must be considered where appropriate. Strict adherence to isolation and infection control precautions has prevented secondary transmission in almost all cases.

2. VHFs are severe febrile illnesses that can be complicated by a haemorrhagic tendency, petechiae, hypotension (and even shock), flushing of the face and chest, and oedema. Constitutional symptoms such as headaches, myalgia, vomiting and diarrhoea may occur. Some VHFs manifest particular features not shared by the others.

3. Once suspected, VHFs are category 4 pathogens, so precautions for healthcare workers must be instituted and the case notified to the proper authorities. Isolation measures and barrier nursing procedures are indicated (Marburg, Ebola, Lassa and Congo-Crimean HF viruses may be particularly prone to aerosol nosocomial spread), usually in a special infectious diseases/tropical medicine unit staffed with clinicians with expertise in the field. Intensive supportive care may be required.

4. Diagnosis requires clinical expertise in infectious diseases/tropical medicine. The differential diagnosis includes malaria, yellow fever, dengue, typhoid/paratyphoid fever, non-typhoidal salmonellae, typhus and other rickettsial diseases, leptospirosis, *shigella* dysentery, relapsing fever (borreliosis), fulminant hepatitis and meningococcal disease. Antigen tests, antibody detection and viral culture are all available for most of the VHFs. The patient should be fully investigated and treated

Fig. 5.11 Investigating a possible VHF case.

the joints (even gout and pseudogout can look like cellulitis) or the bone (osteomyelitis). Ulceration may be present on the legs. Venous and arterial insufficiency may complicate the picture—infected legs in older people can be very difficult to treat with antibiotics alone. Recent long-haul air travel may point more towards thrombosis, but swollen legs with compromised veins easily get infected! Although rare, syphilis, yaws and *Mycobacterium ulcerans* can cause leg ulcers that are potentially amenable to treatment. Pyoderma gangrenosum can resemble infection of the leg, but is associated with non-infectious systemic diseases.

- Establish diagnosis/aetiology:
    1 exclude DVT (and possible embolic disease on occasions),
    2 swabs: from ulcers, between the toes,
    3 blood cultures,
    4 ASO titre, antistaphylococcal titres (on occasions), VDRL,
    5 joint assessment: urate levels for gout, assess (if relevant) for pseudogout, rheumatological screen, synovial fluid analysis (if relevant), Lyme disease titres (depends on the travel history, etc.),

    6 leg ulcers in the young: consider sickle cell disease, hereditary sphe-
      rocytosis.
- Assess clinical status:
  1. white cell count,
  2. inflammatory markers: ESR, CRP,
  3. assess blood vessel integrity: e.g. compression ultrasound for venous problems, lower limb arteriography.
- Assistance with therapy:
  1. exclude diabetes,
  2. x-ray, bone scanning—is osteomyelitis present?
- Prevention:
  1. treat diabetes if present,
  2. treat other underlying conditions if present,
  3. patient advised to take care in future (e.g. DVT avoidance while travelling).

Vesicular rash

Many vesicular rashes are infective, many are not. In particular, the distribution of the rash should be carefully assessed and joint assessment and management with a dermatologist is often valuable. If atopic, eczema herpeticum comes into the picture. Staphylococcal impetigo can cause vesiculation. If there is a relevant travel history, rickettsial pox and monkey pox (and, if militarily-orientated, even smallpox, a known bioterrorism candidate organism!) come into the picture. Erythema multiforme, which often has an infective basis but can also be produced by medications, can produce a vesiculating rash (so check the mouth, eyes and genitalia, and determine the medication history). Non-infective blistering conditions include dermatitis herpetiformis (coeliac disease), pompholyx and pemphigus.

301

- Establish diagnosis/aetiology:
  1. vesicular fluid—EM, culture, etc.,
  2. serology—HSV, HVZ, rickettsial pox, coxsackievirus, ASO titre.
- Assess clinical status:
  1. CXR—chickenpox (if compromised, arterial blood gases will be needed),
  2. EEG if cerebral symptoms present (e.g. cerebellar encephalitis can occur with HVZ),
  3. monkey pox, small-pox, rickettsial pox: the patient will be ill and will require full assessment, even possibly intensive care.
- Assistance with therapy: pregnancy test—HVZ a bigger problem in pregnancy.
- Prevention:
  1. avoid precipitants with erythema multiforme,
  2. manage atopy optimally.

Further reading

Armstrong D, Cohen J, eds. (2000) *Infectious Diseases*, Mosby-Year Book, St Louis.

Caumes E. (1995) Health and travel, in *Manson's Tropical Diseases*, 20th edition, ed Cook GC, WB Saunders, Philadelphia.

Intersep Parasite disc (Winstanley T, Clark T, Green ST, ☞ http://www.instruchemie.nl/parasitology_quality%20controls.htm), 2000.

Mandell GL, Douglas JE, Dolin R, Bennett RE, eds. (1998) *Principles and Practice of Infectious Diseases*, 5th edition, Churchill Livingstone.

Peters W, Pasvol G. (2001) *Color Atlas of Tropical Medicine and Parasitology*, 5th edition, Mosby-Year Book, St Louis.

Shanson DC. (1999) *Microbiology and Clinical Practice*, 3rd edition, Butterworth-Heinemann, Oxford.

Steffen R, Dupont HL. (1999) *Manual of Travel Medicine and Health*, BC Decker.

Chapter 6

Cardiology

303

Ambulatory electrocardiography

Clinical indications

The indications for ambulatory electrocardiography (AECG) or Holter monitoring have broadened with an increasing awareness of the importance of arrhythmias coupled with improved design of the available monitoring devices[1]. AECG recordings can be used to document the presence, complexity or absence of arrhythmias, and their correlation with patient-perceived symptoms. Documenting abnormalities of the ST segment in patients with silent ischaemia and heart rate variability in the risk stratification of patients with CHD may also be clinically useful.

Indications for AECG recording include

Assessment of symptoms that may be related to disturbances of heart rhythm
- Altered consciousness (dizziness, pre-syncope, syncope, other neurological events).
- Palpitation.
- Intermittent breathlessness.
- Unexplained chest pain.
- Fatigue, sweating, etc.

Assessment of risk in patients without symptoms of arrhythmia
- After myocardial infarction.
- Congestive heart failure.
- Hypertrophic cardiomyopathy.
- Systemic hypertension.
- Pre-operative patient assessment.
- Screening in other patients.

Efficacy of anti-arrhythmic therapy
- Assessment of pacemaker and AICD function.
- Monitoring for myocardial ischaemia.
- Assessment of paediatric patients.

Contraindications

None. The use of AECG in asymptomatic patients or routine population testing is not however recommended.

Patient preparation

With devices that require the application of skin electrodes, meticulous preparation of the skin is important if high quality, artefact-free recordings are to be obtained. The skin under the electrode should be shaved if necessary, abraded and cleansed with an alcohol swab in an attempt to reduce the electrical resistance of the skin. The patient is supplied with a diary for recording the temporal relationship and nature of symptoms occurring during the AECG. Typically, a recording continues for 24h, although continuing the recording for up to 72h can increase the yield.

Procedure

Conventional AECG recorders are battery powered, lightweight portable devices that continuously record two or three bipolar leads on conventional magnetic cassette tape. More recently, solid-state memory devices have begun to replace conventional tape technology which is prone to jamming, tape stretch or fracture. Contemporary tape analysis systems are computer based, and allow a trained technician to select segments of ECG that demonstrate abnormalities of heart rhythm (*Fig. 6.1*) or the ST segment which can be correlated with symptoms noted in the dairy by means of an internal timing channel. Additional data generated by current technology include automatic counts of abnormal beats, minimum and maximum rates, incidence and duration of ST segment depression, etc.

Patient-activated 'event recorders' (e.g. Cardiomemo) can be used where symptomatic episodes are rare or infrequent; these usually involve a solid-state loop recording that can be transmitted by the patient to a central (hospital-based) receiving station via a standard telephone line for later analysis. Alternatively, implantable loop recorders (e.g. Reveal) are inserted in a small subcutaneous pocket and can continuously monitor the ECG for period of 1–2 years, without the need for additional electrodes; these devices are particularly useful for discriminating between infrequent episodes of cardiac or neurally mediated altered consciousness (e.g. Stokes-Adams attacks *vs.* epilepsy).

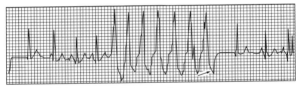

Fig. 6.1   ECG showing ventricular tachycardia.

Possible results
Symptoms (e.g. dizziness, syncope) in association with an arrhythmia suffi-cient to reduce cardiac output and therefore cerebral perfusion allow the patient to be offered specific targeted therapy (e.g. permanent pacing, anti-arrhythmic medication). In the absence of symptoms or demonstrable arrhythmia, it is important to persist with repeated, and if necessary more prolonged, AECG testing. Consideration of using an alternative recording method (e.g. Cardiomemo, Reveal device) may be appropriate. The yield of the AECG in the patient presenting with syncope is low (~5%). Palpitation accounts for 30–50% of indications for outpatient AECG mon-itoring, with an arrhythmia documented in up to 45% of symptomatic recordings. The identification of arrhythmias in high-risk subsets (e.g. post-myocardial infarction, dilated cardiomyopathy) will determine the need for further investigation (e.g. cardiac catheterisation, electrophysiological testing) or treatment (e.g. AICD, drug therapy). Risk stratification fol-lowing acute myocardial infarction can be improved by combining a number of tests (e.g. echo-derived ejection fraction, AECG, SAECG, tread-mill exercise test, etc.).

The AECG is a useful technique to detect and monitor myocardial ischaemia using the analysis of ST segment changes. In that up to 80% of episodes of myocardial ischaemia (ST segment ↓) are asymptomatic, the

AECG is ideally suited to record such episodes, and contemporary play-back machines can analyse and quantitate these changes automatically. There remains doubt as to the importance of such changes when found in the normal population.

Advantages over other tests
Cheap, simple and repeatable. The only method, other than chance observation on a cardiac monitor, of correlating ECG findings and symptoms.

Ancillary tests
In the investigation of the patient with possible arrhythmias, additional treadmill exercise testing, tilt table testing or electrophysiological testing may be helpful.

Pitfalls
Symptomatic correlation of abnormalities recorded on the AECG is an important prerequisite of interpretation of the significance of 'abnormalities' found on the recording. An appreciation of findings frequently seen in a normal population is fundamental if an excess of 'false positive' recordings are to be avoided. Normal findings include sinus bradycardia, particularly during sleep, with rates as low as 30 beats/min, sinus arrhythmia, sinus arrest (with pauses of up to 3s), sinoatrial exit block, second-degree AV (Wenckebach) block, wandering atrial pacemaker, junctional escape rhythm, and premature atrial and ventricular ectopics. In an elderly population the criteria of 'normality' are even broader.

📖 OHCM p90.

1 ACC/AHA. (1999) Guidelines for ambulatory electrocardiography. *J Am Coll Cardiol* **34**, 912–948.

Cardiac enzymes

Clinical indications
Cardiac enzymes (markers of myocardial damage) should be measured in any patient presenting with prolonged (<15min) ischaemic sounding chest pain. The management of patients with acute coronary syndromes (ACS) (Fig. 6.2), and the diagnostic criteria for acute myocardial infarction have recently been redefined [1–4].

Indications for measurement of cardiac enzymes include
- Patients presenting with ACS (unstable angina, non ST-segment elevation myocardial infarction, Q-wave myocardial infarction).
- Patients presenting with chest pain when the diagnosis of ACS is in doubt.
- Routinely following percutaneous coronary intervention (PCI).
- Routinely following surgical revascularisation (CABG).

Procedure
Venous blood is drawn from the patient on presentation and at 12, 24, 48 and 72h after the onset of symptoms.

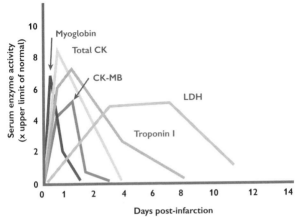

Fig. 6.2

Possible results

Myocyte necrosis is detected biochemically when intracellular macromolecules leak from myocytes into the peripheral circulation. Myoglobin and the creatine kinase MB isoenzyme (CK-MB), both non-specific markers, are released within 2h. CK-MB2, a subform (isoform) of CK-MB 5MHZ has a higher sensitivity and specificity. The troponins (cTnT and cTnI) are part of the calcium-sensitive apparatus that regulates the interaction of actin and myosin within cardiac myocytes; troponins are specific for myocardial cell injury but may not be detectable for 6–12h (Fig 6.2). Other 'classic' markers (AST, LDH) are unreliable and should not be used in the diagnosis of myocardial damage.

307

The most sensitive early marker for myocardial infarction is CK-MB2 (91%) followed by myoglobin (78%), thus a normal CK-MB2 subform at 6h reliably excludes infarction. At 10h, the cTnI sensitivity is 96% with a specificity of 93%.

Interpretation

The diagnosis of ST-elevation myocardial infarction (STEMI) is usually obvious from the appearance of the ECG, and is subsequently confirmed by elevated cardiac enzymes. Formerly, a subgroup of high-risk patients with 'unstable angina' was recognized (also called minimal myocardial damage) with elevated levels of cTnI and cTnT, but normal CK-MB. These have now been reclassified as having sustained a non-ST-elevation myocardial infarction (NSTEMI). It is estimated that ~30% of patients presenting with ACS in the absence of ST elevation would previously have been diagnosed as 'unstable angina', but have in fact suffered myocyte necrosis (NSTEMI) using an elevation in cTnT (>0.1µg/L) as the discriminator.

Advantages over other tests
Cardiac enzyme estimation allows risk stratification in patients presenting with ACS and also determines the need for further inpatient investigation (e.g. diagnostic coronary arteriography). When used in conjunction with serial ECGs, cardiac enzyme elevation is diagnostic of acute myocardial infarction.

Ancillary tests
The results of cardiac enzyme estimations should always be interpreted in conjunction with the clinical history (including the presence of other medical conditions) and serial 12-lead ECGs. Prognostic risk stratification can be improved by combining enzyme estimation with risk factors and findings on clinical examination (Figs. 3 & 4), or with the results of treadmill exercise testing (📖pp314). Myocardial infarction can also be detected by contrast ventriculography, myocardial perfusion imaging (📖p561) and dobutamine stress echocardiography.

Pitfalls
Patients presenting very early following myocardial infarction may have normal cardiac enzymes. Myoglobin and CK-MB may be detected as early as 2h, but cTnI and cTnT may not be significantly increased for 12h. Troponins may also be released in acute myocarditis, pericarditis and in patients with renal failure. Diagnosis of reinfarction (or extension) may be impossible if relying on the troponins alone as they may remain elevated for up to 14 days after the initial attack.

1 ACC/AHA Guidelines for the management of patients with acute myocardial infarction (1999) web version: www.acc.org; 2 ACC/AHA. (2000) Guidelines for the management of patients with unstable angina and non-ST-segment elevation myocardial infarction. *JAC* **36**, 970–1062; 3 ESC/ACC. (2000) Myocardial infarction redefined—A consensus document of The Joint European Society of Cardiology/American College of Cardiology Committee for the redefinition of myocardial infarction. *Eur Heart J* **21**, 1502–1513; 4 (2000) Guidelines for the management of patients with acute coronary syndromes without persistent ECG ST segment elevation. (2001) *Heart* **85**, 133–142; PJLM et al. (2000) The TIMI risk score for unstable angina/non-ST elevation MI. *JAMA* **284**, 835–842.

Echocardiography (transoesophageal)

Clinical indications
Transoesophageal echocardiography (TOE) is undertaken when transthoracic echocardiography (TTE) has failed to provide images of diagnostic quality, or as an adjunct to TTE, improving the sensitivity and specificity of echocardiographic imaging in particular patient subsets.

Indications for TOE include

Non-diagnostic/poor quality TTE images
• Patients with COPD.
• Obese patients.

Source of systemic thromboembolism
• Atrial thrombus.
• Atrial tumour (e.g. myxoma).

- Paradoxical embolism (e.g. PFO, ASD).
- Vegetation arising from the aortic or mitral valve.
- Left ventricular thrombus (e.g. mural thrombus post-AMI).
- Atheroma of the ascending aorta.
- Malignant cardiac tumour.

Atrial pathology
- Atrial septal defect.
- Patent foramen ovale.
- Atrial myxoma.
- Atrial septal aneurysm.

Valve pathology
- Aortic valve abnormalities (bicuspid valve, aortic regurgitation).
- Mitral valve pathology (stenosis, abnormalities of the sub-valve apparatus, prolapse, flail valve, parachute valve, mitral regurgitation).
- Infective endocarditis (small vegetations, perforations, abscess formation).
- Prosthetic valves (thrombosis, para-prosthetic regurgitation, infection, other dysfunction).
- Tricuspid stenosis and regurgitation.
- Pulmonary stenosis and regurgitation.

Coronary pathology
- Congenital abnormalities (anomalous origin).
- Fistulae.
- Proximal stenoses.
- Vasculitis (Kawasaki).

Aortic pathology
- Aneurysm.
- Atheroma.
- Dissection.
- Rupture.
- Mural haematoma.

Congenital heart disease
- Atrial situs.
- Abnormalities of connection (e.g. TGA).
- Abnormalities of valves.
- Pulmonary venous anomalies (e.g. TAPVD).
- Post-operative assessment of surgical results (e.g. Fallot correction, Fontan, Mustard, Senning procedures, valve replacement).

Use in the intensive care unit
- Complications of myocardial infarction (VSD, acute mitral regurgitation, cardiac rupture).
- Acute pulmonary embolism.
- Post-cardiac surgical hypotension (cardiac tamponade).
- Unexplained hypotension.

Use in the operating room
- Assessment of mitral valve repair.

TIMI risk score for ST-elevation MI (STEMI) & unstable angina/non-ST-elevation myocardial infarction (NSTEMI)

TIMI risk score for ST-elevation myocardial infarction (STEMI)

Historical	Points	Risk score	30-day mort (%)*
Age ≥75	3	0	0.8
65–74	2	1	1.6
DM, HTN or angina	1	2	2.2
Examination		3	4.4
SBP <100mmHg	3	4	7.3
HR >100beats/min	2	5	12
Killip II–IV	2	6	16
Weight <67kg	1	7	23
Presentation		8	27
Anterior STE or LBBB	1	>8	36
Time to Rx >4h	1		

Risk score = total points (0–14)

TIMI risk score for unstable angina/non-ST-elevation myocardial infarction (NSTEMI)

Historical	Points	Risk score	Risk of cardiac events by 14 days**	
			Death or MI	Death, MI or Urg ent revasc
Age ≥65	1	0/1	3	5
≥3 CAD risk factors	1	2	3	8
(F/H, HTN, ↑chol, DM, smoker)		5	13	
Known CAD (stenosis ≥50%)	1	4	12	26
ASA use in last 7 days	1	6/7	19	41
Presentation	3			
Recent (≤24h) severe angina	1			
↑ cardiac markers	1			
ST deviation ≥0.5mm	1			

Risk score = total points (0–7)

*Data from TIMI II. Entry criteria: CP >0min, ST↑, Sx onset <6h, fibrinolytic eligible[5].
**Data from TIMI IIB. Entry criteria UA or NSTEMI defined as ischaemic pain at rest within past 24h, with evidence of CAD (ST deviation or +ve markers)[6].

5 Morrow DA, Antman EM, Charlesworth A et al. TIMI risk score for ST-elevation myocardial infarction: a convenient, bedside, clinical score for risk assessment at presentation. Circ 102, 2031–2037 (web version: www.timi.org); 6 Antman EM, Cohen M, Bernink

- Quantifying the severity of valve pathology in a patient undergoing CABG.

Interventional procedures
- Mitral balloon valvuloplasty.
- Device closure (PFO, ASD, VSD).

Contraindications

With experienced operators, there are few contraindications to TOE; they include:
- Oesophageal pathology:
  - Stricture (undilated).
  - Tumour.
  - Tear, fistula, rupture.
  - Severe oesophagitis.
  - Varices.
- Dysphagia of unknown origin.
- Instability of the cervical vertebrae.
- Uncooperative patient.
- Fasting <4h (relative).

Patient preparation

Patients should be fasted for at least 4h. A detailed history is obtained from the patient, including previous difficulties with swallowing, the presence of oesophageal or other upper gastrointestinal pathology, or drug allergy. Dentures and other dental prostheses are removed, and intravenous access obtained. O_2 saturation, ECG and blood pressure are monitored throughout the procedure, and full resuscitation facilities should be available. The larynx is sprayed with xylocaine 4% and the patient is sedated with intravenous midazolam (2.5–7.5 mg). Routine antibiotic prophylaxis is not recommended for TOE.

311

Procedure

Following patient preparation, the TOE probe is introduced through the pharynx and down the oesophagus via the mouth. Once the probe passes the pharynx, passage through the oesophagus and on to the stomach is usually achieved without difficulty. The TOE probe is interfaced with a conventional cardiac ultrasound machine. In structure, the probe is somewhat similar to an endoscope, without the fibreoptic cables and suction channel. Adult probes vary from 27 to 45cm in length, with a diameter of 10–14mm. The ultrasound transducer is situated at the tip of the probe, typically a 5mHZ multi-element array, capable of rotation, flexion, advance and withdrawal. Images are recorded in standard views from the oesophagus and stomach.

Possible results

With the wide variety of indications for TOE, a detailed description of the imaging results obtained is beyond the scope of this book. TOE is invaluable in the assessment of the patient with valvular heart disease (particularly those with infective endocarditis), identifying sources of systemic embolism, confirmation of complex anatomy in congenital heart disease, and the analysis of results from surgical procedures. Serial examinations allow the natural history of a condition to be followed, and intervention to be timed with confidence.

Interpretation
▶Training and accreditation in TOE is a necessary prerequisite to skilful and safe performance. Operators should be skilled in TTE, and then introduced to the technique of oesophageal intubation. Specialist training in cardiology (UK) requires a minimum of 500 TTE and 75 TOE studies.

Advantages over other tests
TOE is the most sensitive test for detecting the source of systemic thromboembolism; despite the frequent request for a TTE, this investigation has such a low sensitivity for this indication that such a request should be declined. There are no competing techniques offering advantages in the assessment of atrial and valvular pathology. Aortic pathology (e.g. dissection) can also be investigated using CT scanning (📖pp521), MR scanning (📖p522), or aortography. TOE offers high sensitivity and specificity, portability, rapid acquisition speed, no contrast, no radiation and low cost compared with the other imaging modalities, although this group of patients requires a high degree of operator skill and expertise.

Pitfalls
Successful intubation and imaging is achieved in at least 98% of patients; an inability to pass the probe is most commonly related to operator inexperience or lack of patient cooperation, rather than oesophageal pathology. Major complications (death, oesophageal perforation, malignant arrhythmia, congestive heart failure, laryngospasm) occur in less than 0.3% of patients, and often result from the presence of unexpected oesophageal pathology (e.g. tumour). Minor complications (transient hypoxia, hypotension, bronchospasm, arrhythmia) occur in less than 3% of patients.
📖OHCM p94.

Electrophysiological testing

Clinical indications
Electrophysiological (EP) testing is used as an adjunct to non-invasive tests (e.g. resting and exercise electrocardiography, AECG) in the diagnosis of arrhythmias, the assessment of drug and device therapy, and as an integral part of therapeutic radiofrequency catheter ablation procedures[1].

Indications for EP testing include:
- Bradyarrhythmias: assessment in the following symptomatic patient groups:
  - Sinus node dysfunction.
  - AV (His-Purkinje) block.
  - Intraventricular conduction delay.
  - Left or right bundle branch block.
  - Guide to device therapy (permanent pacing).
- Tachyarrhythmias:
  - Narrow QRS complex tachycardia (e.g. atrial flutter, AVRT, AVNRT).
  - Broad QRS complex tachycardia (e.g. VT).

- Non-sustained ventricular arrhythmias (e.g. VPBs, non-sustained VT).
- Prolonged QT syndrome.
- Unexplained syncope.
- Survivors of cardiac arrest (near-miss sudden death).
- Guide to drug therapy.
- Guide to device therapy (AICD).
- During radiofrequency ablation.

Contraindications

EP testing is not indicated in patients in whom more simple tests (e.g. ECG, AECG) have documented an abnormality that correlates with symptoms or is in itself worthy of intervention. EP testing is rarely indicated in asymptomatic patients unless there is a significant family history (e.g. arrhythmogenic right ventricular dysplasia).

Patient preparation

EP testing in adults is usually undertaken with a combination of sedation and local anaesthesia. As the procedures may be prolonged (>6 h), intravenous access should be available for rehydration. In the absence of an indwelling arterial line, non-invasive blood pressure is monitored, together with oxygen saturation via a finger probe. EP procedures are performed in a fully equipped (preferably bi-plane) cardiac catheterization laboratory with experienced personnel, full resuscitation facilities, and a computer-based EP machine capable of displaying and storing data.

Procedure

Under fluoroscopic guidance, multipolar electrode catheters are introduced into the heart via the femoral and/or the subclavian vein (Fig. 6.3). Electrodes are positioned adjacent to various structures within the cardiac chambers to record local electrical activity. Signals from multiple leads are recorded simultaneously to demonstrate the activation sequence and to determine the effect of extra stimuli on the genesis of arrhythmias. Once an arrhythmia is induced, the activation sequence can be mapped with a view to radiofrequency accessory pathway ablation or modification.

313

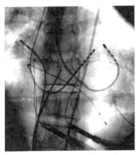

Fig. 6.3 Intracardiac electrodes.

Possible results

By measuring conduction times, refractory periods and the effects of extra stimuli, atrial and ventricular pacing, the anatomic substrate for arrhythmias can be determined; for example, the presence of an AV nodal re-entry pathway. Programmed electrical stimulation techniques are used to determine the likelihood of an underlying ventricular arrhythmia causing symptoms.

Advantages over other tests

The role of EP testing in the management of bradyarrhythmias is limited and offers little over and above more simple investigations (e.g. AECG, tilt testing). EP testing is unique in correlating electrical activity with intracardiac anatomy prior to therapeutic ablation. The initiation and termination of ventricular arrhythmias determines the applicability of device technology (e.g. AICD) to a particular patient.

Ancillary tests

EP testing usually follows assessment by more simple investigations (e.g. resting and exercise ECG, AECG). In many patients structural heart disease is excluded or confirmed by means of echocardiography, MR imaging, cardiac catheterization and coronary arteriography.

Pitfalls

EP testing now tends to be focused on identifying a specific problem, which frequently involves identifying and treating an arrhythmia substrate with guided radiofrequency catheter ablation. The limitations and reproducibility of tests of conduction and refractoriness, as well as extra stimulus and serial drug testing are well appreciated.

1 ACC/AHA Task Force Report. (1995) Guidelines for clinical intracardiac electrophysiological and catheter ablation procedures. *J Am Coll Cardiol* **26**, 555–573

Exercise testing

Clinical indications

Exercise testing[1] is the most frequent non-invasive test used in the assessment of the patient presenting with chest pain: more particularly, to determine the presence or absence of prognostically important coronary heart disease. The exercise test should be regarded as a natural extension of the clinical examination, allowing the physician to assess the overall physiological response to exercise including the appearance of the patient during exercise, the time of onset and the development of symptoms, the haemodynamic response to exercise, and observed changes on the ECG provoked by exercise.

Indications for exercise testing include

- Assessment of objective exercise tolerance.
- Nature of symptoms limiting exercise (chest pain, fatigue, breathlessness, etc.).
- Evaluation of haemodynamic response to exercise.
- Document ST segment changes occurring with exercise or during the recovery period.
- Evaluation of exercise-induced arrhythmias.

- Document beneficial effects of surgical revascularisation, PCI or medical therapy in patients with angina.
- Quantify the beneficial effects of treatment in patients with heart failure.
- Risk stratification following acute myocardial infarction.
- Guide to rehabilitation following acute myocardial infarction.
- Risk stratification in patients with hypertrophic cardiomyopathy.
- Evaluation of functional capacity in selected patients with valvular heart disease (e.g. aortic and mitral regurgitation).
- Risk stratification of patients with ventricular ectopy in patients at rest.

Contraindications to exercise testing include
- Unstable angina.
- Very recent (<5 days) following acute myocardial infarction.
- Acute pericarditis.
- Acute myocarditis.
- Uncontrolled systemic hypertension (resting diastolic BP >100mmHg).
- Uncompensated heart failure.
- Critical aortic stenosis.
- Sustained ventricular arrhythmias at rest.
- High-grade atrioventricular block.
- Acute systemic illness, fever, anaemia, etc.

Patient preparation
Patients are advised not to smoke, eat or drink for 3h prior to the test. In most patients, cardioactive medication (e.g. β-blockers, calcium antagonists, long-acting nitrates) should be discontinued 48h before exercise testing. Patients are advised to wear comfy clothes and shoes (e.g. trainers).

Procedure
Both the bicycle ergometer and treadmill exercise testing have been used in the assessment of cardiac patients; disadvantages of the bicycle include an inability to cycle in some patients, premature muscle (quadriceps) fatigue, and the relatively low level of exercise achieved. Most of the data from cardiac patients relate to treadmill testing, using either the Bruce or modified Bruce protocol (see table below). Treadmill testing is applicable to a wide variety of patient groups including children and the elderly, and it also allows the physician rather than the patient to control the time of completion of the test, and therefore the amount of work achieved. Exercise tests should be supervised by experienced personnel (e.g. technician, nurse practitioner, physician) trained in advanced cardiopulmonary resuscitation. A resting supine and standing ECG is recorded, together with the resting blood pressure. Exercise is increased in 3min increments, with further recordings of the ECG, pulse rate and blood pressure up to and including symptom-limited peak exercise. Further recordings are made each minute during the recovery period until the ECG, heart rate and blood pressure have fallen back to pre-test levels. The exercise test laboratory should be equipped with full resuscitation equipment including a defibrillator.

Full (standard) Bruce protocol

Stage	Speed (mph)	Gradient	Duration (min)
I	1.7	10	3
II	2.5	12	3
III	3.4	14	3
IV	4.2	16	3
V	5.0	18	3
VI	5.5	20	3
VII	6.0	22	3

Modified Bruce protocol

Stage	Speed (mph)	Gradient	Duration (min)
I	1.7	0	3
II	1.7	5	3
III	1.7	10	3
IV	2.5	10	3
V	3.4	14	3
VI	4.2	16	3
VII	5.0	18	3

Reasons for terminating an exercise test
- Symptomatic (chest pain, breathlessness, exhaustion).
- Progressive fall in systemic blood pressure.
- Peripheral circulatory insufficiency (claudication).
- Sustained ventricular arrhythmia (e.g. ventricular tachycardia).
- Symptomatic heart block.
- Failure of treadmill or ECG apparatus.
- Diagnostic ST segment shift.
- Target heart rate or grade of exercise achieved.
- Extreme elevation of blood pressure (>250mmHg systolic).

Possible results
In patients with significant coronary heart disease, myocardial ischaemia is reflected in ST segment depression, defined as horizontal (planar) or downsloping ST segments D1 mV (100mV) or 1mm, 80ms after the J point (Fig. 6.4). These changes are usually most apparent in the lead with the tallest R wave, commonly V5. Upsloping ST segment depression, J point depression, changes in T wave morphology and rate-dependent aberrancy, do not reliably indicate ischaemia. Other indicators of myocardial ischaemia include ST segment elevation, 'pseudo-normalization' of inverted T waves and an increase in R wave amplitude; some patients also exhibit a flat heart rate response to exercise (chronotropic incompetence).

Interpretation
The earlier and more dramatic the ST segment shift, the more severe the coronary disease, especially if the ECG changes occur in association with symptoms (chest pain) or a fall in blood pressure. For the identification of coronary heart disease, a 'positive' test (using ST segment depression of D1 mV) has a specificity ~77% and a sensitivity of ~68% for identifying a 50% luminal obstruction of a coronary artery. Exercise testing is useful in

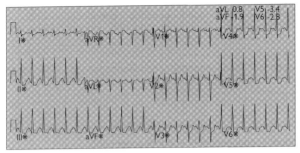

Fig. 6.4 Exercise testing: ST segment depression occurring during exercise.

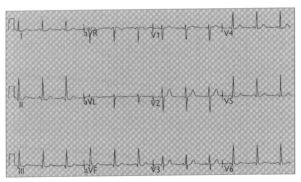

Fig. 6.5 ST segment depression at rest.

the identification of 'high-risk' coronary disease, with a specificity of ~66% and a sensitivity of ~81% for multivessel disease, and a specificity of ~53% and a sensitivity of ~86% for left main stem disease. The prognostic value of exercise testing early after acute myocardial infarction is well validated with a poor exercise performance, ST segment depression at a low workload and an abnormal blood pressure response all indicators of an adverse prognosis. Many contemporary treadmill machines offer additional parameters (e.g. ST/HR slope, ST/HR index), which may significantly increase the sensitivity of the test.

The relationship between the level of ST segment depression deemed 'significant' and the likelihood of CHD is shown in Fig. 6.5. If 2mm ST segment depression is taken as 'positive', rather than the standard 1mm, the sensitivity of the test is reduced, but the specificity is increased.

Advantages over other tests

Cheap, simple, non-invasive, reproducible and applicable to a wide population.

Ancillary tests

The sensitivity and specificity of routine treadmill exercise testing can be increased by combining exercise with myocardial scintigraphy; or, alternatively, undertaking dobutamine stress echocardiography.

Pitfalls

In patient subsets with a low incidence of coronary heart disease (e.g. routine testing in asymptomatic individuals including the normal population, as part of an 'insurance' medical, pilots, etc,), the number of 'false positive' responses become significant, thereby reducing the specificity of the test. 'False positive' tests are also more common in young women.

Causes of a 'false positive' exercise test result

- Systemic hypertension.
- Aortic stenosis.
- Cardiomyopathy.
- Valve disease (e.g. mitral valve prolapse, mitral and aortic regurgitation).
- Bundle branch block (LBBB, RBBB).
- Pre-excitation.
- Hyperventilation.
- Hypoglycaemia.
- Hypokalaemia.
- Drugs (e.g. digoxin).
- Anaemia.

Most of the post-infarct exercise test data relate to the pre-thrombolytic era; there is some doubt as to the validity of these studies in determining prognosis with contemporary treatment.

Exercise testing is safe with a major complication rate of 0.03% (including death from fatal myocardial infarction or cardiac rupture); non-fatal events occur in ~0.09% (myocardial infarction, successful resuscitation from VF), and complex arrhythmias including VT in 1.4%. Complications are more common in patients studied earlier after myocardial infarction.

OHCM p90.

1 ACC/AHA. (1997) Guidelines for exercise testing. *J Am Coll Cardiol* **30**, 260–315.

Signal-averaged electrocardiography

Clinical indications

Risk stratification of patients recovering from acute myocardial infarction in terms of likelihood of developing sustained ventricular arrhythmias.

Signal-averaged electrocardiography (SAECG)[1] has also been used to investigate the presence of inducible sustained ventricular tachycardia in patients with known coronary heart disease or cardiomyopathy and unexplained syncope.

Procedure

A resting ECG is recorded in the supine position using an ECG machine equipped with a SAECG capability. Signal averaging improves the signal to noise ratio when the signals are recurrent and the noise is random; hence muscle potentials can be removed with appropriate filtering. The SAECG is commonly used to interrogate late ventricular potentials, typically 1–25mV in amplitude, which are in continuity with, and follow, the QRS complex (Fig. 6.6); these late potentials are thought to represent delayed and fragmented ventricular activation which may be the substrate for micro re-entry leading to ventricular arrhythmias.

Possible results

Late potentials may be recorded in 0–10% of normal volunteers, 15–30% of patients early after a myocardial infarction with ventricular tachycardia, and in 50–90% of patients with a myocardial infarction complicated by ventricular tachycardia. Early use of thrombolytics may reduce the incidence of late potentials.

Interpretation

The prognostic value of the SAECG in defining risk for development of ventricular tachycardia or sudden death following myocardial infarction gives a sensitivity of ~72%, a specificity of ~75%, a positive predictive value of ~20% and a negative predictive value of ~96%.

1 ACC Expert Consensus Document. (1996) Signal-averaged electrocardiography . J Am Coll Cardiol 27, 238–249.

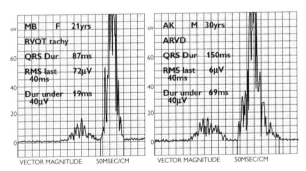

Fig. 6.6   Signal-averaged ECG.

Swan-Ganz catheterisation

Clinical indications

Although the safety of bedside right heart catheterization has recently been questioned[1], the application and indications for the technique have been confirmed by the American College of Cardiology[2].

There is general agreement that bedside right heart catheterization is warranted in the following:

- Differentiation between haemodynamic and permeability pulmonary oedema.
- Determining the contribution of impaired cardiac output in the patient with concomitant COPD.
- Differentiation between cardiogenic and non-cardiogenic shock when volume expansion has failed or is considered to be high risk.
- Determining the optimum management of patients in heart failure (e.g. volume replacement, inotropic support, intra-aortic balloon counter-pulsation.
- Guidance of management of patients with right ventricular infarction.
- Determining the optimum fluid loading in patients undergoing major surgery.
- Establishing the presence (and quantification) of left to right shunting in infarct-related ventricular septal defect.
- Confirmation of cardiac tamponade in patients in whom echocardiography is non-diagnostic.
- Confirmation of the presence of pre-capillary (primary) pulmonary hypertension.
- Detection and reversibility of pulmonary hypertension in patients undergoing assessment as potential heart transplant recipients.

In excess of 1.5 million Swan-Ganz catheters are sold annually in the USA; 30% are used in cardiac surgery, 30% in cardiac catheterisation laboratories or CCUs, 25% in high-risk surgery or trauma, and 15% in medical intensive care units.

Contraindications

- Right-sided endocarditis.
- Mechanical tricuspid or pulmonary valve prosthesis.
- Right heart tumour or thrombus visible on echocardiography.
- Swan-Ganz catheterisation cannot be recommended in the routine management of patients with:
  - Heart failure.
  - Acute myocardial infarction.
  - Patients undergoing surgery.

Procedure

- A 6F sheath is inserted into a central vein (e.g. subclavian, internal jugular, femoral) over a guide wire similar to the technique used for the insertion of a CVP line.
- Prior to insertion through the sheath, the triple lumen (Swan-Ganz) catheter is flushed with 0.9% saline and the balloon inflated to check integrity (see instructions for use). Typical catheters have one lumen for balloon inflation, and two lumens to measure pressure and obtain blood samples (one at the tip of the catheter and one 25–30cm more

proximal), together with a thermistor at the tip for measuring cardiac output. Bedside insertion of the catheter is usually performed without fluoroscopic guidance.

- The catheter is then attached to a pressure transducer, and then gently advanced through the sheath for 20cm.
- Blood is aspirated to confirm intravascular placement, and the balloon is gently inflated with 1.5mL of air.
- Pressure is monitored through the port connected to the tip, with confirmation on the monitor of the characteristic pressures in the right atrium, right ventricle, pulmonary artery (PA) and pulmonary artery capillary wedge pressure (PACWP) (Fig. 6.7).
- The catheter is advanced and secured in such a position to demonstrate the PA pressure when the balloon is deflated and the PACWP when the balloon is inflated.
- Blood samples for O_2 saturation can be withdrawn from either the proximal or distal port, and cardiac output calculated via the thermistor using the thermodilution technique.
- Contemporary systems provide an interface that displays cardiac output, cardiac index, systemic and pulmonary vascular resistance, etc.

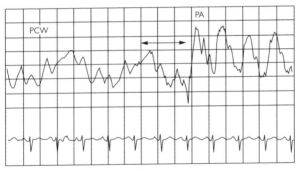

Fig. 6.7 Intracardiac pressure wave forms.

Possible results

The principle use of Swan-Ganz catheterisation is in the management of the patient with heart failure, distinguishing between cardiogenic and non-cardiogenic (hypovolaemic) shock. By measuring the indirect left atrial pressure, left ventricular pre-load can be accurately determined following which appropriate treatment can be instituted. The PACWP waveform is similar in appearance and magnitude to the left atrial pressure, with a and v waves and x and y descents. Volume expansion is appropriate if the cardiac index is low (normal range 2.5–4.2 L/min/m^2) in association with a low PACWP (normal mean 9mmHg, range 4–12mmHg). If the cardiac index is low and the PACWP is high (>15mmHg), the administration of diuretics, vasodilator therapy, often in combination with inotropic support, is appropriate. The systemic vascular resistance determines the choice of pressor agent (e.g. dobutamine, adrenaline(epinephrine), noradrenaline(norepinephrine)).

Advantages over other tests
Swan-Ganz catheterisation provides unique haemodynamic data that can be continuously measured, thereby monitoring the response to treatment or other intervention.

Ancillary tests
Echocardiography (TTE & TOE) is the most important alternative or complimentary test to Swan-Ganz catheterisation. Echocardiography can give important information on chamber dimensions, ventricular contractility, valve dysfunction and septal rupture (📖OHCM pp84–89).

Pitfalls
Complications include those related to central venous access, catheter-related infection, venous or intracardiac thrombus formation, infective endocarditis and pulmonary infarction (0–1.3%). Minor arrhythmias (ectopic activity) have been reported in 30–60% of patients; sustained ventricular arrhythmias are rare, usually occurring in patients with myocardial ischaemia or infarction. The risk of infection increases significantly if catheters are left *in situ* for more than 4 days.

1 Connors AF, Speroff T, Dawson NV et al. (1996) The effectiveness of right heart catheterization in the initial care of critically ill patients (SUPPORT Investigators). JAMA **276**, 889–897;
2 ACC Expert Consensus Document. (1998) Present use of bedside right heart catheterization in patients with cardiac disease J Am Coll Cardiol **32**, 840–864.

Tilt test

Clinical indications
Tilt testing[1] is the only effective non-invasive technique available for investigating the patient with neurally mediated syncope (vasovagal syncope, carotid sinus syndrome, micturition syncope) occurring in the absence of structural heart disease. It may also be used when structural heart disease is present, but is not thought to be the cause of the symptoms.

Patient preparation
Patients are fasted overnight, or for several hours before the procedure. Venous access should be in place and parenteral fluids (0.9% saline) administered if necessary in an attempt to reduce 'false positive' results from postural hypotension. Cardioactive drugs should be omitted for at least 24h.

Procedure
The procedure is carried out in a specially equipped laboratory which is quiet, comfortable and dimly lit. The patient rests supine on the specifically designed tilt table (with foot support) for 20–45min, during which time a resting pre-test ECG is recorded in at least three leads, together with non-invasive beat-to-beat blood pressure recordings. The patient is then tilted head-up to 70° for a period of 45min, during which time symptoms, ECG and blood pressure are monitored continuously. In the absence of a response, provocation with isoprenaline (as an intravenous infusion starting at 1mg/min, increasing to 5mg/min if necessary) may

increase sensitivity. All tilt tests should be supervised by trained personnel (e.g. technician, nurse practitioner, physician).

Possible results

A positive test is defined as syncope occurring as a result of neurally mediated hypotension and/or bradycardia. The temporal association between altered consciousness and the haemodynamic change is fundamental to a positive result. In the absence of symptoms, heart rate or blood pressure changes alone do not constitute a positive result.

Responses include a fall in heart rate or asystole (cardioinhibitory response); blood pressure fall with no associated bradycardia (vasodepressor); or both heart rate and blood pressure fall (mixed response).

Interpretation

Tilt testing is highly specific (~90%) for identifying neurally mediated syncope, but the specificity is variable (~75%); reproducibility is in the range 65 to 85%.

Ancillary tests

A typical clinical history (fainting in an emotional setting with warning in a patient <60 years old in association with other autonomic symptoms, e.g. sweating, nausea) has a low sensitivity in comparison with tilt testing. Occasionally, ambulatory ECG or blood pressure monitoring may capture spontaneous attacks of neurally mediated syncope; heart rate variability and response to carotid sinus massage may also be used in assessing this group of patients.

1 ACC Expert Consensus Document. (1996) Tilt table testing for assessing syncope. *J Am Coll Cardiol* **28**, 263–275.

Other key cardiology topics

323

The following are discussed in detail in the *Oxford Handbook of Clinical Medicine*, 5th edition:

Electrocardiography
📖OHCM p84–89.

Cardiac catheterisation
📖OHCM p92.

Coronary arteriography
📖OHCM p93.

Transthoracic echocardiography
📖OHCM pp94–95.

Gastroenterology

325

Basic liver 'function' tests

Bilirubin

Breakdown product of haem. Serum estimations are mostly based on the depth of a violet colour reaction when a diazo reagent is added to serum, with (total bilirubin) and without ('direct' or conjugated bilirubin) the presence of an accelerator, e.g. ethanol. 'Indirect' or unconjugated bilirubin is the difference between the total and direct values.

Isolated ↑ bilirubin may be

Unconjugated
- Haemolysis.
- Ineffective erythropoiesis.
- Immature bilirubin metabolism:
  - E.g. physiological jaundice in neonate.
  - Inherited defects in uptake or conjugation, e.g. Gilbert and Crigler-Najjar syndromes.

Conjugated
- Inherited defects in excretion:
  - E.g. Dubin-Johnson and Rotor syndromes.
- ↑Bilirubin also results from hepatocellular disease and post-hepatic or cholestatic disease (intrahepatic and extrahepatic), including drug toxicity.

Aminotransferases

Aspartate aminotransferase (AST) is a mitochondrial and cytoplasmic enzyme in liver, and is also present in high concentration in cardiac and skeletal muscle, kidney, pancreas and red cells. Alanine aminotransferase (ALT) is a cytoplasmic enzyme in liver, and as it is present in a higher concentration here than in other tissues it is considered more specific for liver damage. Aminotransferases are most useful in the diagnosis (e.g. early stages of viral hepatitis) and monitoring of hepatocellular disease, but can also be very high in acute cholestatic disease (especially choledocholithiasis). Marked elevations may also be seen in acute profound hypotension and acute cardiac failure. Levels may be normal in compensated cirrhosis, chronic hepatitis C and chronic incomplete biliary obstruction. As a rough guide, AST>ALT in alcoholic hepatitis and cirrhosis, infiltrative liver disease and non-biliary cirrhosis, while ALT>AST in viral and drug hepatitis, chronic hepatitis C and cholestasis. AST increases in many non-hepatobiliary diseases.

Alkaline phosphatase (ALP) is present as a number of isoenzymes and is found in the highest concentrations in bone, liver, kidney, intestine and placenta. In liver, it is located in the microvilli of canaliculi and on the sinusoidal surface of hepatocytes. ALP elevations are highest in cholestatic disease and infiltrative disease; lower levels are seen in hepatocellular disease. Isoenzymes can be distinguished, but a concomitant rise in γGT also indicates that the likely source of a high ALP is hepatobiliary. ALP rises in many diseases other than those involving the liver, e.g. bone lesions.

γ-glutamyl transpeptidase (γGT) is a membrane-bound enzyme in many tissues. It rises in almost all types of liver disease, and is highest in intrahepatic cholestasis and hepatic malignancy (primary or secondary). γGT is useful in alcohol abuse, where an isolated elevation may occur (presumably as a result of enzyme induction) even in the absence of significant liver disease. Levels return to normal within 1 month of abstinence. However, sensitivity is limited (one-third of alcoholics may have normal γGT), and there is poor correlation between alcohol intake and serum level.

Albumin can be a sensitive marker of hepatic functional capacity in chronic disease, but it has a long half-life (~20 days) and many other conditions are associated with low levels.

Other common liver biochemical tests

Globulins

α₁-globulins tend to be ↓ in chronic hepatocellular disease. Most are α₁-antitrypsin and ↓↓ or absent levels suggest AAT deficiency. α₂- and β-globulins include lipoproteins and ↑ in cholestatic disease; they may help in distinguishing biliary and non-biliary cirrhosis. Polyclonal ↑ γ-globulin is common in chronic liver disease (especially autoimmune hepatitis).

Immunoglobulins: IgG is ↑ in viral hepatitis, and ↑↑ in chronic hepatitis and cirrhosis. IgM is ↑↑ in primary biliary cirrhosis, and ↑ in viral hepatitis and non-biliary cirrhosis. IgA is ↑↑ in alcoholic cirrhosis, and this results in 'bridging' or 'fusion' of the β and γ bands on an electrophoretic strip.

Caeruloplasmin is an α₂-globulin. It is the main copper-containing plasma protein and has oxidase activity. It is also an acute phase protein. Serum caeruloplasmin is an important diagnostic test in Wilson's disease (hepatolenticular degeneration): ↓ in 95% homozygotes and 10% heterozygotes. Related biochemical diagnostic tests are serum copper (↓ total, ↑ free fraction) and ↑ 24h urine copper. ↓ caeruloplasmin also occurs in severe non-Wilson's hepatic failure, severe malnutrition, protein-losing enteropathy and nephrotic syndrome. ↑ levels are found in pregnancy, oestrogen therapy, active non-Wilson's liver disease, biliary obstruction, some inflammatory and malignant disorders.

α₁-antitrypsin (AAT) is the main α₁-globulin. It is a serine proteinase inhibitor (especially of elastase), and is also an acute phase protein. ↓ levels result from a number of gene mutations by several mechanisms, but liver damage only occurs in those phenotypes associated with accumulation of AAT in hepatocytes—classically Pi (proteinase inhibitor) Z, but also Pi M_malton and Pi M_duarte. ↑ levels are seen in pregnancy, oestrogen therapy, inflammatory disorders.

α-fetoprotein—📖OHCM pp496, 706.

Urinary bilirubin: bilirubinuria is normally absent and is also absent in unconjugated ↑ bilirubin; its presence suggests cholestasis or liver disease, but there is a significant false −ve rate. In acute viral hepatitis, bilirubin may appear in the urine before the onset of jaundice. Dipsticks impregnated with a diazo reagent allow rough and ready quantification.

Urinary urobilinogens are a product of the enterohepatic circulation; give a purple colour with Ehrlich's aldehyde reagent (dipsticks containing this reagent are available); and may be absent in complete biliary obstruction. This test has been superseded by other serum tests and imaging.

Tumour markers

α-fetoprotein (αFP)
A major plasma protein in the fetus, αFP is present in very low levels in the normal non-pregnant adult. ↑ and ↑↑ levels occur in >90% of hepato-cellular carcinoma (HCC). ↑ levels also occur in other liver diseases, e.g. cirrhosis (~15%), HBsAg −ve chronic hepatitis B, regeneration following acute viral hepatitis, hepatic metastases, and in pregnancy (marked eleva-tions may be seen in trisomy 21 and neural tube defects), choriocarcinoma and gonadal teratoma. αFP is useful in diagnosis and monitoring of response to treatment of HCC, and in monitoring patients with chronic hepatitis B or cirrhosis for development of HCC.

Carcinoembryonic antigen (CEA)
CEA is high in ~60% of colorectal carcinoma, especially in advanced disease (80–100% if metastasised to liver). It may also be high in bronchial carcinoma, breast carcinoma and a variety of non-malignant conditions including inflammatory bowel disease, liver disease, pancreatitis, and in some heavy smokers. It is insufficiently sensitive or specific for screening for colorectal cancer, and has no diagnostic value. Levels tend to correlate poorly with tumour bulk, which limits usefulness in monitoring, although a rising level after a potentially curative procedure suggests recurrence.

Carbohydrate antigen (CA) 19-9
CA19-9 may be useful in monitoring effects of treatment in pancreatic car-cinoma, and possibly colorectal and gastric carcinomas.

Faecal occult blood

Indications
Suspected occult gastrointestinal haemorrhage (including potential screening test for colorectal carcinoma).

Procedure
The most common method is a simple and inexpensive qualitative chem-ical test using guaiac-impregnated paper. Haem (in faecal blood) has pseudoperoxidase activity and catalyses the release of a free oxygen radical from hydrogen peroxide (in the developing solution), resulting in the oxidation of phenolic chromogens (in guaiac) to quinones, and the production of a blue colour. Faecal samples are collected from several (e.g. three, consecutive) bowel actions, or following rectal examination.

Precautions
Avoid sample collection during menstruation, active haemorrhoids, anal fissures, etc.

Results
In trials of faecal occult blood screening for colorectal carcinoma, the sensitivity of tests for detecting cancer presenting within 2 years was 37–79%, and the specificity was as low as 87%. More sensitive but less specific kits are now available (e.g. Haemoccult Sensa®, Haema-screen stat®).

False positives
- Diet containing animal haemoglobin or vegetable peroxidase (tests may recommend exclusion of red meat and certain uncooked fruits and vegetables for 3 days before and during collection period).
- Aspirin and NSAIDs; use of rectal drugs (*Note:* iron therapy should not affect guaiac-based tests).

False negatives
- GI lesions, including carcinoma, may bleed intermittently or not at all.
- Insensitive for blood loss from upper GI tract, unless considerable (haem is metabolised in the small bowel).
- High dose vitamin C intake (reducing agent).

Other methods of detecting faecal occult blood

Qualitative immunochemical tests (e.g. HemeSelect®) are specific for human haemoglobin, thus minimizing dietary false +ves, but nevertheless have a significant false +ve rate as they tend to react to 'physiological' quantities of faecal blood. They are also more expensive and more complicated.

Quantitative tests include ^{51}Cr-labelled red cells and radioassay of faecal samples. The upper limit of normal is ~2mg Hb/g faeces.

Faecal osmotic gap

Indication
Unexplained chronic diarrhoea (not commonly used).

Principle
Diarrhoea may be divided pathophysiologically into *secretory* ('pure' examples: stimulant laxative abuse; some GI infections, e.g. *E. coli*, cholera; hormonal causes, e.g. VIPoma, carcinoid syndrome) and *osmotic* ('pure' examples: osmotic laxative abuse, e.g. magnesium, lactulose; carbohydrate maldigestion/absorption, e.g. lactose intolerance). Diarrhoea associated with most GI diseases often results from a combination of both mechanisms. Faecal osmotic gap (FOG) is ↓ in secretory diarrhoea and ↑ in osmotic diarrhoea.

Procedure

Faecal water is prepared from a stool sample by filtration or centrifugation.

$$\textbf{FOG} = 290 - 2 \times (\text{faecal}\,[Na^+] + \text{faecal}\,[K^+])$$
where 290 is the assumed plasma osmolality

FOG*	Interpretation	Examples of further tests
<0	Secretory diarrhoea, excludes osmotic diarrhoea	Laxative screen Gut hormone screen
0–50	Excludes osmotic diarrhoea, hormonal causes	Laxative screen
50–100	Excludes osmotic diarrhoea, hormonal causes, stimulant laxative abuse	
>100	Possible osmotic diarrhoea, excludes secretory diarrhoea	Faecal water magnesium Lactose intolerance tests

* in mOsmol/kg.

Tests for laxative abuse

Thin layer chromatography (TLC)

TLC of a random urine sample or loose faeces sample can detect anthraquinone (sennosides, danthron, aloin) and diphenylmethane (phenolphthalein, bisacodyl) laxatives or their metabolites.

Phenolphthalein can also be detected by *alkalinisation of urine or faecal water* with sodium hydroxide (production of red colour), but false −ve rate is high.

If faecal osmotic gap >100mOsmol/kg, measure faecal water magnesium (>30mmol/L suggests magnesium abuse). Faecal water sulphate and phosphate may also be measured.

Diagnostic paracentesis

Indication
Ascites.

Procedure
20–50mL of ascitic fluid is aseptically aspirated through a needle inserted preferentially into the left lower quadrant of the abdomen below the border of shifting dullness. Local anaesthetic may be used. Ultrasound guidance may help in difficult cases. Complications (e.g. bowel perforation, haemorrhage, infection) are rare.

Typical ascitic fluid characteristics in a variety of conditions

	WBC (mm³)	Protein (g/L)	Other characteristics
Portal hypertension (e.g. cirrhosis)	<500, predom mono	<25	albumin gradient >11g/L
Cardiogenic ascites (right heart failure; constrictive pericarditis)	<500, predom mono	>25	albumin gradient <11g/L
Peritoneal carcinomatosis	variable, predom mono	>25	↑LDH; ↑↑CEA; cytology positive
Hepatocellular carcinoma	<500, predom mono	<25 (usually)	cytology negative
Pancreatic ascites (acute pancreatitis)	<500, predom mono	>25	↑↑amylase, lipase
Tuberculous peritonitis	>500, predom mono	>30	↑LDH; AAFB on culture
Spontaneous bacterial peritonitis	>250 poly or >500 predom poly	<25	↑LDH; usually 1 organism on culture; →glucose
Secondary bacterial peritonitis (post-paracentesis; any intra-abdominal source of infection)	>1000 poly (usually)	>25	↑LDH; usually >1 organism on culture; ↓glucose

predom, predominantly; mono, mononuclear leucocytes; poly, polymorphonuclear leucocytes (neutrophils); LDH, lactate dehydrogenase; CEA, carcinoembryonic antigen; AAFB, acid/alcohol fast bacilli.

331

Routine tests on ascitic fluid include

- **Appearance.** *Straw-coloured*; *bloody* (malignancy, abdominal trauma including recent surgery or invasive procedures such as paracentesis or liver biopsy, or catastrophe, 'bloody tap'); *milky* (chylous ascites—confirm if fat floats on standing and high triglyceride content: malignant or inflammatory lymphatic duct obstruction, trauma, may be seen in advanced cirrhosis or nephrotic syndrome). *Turbid* fluid may indicate infection.
- **Cell count.**
- **Gram stain** and **bacterial culture.** Yield is markedly improved if fluid is inoculated into blood culture bottles at bedside.
- **Ziehl-Neelsen** or **auramine stain**, and **acid/alcohol-fast bacilli culture.**
- **Protein** <25g/L suggests 'transudate' (e.g. portal hypertension, ↓albumin), >25g/L suggests 'exudate' (e.g. malignancy, pancreatitis, tuberculosis), but this is an unreliable method of classification. Hepatic venous occlusion (Budd-Chiari syndrome) is usually associated with a ↑↑ protein.
- **Albumin.** Serum-ascites albumin gradient (serum albumin *minus* ascites albumin) >11g/L suggests 'transudate'.
- **Amylase.**
- **Cytology.**

Percutaneous 'blind' liver biopsy[1]

Do benefits of knowing histology (?alters treatment, ?clarifies prognosis) outweigh risks to patient?

Indications
- Acute hepatitis including ?drug-related (biopsy not usually needed in typical acute viral hepatitis).
- Chronic liver disease for diagnosis and monitoring.
- Alcoholic liver disease.
- Primary biliary cirrhosis and primary sclerosing cholangitis (especially for more advanced disease).
- Focal liver lesion (avoid if resection considered).
- Unexplained persistently abnormal LFT (isolated ↑γGT is not associated with major liver disease and is *not* an indication).
- Unexplained hepatomegaly.
- Liver transplantation, e.g. routine monitoring, rejection, recurrent disease, CMV infection.
- Pyrexia of unknown origin.
- Infections, e.g. tuberculosis.
- Storage disorders.

Contraindications
- Uncooperative patient—consider sedation or general anaesthesia.
- Extrahepatic cholestasis (risk of biliary peritonitis)—transvenous biopsy may be performed if doubt about diagnosis and benefits outweigh risks.
- Bacterial cholangitis (risk of peritonitis).

- Coagulopathy—percutaneous biopsy considered safe if platelets $\geq 60 \times 10^9/L$ and PT <4s prolonged (or INR <1.5). Outside these limits, consider platelet transfusion, vitamin K IV and FFP, as appropriate, or other methods of biopsy (transvenous, plugged or laparoscopic). Biopsy safe in haemophilics if factor deficiency corrected pre- and for 24h post-biopsy.
- Tense ascites (high probability of failure, risk of uncontrollable haemorrhage into ascites)—consider total paracentesis, or image-guided (no increase in complication rate in presence of ascites), transvenous or laparoscopic biopsy.
- Hydatid cysts (risk of abdominal dissemination, risk of anaphylaxis)—USS-guided aspiration with small needle under albendazole cover appears safe.
- Amyloidosis (▶▶risk of haemorrhage).

Patient preparation
- Liver imaging ≤1 month (identifies abnormal anatomy and focal lesions, and defines borders in difficult cases, e.g. obesity, emphysema, cirrhosis).
- FBC, coagulation profile, G&S (preferably ≤24h; ≤1 week if stable liver disease); consider bleeding time (e.g. aspirin/NSAIDs, uraemia, paraproteinaemia).
- Informed consent.
- Prophylactic antibiotics for valvular heart disease or risk of septicaemia (e.g. biliary sepsis).
- Consider sedation (e.g. midazolam, diazepam), atropine.

Procedure
1. The liver borders of the supine patient are defined by percussion or ultrasound.
2. Local anaesthetic is infiltrated in the mid-axillary line through the 8th or 9th intercostal space down to the liver capsule (intercostal or transthoracic approach).
3. The site of entry may be subcostal in hepatomegaly.
4. A small incision is made, and the biopsy needle is inserted and advanced (slightly superoposteriorly to avoid the gallbladder) while the patient holds his/her breath in expiration.
5. There are two main types of biopsy needle: cutting (e.g. Tru-cut®) and suction (Menghini); the latter is cheaper, smaller and involves less time within the liver, with a lower complication rate but has a lower yield.
6. For histology, one sample is usually sufficient, but in situations where the probability of sampling error is high, e.g. macronodular cirrhosis, two samples may be taken without significantly increasing complications.
7. Post-biopsy, the patient lies on his/her right side or supine, and observations typically involve monitoring vital signs every 15min for 2h, then every 30min for 2h, and then hourly for 2h.
8. If there are no problems at the end of this 6h period (most complications occur in the first 3h), the patient may be discharged, but should have a responsible person to stay on the first night and should be able to return to hospital within 30min.

9. Low-risk patients may thus be suitable for 'day case' biopsy.

Complications

Mortality (0.01–0.1%)
- Intraperitoneal haemorrhage (main cause; cirrhosis and malignancy increase risk).
- Gallbladder puncture with biliary peritonitis.

Morbidity
- Pain 30%.
- Significant haemorrhage (↓Hb >2.0g/dL) 0.5%; intrahepatic/subcapsular haematoma (23%) is often subclinical.
- Haemobilia (biliary pain, jaundice, melaena) 0.05%.
- Puncture of other viscera (lung, colon, kidney, gallbladder) 0.01–0.1%; intervention is rarely required.
- Others: sepsis, anaesthetic reaction, biopsy needle breakage, intrahepatic arteriovenous fistula, seeding of tumour down biopsy track.

Ancillary tests
Special stains/dry weight estimations, e.g. for copper or iron overload.

Other methods of liver biopsy

Percutaneous guided liver biopsy
Undertaken during real time imaging of the liver by USS (or CT, MNR). It is used in focal disease but its use in diffuse disease is more debatable: it should enable sampling of thicker parenchyma and result in fewer complications.

Percutaneous plugged liver biopsy
Modification of a conventional biopsy using a Tru-cut® needle, in which the obturator containing the sample is removed, and gelatin or gel foam is injected down the sheath as it is withdrawn. It is a safer alternative in patients with significant coagulopathy where transjugular biopsy is unavailable.

Transvenous (transjugular) liver biopsy
A catheter introduced into the right internal jugular vein using the Seldinger technique is guided under fluoroscopic control and cardiac monitoring through the right atrium and inferior vena cava into the hepatic veins. The biopsy needle is then inserted into the catheter and, with the patient holding his/her breath, rapidly advanced 1–2cm beyond the tip into the liver. Tissue is retained by suction. Although usually performed via the transjugular route, it may be done via a *transfemoral* approach. Transvenous biopsy is remarkably safe.

Laparoscopic liver biopsy
Liver lesions found may be found incidentally at laparoscopy, but it is also used in patients with significant coagulopathy where transjugular biopsy is unavailable, and in patients with the combination of a focal liver lesion and deranged coagulation.

Grant A, Neuberger J. (1999) Guidelines on the use of liver biopsy in clinical practice. *Gut* **45**, (suppl IV).

Carbohydrate maldigestion & absorption tests

D-xylose absorption test
No longer routinely used.

Indication
?Small bowel malabsorption.

Principle
D-xylose is a sugar that is normally almost completely absorbed in the proximal small bowel, minimally metabolised by either the normal microflora of the small bowel of man, and excreted unaltered in urine.

Procedure
An oral dose of D-xylose is given and urine is collected for 5h.

Results/Interpretation
Excretion of <22% of 5g dose (or <17% of 25g dose) is abnormal. The test is sensitive for small bowel mucosal disease (e.g. coeliac disease) and rarely gives false +ves in pancreatic disease (false +ves may however occur as result of delayed gastric emptying, poor renal function or poor urine output).

Disaccharidase (lactase) deficiency test

Lactose breath H_2 test
Lactose maldigestion occurs as a result of lactase deficiency, which may be primary (congenital or acquired) or secondary to a structurally abnormal small bowel with loss of brush border membrane disaccharidases (e.g. gastroenteritis, coeliac disease, inflammatory bowel disease). It may also occur as a result of a short gut, enterocolic fistula or Billroth II anastomosis. *Note*: Most of the world's adults (especially non-whites) are lactose deficient but not intolerant.

335

Procedure
Test substrate: 50g lactose ($\cong$ 2pints of milk; lower, more physiological, doses have been suggested). Breath H_2 is measured and the patient is also monitored for the symptoms of lactose intolerance (bloating and distension, pain, borborygmi, flatulence, diarrhoea).

Advantages
- Inexpensive.
- Sensitive (≥90%).
- Specificity may be ≥90%, especially if cut-off is increased from 20 to 30PPM.

Lactose tolerance test
Lactose (2mg/kg up to max. 50g) is given orally to fasted patient. Plasma glucose is measured at baseline and at 30min intervals for 2h, and the patient is monitored for provocation of symptoms. Failure of plasma glucose to rise by ≥1.1mmol/L indicates a positive test, especially if accom-

panied by symptoms (repeat test with glucose/galactose to exclude monosaccharide malabsorption). Sensitivity and specificity are lower than breath H_2 test. Test may be used with other disaccharides, e.g. sucrose.

Small bowel disaccharidase activity

Activity of lactase (and that of other disaccharidases, e.g. sucrose, maltose) may be quantified directly in small bowel biopsy specimens. Test is limited by considerable individual variation, and hypolactasia does not necessarily mean lactose intolerance.

Breath hydrogen tests

Principle

H_2 is normally derived exclusively from the metabolism of unabsorbed carbohydrates by colonic bacteria and some yeasts (the normal bacterial density of the small bowel does not produce significant amounts of H_2). ~20% is absorbed across the mucosa and excreted in expired air.

Procedure

A carbohydrate substrate is administered orally. End-expiratory (alveolar) air is sampled basally and at intervals (e.g. 20–30min) for up to 3h, and analysed using a H_2 sensor.

Results/Interpretation

Basal breath H_2 is usually ≤5ppm. A rise of ≥20ppm above basal is regarded as a positive test. High basal concentrations may prohibit the detection of significant H_2 production from the test substrate, and may occur as a result of fermentation of unabsorbed carbohydrate consumed the previous evening, poor oral hygiene, malabsorption, small bowel bacterial overgrowth and pneumatosis cystoides intestinalis.

Precautions
- 12h fast.
- Careful oral hygiene, including no smoking.

Indications
- Carbohydrate malabsorption (lactose).
- Small bowel bacterial overgrowth (glucose, lactulose).
- Measurement of mouth-to-caecum transit time (lactulose).

Fat maldigestion/absorption tests

Faecal fat

Procedure

Faeces are collected for several days: at least 3 days, preferably 5 days (to account for considerable variation in day to day faecal output). Faecal mass/volume and fat are quantified. Dietary fat intake should be known or standardised, e.g. 70–100g/day (individual fat intake varies enormously). Faecal markers (isotopic or radio-opaque) improve accuracy and allow reduction in collection period.

Results/Interpretation

Faecal fat of >6g/day (>18mmol/day) or dietary fat absorption of <93% indicates fat maldigestion (parenchymal liver disease, biliary obstruction, excess gastric acid, pancreatic disease, bile acid deconjugation by small bowel bacterial overgrowth, bile acid malabsorption due to terminal ileal disease/resection or cholestyramine) or fat malabsorption (small bowel mucosal disease, abetalipoproteinaemia, lymphatic obstruction).

Advantages
● Direct.
● Quantitative.
● Simple.

Disadvantages
● Unpleasant for all concerned.
● Needs to be conducted rigorously.
● Cannot distinguish maldigestion and malabsorption.
● Insensitive for mild pancreatic disease.

$^{14}CO_2$ fat breath tests

Principle
Triglycerides are hydrolysed by pancreatic lipase into monoglycerides and fatty acids. These are then incorporated into mixed micelles with bile constituents, absorbed, metabolised, and ultimately excreted as CO_2.

Procedure
A ^{14}C-labelled triglyceride (e.g. [^{14}C]triolein) is ingested and breath $^{14}CO_2$ is measured at intervals. With intact fat digestion and absorption, there is a peak in breath radioactivity at 5–7h. This is repeated 2 weeks later with a ^{14}C-labelled free fatty acid (e.g. [^{14}C]oleic acid) to differentiate between maldigestion and malabsorption.

Advantages
● Can distinguish maldigestion and malabsorption.
● Good correlation with faecal fat test.

Disadvantages
● Indirect.
● Qualitative.
● Involves radioisotope.
● Insensitive for mild pancreatic disease.

Faecal microscopy
Faecal microscopy (for fatty acid crystals, neutral fat, soaps) is poorly validated and of dubious value.

Small bowel bacterial overgrowth tests: 1

Glucose breath H_2 test

Principle
Glucose is normally completely absorbed in the proximal small bowel, and any rise in breath H_2 is indicative of bacterial overgrowth.

Procedure
Test substrate: 50–75g glucose.

Results/Interpretation
Variable sensitivity (65–90%) and specificity (75–100%). False −ves presumably result from variations in the particular microflora present, with differing capacities for the metabolism of glucose (and other substrates, e.g. lactulose, glycocholic acid and xylose, in other tests). False +ves may occur in glucose malabsorption.

Lactulose breath H_2 test

Test substrate: 10–15g lactulose, a non-absorbed disaccharide. In bacterial overgrowth, fermentation occurs not only in the colon but also in the small bowel, resulting in an early (e.g. 40min) peak in breath H_2. The test may has also been used to measure oro-caecal transit time (reference range: 30–140min).

[^{14}C]glycocholate breath $^{14}CO_2$ test

A conjugated bile acid with the amino acid portion labelled ([^{14}C]glycine in glycocholate) is administered orally. Breath $^{14}CO_2$ is measured discontinuously. Normally very little deconjugation occurs and the bile acid is absorbed intact in the terminal ileum. In small bowel bacterial overgrowth, deconjugation by anaerobic bacteria occurs, liberating [^{14}C]glycine which is absorbed and rapidly metabolised in the liver to $^{14}CO_2$, which is then excreted and detected in the breath. Sensitivity is similar to the glucose breath H_2 test, and the latter does not involve radioactivity. In terminal ileal disease/resection, glycocholate reaches the colon where it is deconjugated by colonic bacteria. This false +ve result may be recognized by a delayed breath radioactivity peak and the presence of faecal radioactivity.

[^{14}C]D-xylose breath $^{14}CO_2$ test

In bacterial overgrowth, a significant amount of a 1g oral dose of [^{14}C]D-xylose is metabolised by aerobic Gram −ve bacteria to $^{14}CO_2$. This is absorbed and excreted in breath. Again, this has no advantage over the glucose breath H_2 test, and involves the use of a radioisotope.

Small bowel bacterial overgrowth tests: 2

Duodenal/jejunal juice aspiration

Procedure
Duodenal contents can be aspirated at gastroscopy (or jejunal contents at enteroscopy), but this may miss bacterial overgrowth confined to the distal small bowel. Jejunal and even ileal intubation, under fluoroscopic control, may be required. Aspirated juice is cultured (anaerobic and aerobic) and may be assayed for deconjugated bile acids or short-chain fatty acids. Normal total bacterial count: <10^4–10^5 cfu/mL in duodenum and jejunum, <10^5–10^9 cfu/mL in ileum (cfu: colony-forming units).

Advantages
• 'Gold standard' (but not without problems).

- Direct.
- High specificity, but sensitivity <60% (missed distal disease).

Disadvantages
- Invasive.

Urinary indican
This test involves measurement of urinary excretion of indoxylsulphate (indican), a bacterial metabolic product of dietary tryptophan. An alternative is phenols from dietary tyrosine. These tests cannot distinguish bacterial overgrowth from other causes of malabsorption.

Pancreatic exocrine function tests: 1

Pancreatic function tests are indicated when there is a clinical suspicion of chronic pancreatic disease but imaging (AXR, USS, CT, ERCP) is normal or equivocal. Currently no test is able to detect the earliest stages of pancreatic insufficiency. Invasive ('tube') tests have largely been superseded by simpler, safer, non-invasive ('tubeless') tests.

Secretin and related tests

Principle
Maximal secretion of pancreatic juice and output of bicarbonate and enzymes is related to the functional mass of pancreas.

Procedure
A tube is passed into the duodenum (beyond the ampulla of Vater) of the fasted patient under fluoroscopic control. Suction is applied until the duodenal content is clear. Secretin is administered IV and is usually followed by cholecystokinin-pancreozymin, CCK-PZ (or its cheaper amphibian analogue, cerulein). Bile may also be administered by tube into the duodenum. Duodenal juice is collected.

Stimulation by secretin alone allows measurement of volume and bicarbonate secretion (enzyme secretion is inconsistent), but co-stimulation with PZ also allows assay of pancreatic enzymes (e.g. trypsin). Bile administration prevents false +ve results caused by inadequate gallbladder contraction.

Results
Secretin-PZ test can have a sensitivity of >90%, and specificity of ≤90%.

Advantages
- 'Gold standard'.
- Direct assessment of pancreatic function.

Disadvantages
- Invasive.
- Time-consuming, labour-intensive.
- Expensive.

339

Lundh test

Procedure

Similar to secretin test except that stimulus is the Lundh test meal (15g protein, 40g glucose, 18g fat, 300mL water). Activity of one or more enzymes (e.g. trypsin, lipase) in duodenal juice is assayed.

Advantages
- Physiological stimulus with integrated response.
- Easier and cheaper than secretin-PZ.

Disadvantages
- Less sensitive and less specific (false +ves may occur in small bowel mucosal disease) than secretin-PZ test.

Pancreatic exocrine function tests: 2

BT-PABA test

Principle

N-benzoyl-l-tyrosyl-p-aminobenzoic acid (bentiromide, BT-PABA, BTP) is a synthetic tripeptide that is specifically hydrolysed by pancreatic chymotrypsin in duodenum to yield p-aminobenzoic acid (PABA). PABA is absorbed and partly conjugated in the liver to various arylamines, which are excreted by the kidneys.

The percentage recovery of PABA metabolites in the urine following oral bentiromide is an indirect measure of chymotrypsin activity and thus pancreatic function. Recovery is also affected by individual variations in rate of gastric emptying, small bowel absorption, hepatic conjugation and renal excretion, and to control for these, PABA recovery is compared with recovery of radiolabelled free PABA (or unlabelled p-aminosalicylic acid) administered at the same time (or unlabelled free PABA administered on a separate day).

Patient preparation

For 2–3 days beforehand: no pancreatic enzyme supplements; avoid certain drugs (e.g. paracetamol, thiazides, sulphonamides, benzodiazepines), and certain fruits and vegetables (e.g. apples, cranberries, prunes, beetroot) that can interfere with the test.

Procedure

Patient is fasted from the night before and during the test, but a high water intake is encouraged to ensure adequate urine output. Bentiromide tablets (in a standard meal, e.g. Lundh, to stimulate pancreatic secretion) and free [^{14}C]PABA (in a drink) are ingested. Urine is collected for 6h.

Results/Interpretation

Excretion index (or T/K ratio) is calculated as ratio of PABA recovery ('Test') to free [^{14}C]PABA recovery ('Kontrol'). >0.75 is normal, 0.60–0.75 is equivocal (repeat or consider 'tube' test), <0.60 is abnormal. Sensitivity is ~75% (moderate and severe insufficiency), specificity is ~90%.

Advantages
- Non-invasive.
- Relatively simple.

Disadvantages
- Indirect.
- May involve radioisotope.

Pancreatic exocrine function tests: 3

Pancreolauryl test

Principle
This is similar to PABA test. Fluorescein dilaurate (pancreolauryl) is an ester that is specifically hydrolysed by pancreatic arylesterases, in the presence of bile acids, to release fluorescein, which is then absorbed, conjugated and excreted in urine.

Patient preparation
Patient need not fast, but must avoid pancreatic enzyme supplements, vitamin B and some other drugs for 2 days beforehand.

Procedure
Pancreolauryl capsules ('Test') are ingested in the middle of a standard breakfast (50g white bread, 20g butter, one cup of liquid). A high liquid intake is maintained. Urine is collected for 10h, and fluorescein recovery is measured spectrophotometrically. The test is repeated one or more days later with capsules of free fluorescein ('Kontrol').

Results/Interpretation
T/K ratio of >0.30 is normal, 0.20–0.30 is equivocal (repeat or consider 'tube' test), and <0.20 is abnormal. Sensitivity and specificity are similar to PABA test, but false +ves may also occur in the presence of hepatobiliary disease as bile acids are necessary for pancreolauryl digestion, and bacterial hydrolysis may result in a false –ve in overgrowth. A disadvantage is that it is a two stage test.

Faecal enzymes

Elastase-1 (E1) is a proteinase secreted by pancreatic acinar cells. It remains largely undegraded during gut transit.

Procedure
E1 concentration in a random faecal sample is measured using an immunoassay.

Results/Interpretation
Normal >200µg E1/g faeces; moderate insufficiency 100–200µg/g; severe insufficiency <100µg/g. Good sensitivity. High specificity. Concentration may be lowered in voluminous, watery faeces (false +ve).

Advantages
- Non-invasive.
- Simple.
- Unaffected by pancreatic supplements.

Disadvantages
- Indirect.
- Faecal test.
- Expensive.

Chymotrypsin is another such stable pancreatic proteinase. Its activity in faeces is measured by spectrophotometric assay of 4-nitroaniline released from a synthetic pentapeptide. It is cheaper than faecal E1, but has lower sensitivity and cannot be used if on pancreatic enzyme supplements. It is a common screening test in children with cystic fibrosis.

Fat maldigestion tests
📖p336

Invasive *Helicobacter pylori* tests

Indications
Assessment of *H. pylori* infection and antibiotic sensitivity. Invasive tests are employed when endoscopy is to be performed on a patient to establish the underlying disease, e.g. peptic ulcer.

Patient preparation
For gastroscopy (📖p346).

Procedure
Biopsies taken from within 2cm of the pylorus and also from the body of the stomach if patient on proton pump inhibitor treatment. In general two of the following tests are performed.

Rapid urease or CLO test
A biopsy sample is placed in urea solution containing phenyl red pH indicator changing colour from straw to purple when *H. pylori* infection is present. It takes 24h before result can be said to be definitely −ve, but advantage is that a +ve result is often available within an hour before the patient leaves the endoscopy unit.

Histology
Two samples fixed in formalin and stained with haematoxylin and eosin or modified Giemsa stain. Characteristic spiral/curved shaped Gram negative organisms seen in mucus layer. Useful where histological information of mucosa also desired.

Culture
In micro-aerophilic conditions using chocolate agar. Can take several days for *H. pylori* to grow in tiny opalescent colonies. Transport of biopsy to culture plate within 30min is desirable. Useful where bacterial sensitivity to antibiotics is required in treatment of resistant strains.

Pitfalls
False −ve results occur in patients who recently (within 2 weeks) have been taking antibiotic or proton pump inhibitor treatment.

Non-invasive *H. pylori* tests

Serology

Indications
Initial diagnosis of *H. pylori* infection.

Patient preparation
10mL venous serum sample.

Procedure
This is an enzyme-linked immunosorbent assay (ELISA) measuring IgG to *H. pylori* antigens. Several kits are available which allow 40 patient samples to be assessed at the same time with the results being available in 3h.

Possible results/Interpretation
See table (p344) for test performance. Local validation recommended due to regional variation of cut-off point.

False positives occur where patients have had successful *H. pylori* eradication therapy within the last 2 years and also due to cross-reactivity with antibodies to other organisms.

False negatives occur in elderly and immunocompromised patients.

Pitfalls
Avoid use in assessing eradication of *H. pylori*.

Ancillary tests

Rapid whole blood test and saliva test: useful in epidemiological studies and in children although performance is poorer.

Faecal antigen test: measures *H. pylori* antigens in stool but its role and value is under trial.

Urea breath test

Indications
• Initial diagnosis of infection.
• Assessment of eradication of *H. pylori*.

$$(2NH_2)\text{-}CO + 2H_2O + H^+ \leftrightarrows 2NH_4^+ + HCO_3^- \leftrightarrows 2NH_3 + H_2O + CO_2 + H^+$$

rapid urease test   urea breath test

Helicobacter pylori urease catalyses the hydrolysis of urea to produce ammonium ions and carbon dioxide.

343

Patient preparation and procedure
Two tests are available ^{13}C (stable isotope) and ^{14}C (unstable isotope).
^{13}C test (most commonly used):
- Citrus drink given to delay gastric emptying followed by breath sample collection into a test tube.
- Carbon-labelled urea ingested with repeat breath sample half an hour afterwards. The increase in labelled carbon dioxide exhaled is measured and indicates *H. pylori* infection.
- Carbon dioxide measurements are performed by mass spectrometer, but commercial laboratories will analyse breath samples sent by post.

Possible results/Interpretation
+ve test indicates *active* infection.

Pitfall
Assessment of eradication can only be carried out at least 1 month after eradication therapy by definition. False −ve results occur in patients recently on antibiotics or proton pump inhibitor treatment within 2 weeks and also in patients with previous gastric surgery.

Test	Invasiveness	Sensitivity (%)	Specificity (%)	Use
Culture	Invasive	65	100	Antibiotic sensitivity
Histology	Invasive	97	100	Initial & post eradication
CLO/urease	Invasive	91	100	Initial & post eradication
Urea breath	Non-invasive	100	100	Initial & post eradication
Serology	Non-invasive	95	70	Initial

Gastrointestinal endoscopy check-list

Long before procedure
- General fitness particularly cardiorespiratory state.
- Check pacemaker function.
- Can patient adopt position during endoscopy?
- Can patient open mouth sufficiently to allow insertion of mouth guard?
- Informed consent.
- Check relevant blood test are satisfactory:
  - E.g. INR <1.2 and platelets >80×10^9/L and correct accordingly.
- Continue essential medication.

Just before procedure
- Check pulse and BP.
- Site IV cannula in right hand.

Reilly TG *et al.* (1997) Comparison of serum, salivary, and rapid whole blood diagnostic tests for *Helicobacter pylori* and their validation against endoscopy based tests. Gut **40**, 454–488.

- Give prophylactic antibiotics for heart valve disease valves (gentamicin 80mg and ampicillin 1g IV or vancomycin if allergic).
- Remove spectacles and dentures and metallic objects, e.g. earrings.

During procedure
- LA throat spray or intravenous benzodiazepine + pethidine + buscopan.
- Monitor with pulse oximetry, pulse and BP.
- Keep airway clear, e.g. suction.

After procedure
- Keep airway clear if reduced conscious level, e.g. position in semi-prone position.
- If necessary use flumazenil/naloxone to reverse sedation.
- Monitor pulse and blood pressure.
- If perforation suspected obtain erect CXR.
- Antibiotics may be required post-ERCP.
- Check function of pacemaker.
- If patient has had sedative advise not to drive/operate machinery/sign legal document for 24h.

Special preparation

Patients on warfarin should be admitted and converted to IV heparin before procedure, e.g. mechanical heart valves. Some patients at reduced risk of thrombosis may be allowed to stop warfarin 3 days before procedure without the need to convert to heparin.

Diabetic patients should be first on the procedure list and may require admission and special preparation:
- Diet controlled only—no special preparation.
- Tablet controlled—omit last dose.
- Insulin controlled—reduce/omit last dose and if unstable may need to admit and convert to intravenous insulin.

345

Endoscopy-related complications

Endoscopy carries a small but significant morbidity and mortality which should be appreciated and considered along with the indication. Proper staff training, equipment and monitoring is essential to minimise serious complications.

Froehlich F. *et al.* (1999) Appropriateness of gastrointestinal endoscopy: risk of complications. *Endoscopy* **31**, 684–686; Freeman ML *et al.* (1996) Complications of endoscopic biliary sphincterotomy. *NEJM* **335**, 909–918.

Procedure	Mortality (%)	Perforation (%)	Bleeding (%)	Other (%)
Diagnostic OGD	0.01	0.04	0.02	0.05*
Therapeutic ERCP	0.4	0.3	2.0	5.4**
Diagnostic colonoscopy	0.02	0.2	0.03	0.02
Therapeutic colonoscopy	0.04	0.46	1.16	0.03

Well published figures for enteroscopy and endosonography are not currently available.
*Cardiorespiratory.
**Acute pancreatitis.

Oesophagogastroduodenoscopy (OGD)

Principle
Examination from cricopharyngeus to second part of duodenum

Indications

Symptoms
- Persistent dyspepsia despite appropriate drug therapy *or with*
- Sinister symptoms of dysphagia, vomiting, weight loss.
- Haematemesis, melaena, iron deficiency anaemia.
- Abnormal barium swallow or meal examination.
- For biopsy assessment of *H. pylori*, giardiasis and coeliac disease.

Surveillance
- Oesophageal, pyloric and gastric ulceration.
- Surveillance for Barrett's oesophagus.
- Response to gluten-free diet in coeliac disease.

Screening
- Polyps/papillary tumour in GI cancer family syndromes.

Therapeutic
- Bleeding lesions, e.g. ulcer, vascular malformation or varices.
- Dilatation of oesophageal and pyloric strictures.
- Palliation of dysphagia for oesophageal tumours, e.g. insertion of stent.
- Polypectomy.
- Insertion of percutaneous gastrostomy/jejunostomy feeding tube.
- Removal of foreign body.

Patient preparation
Stop acid suppression therapy for 2 weeks. Nil by mouth 4–6h prior. The procedure takes approximately 15min. Sampling with biopsy or therapy can be carried during the same procedure.

Results
The findings from a series of ~1000 patients attending for open access OGD is shown in the table below.

Finding	%
Normal	34.1
Major abnormalities	
Duodenal ulcer	18.2
Oesophagitis/Barrett's	13.7
Gastric ulcer	3.7
Carcinoma	0.4
Minor abnormalities	
Hiatus hernia	15.3
Gastritis	8.1
Non-erosive duodenitis	2.6
Miscellaneous	5.9

Hungin APS *et al.* (1994) What happens to patients following open access gastroscopy? An outcome study from general practice. *Br J Gen Pract* **44**, 519–521.

Advantages over barium studies include greater accuracy and ability to take samples for histology and provide therapy at the same time.

Ancillary tests
- Biopsy for histology/culture.
- Dye staining to identify abnormal epithelium.
- Aspirate for pathogens, e.g. *Giardia*.

Complications
📖p345.

Flexible sigmoidoscopy & colonoscopy

347

Principle
- *Sigmoidoscopy* is examination from anus to splenic flexure.
- *Colonoscopy* is examination from anus to caecum/terminal ileum.

Indications

Symptoms
- Rectal bleeding:
  - Dark red blood (colonoscopy).
  - Bright red blood (flexible sigmoidoscopy).
- Positive FOBs.
- Pathological diarrhoea.
- Abnormalities on barium enema.
- Unexplained iron deficiency anaemia.

Surveillance
- Known multiple or large adenomas.
- Long-standing colitis >8 years.

Screening
- Familial adenomatous polyposis (FAP) syndrome.
- Hereditary non-polyposis colorectal cancer (HNPCC) syndrome.
- Other cancer family syndromes.

Therapeutic
- Polypectomy.
- Diathermy of vascular abnormalities, e.g. angiodysplasia.
- Dilatation of benign strictures.
- Stenting of malignant strictures.
- Decompression of acute non-toxic megacolon and colonic volvulus.
- Contraindications:
  - Severe colitis.
  - Acute diverticulitis.
  - Suspected perforated bowel.

Patient preparation
Obtain informed consent and check.

Flexible sigmoidoscopy
Give phosphate enema 30–60min before procedure.

Colonoscopy
4 days before examination stop iron tablets. Restrict to light meals with low fibre, e.g. pasta, rice, egg, fish, poultry, yoghurt, mashed potato, jelly, etc. Plenty of clear fluids but no food 24h before the procedure. Bowel clear out is achieved with Picolax, 3 sachets taken divided throughout the day before the morning procedure or 2 sachets the day before and 1 sachet in the morning of the afternoon procedure. In patients with severe rectal bleeding, bowel preparation may not be required/desirable.

Procedure
The procedure is carried out in the endoscopy unit with the patient in left lateral position and takes approximately 15min (flexible sigmoidoscopy)/30min (colonoscopy) to complete.

Findings
The table below shows the diagnoses made at colonoscopy (selected group showing greater yield in pathology than would be expected).

Diagnosis	%
Haemorrhoids	28
Polyps	25
Diverticular disease	16
Inflammatory bowel disease	11
Carcinom	8
Normal	12

Metcalf JV et al. (1996) Incidence and causes of rectal bleeding in general practice as detected by colonoscopy. *Br J Gen Pract* **46**, 161–164.

Advantages over barium enema are: greater yield in pathology, ability to obtain histological biopsies and application of therapy although virtual colonoscopy which is currently under development may become useful for screening and surveillance of polyps/cancer.

Pitfalls
- These tests do not preclude PR examination. Need to differentiate which patients need colonoscopy, flexible sigmoidoscopy or barium enema.
- Failure to take biopsies in patients with diarrhoea but normal-looking mucosa may miss microscopic colitis.
- Risk of perforation if barium enema carried out within a few days after biopsy of rectum/colon.

Other lower GI investigations

Proctoscopy is examination of the lower rectum and anal canal, e.g. for haemorrhoids, fissures, fistulae.

Rigid sigmoidoscopy is used for examination of rectum for proctitis/polyps or carcinoma. This procedure is commonly used in outpatients but is greatly underused as an initial inpatient investigation for diarrhoea or rectal bleeding. This is a simple procedure that can be performed at the bedside and allows biopsy of the rectal mucosa. The patient is positioned on the left side with knees drawn up. The instrument is inserted into the anus in the direction of the umbilicus with the aid of a lubricant for a few centimetres. Air is insufflated and the instrument is guided by direct vision and directed towards the sacrum and advanced usually to 15cm.

📖OHCM p212.

Enteroscopy

Principle
- *Push enteroscopy* allows examination to the jejunum.
- *Sonde enteroscopy* allows examination to the ileum.
- *Intraoperative enteroscopy* allows complete examination of jejunum and ileum.

349

Indications
- Obscure GI bleeding or severe unexplained iron deficiency anaemia.
- Abnormality found in jejunum/ileum on barium follow-through examination or abdominal CT scan.
- Selected cases of chronic diarrhoea/malabsorption syndrome.
- Selective indication as pathology in small bowel rare.

Preparation and procedure
As for OGD, but may need mild bowel clear-out in some cases.
- Push enteroscopy (commonest procedure): allows tip angulation, biopsy and therapy.
- As per gastroscopy but position of patient as per ERCP. Use of over-tube allows better intubation and procedure takes 30–40min.
- Sonde enteroscopy: slimmer endoscope without tip angulation or therapy. Passed to second part of the duodenum with the aid of gas-

troscope. Balloon tip of endoscopy inflated which passes down the small bowel with the aid of peristalsis. This can take several hours, after which the balloon is deflated and withdrawn and examination is performed which allows approximately 50% of the bowel lumen to be viewed.

- Intraoperative enteroscopy: under general anaesthetic with a push enteroscope. The small bowel is concertined over the endoscope allowing full examination down to the terminal ileum.

Advantages over barium examination include detection of vascular and fine mucosal lesions which can be missed on barium examination and also allows therapeutic intervention.

Results

The table shows the yield in small bowel pathology and missed lesions elsewhere in patients with unexplained GI bleeding when enteroscopy was carried out.

Lesion	%
Arteriovenous jejunal malformations	15.0
Jejunal metastases	2.5
Jejunal leiomyoma	2.5
Radiation enteritis	2.5
Ulcerative ileitis	2.5
Missed lesions found during enteroscopy	24.0
Normal	51.0

Landi B et al. (1998) Diagnostic yield of push-type enteroscopy in relation to indication. Gut **42**, 421–425.

Endoscopic retrograde cholangiopancreatography (ERCP)

Principle

Examination of the duodenum, accessory papilla, major papilla, biliary and/or pancreatic ducts.

Diagnostic ERCP

- Pre-operative evaluation of patient with chronic pancreatitis/pancreatic pseudocyst.
- Evaluation of the sphincter of Oddi by manometry.
- Use of duodenoscope to screen patients with suspected papillary tumour and familial adenomatous polyposis (FAP) syndrome. (This is technically not ERCP.)

Therapeutic

Biliary sphincterotomy
- Choledocholithiasis.
- Ampullary carcinoma.
- Severe acute biliary pancreatitis.

- Papillary stenosis.
- Sphincter of Oddi dysfunction.
- Biliary leak.
- Prior to placement of biliary stent/balloon dilatation or providing access for choledochoscope.
- Sump syndrome.

Biliary stent placement
- Palliation of malignant biliary stricture due to pancreatic, ampullar or biliary tumour.
- Benign biliary stricture after balloon dilatation.
- Biliary leak.

Pancreatic sphincterotomy
- Pancreatic stone causing obstruction/pain.
- Prior to placement of stent.
- Distal fistula communicating with ascites or pseudocyst drainage.
- Minor duct papillotomy for pancreatitis due to pancreas divisum.

Pancreatic stent placement
- Drainage of pseudocyst (via stomach).
- Post-dilatation of stricture (temporary).

Preparation
As for OGD. All cases must be discussed with endoscopist with prior imaging or at least ultrasound ± CT scan prior to procedure.

Procedure
Carried out with x-ray screening facilities either in radiology department or dedicated endoscopy suite. Patient left side prone. Side viewing duodenoscope used to identify papilla. Fine cannulae used to selectively intubate the common bile duct/pancreatic duct with abnormalities identified on fluoroscopy after injection of contrast.

Results
The table shows findings in a series of patients undergoing ERCP.

Findings in biliary system	%	Pancreatic system	%
Cholangiocarcinoma	15	Chronic pancreatitis	32
Papillary stenosis	8	Pancreatic carcinoma	13
Choledocholithiasis	7	Pancreas divisum	4
Liver metastasis	7	Pancreatolithiasis	3
Juxtapapillary diverticulum	7	Acute pancreatitis	2
Primary sclerosing cholangitis	3	Pancreatic lymphoma	1
Surgical ligation of bile duct	2	Normal findings	7
Caroli syndrome	1		
Ischaemic biliary lesion	1		
Normal findings	8		

Hintze RE et al. (1997) Clinical significance of magnetic resonance cholangiopancreatography (MRCP) compared to endoscopic retrograde cholangiopancreatography (ERCP). *Endoscopy* **29**, 182–187.

Advantages
- Has replaced previous surgical intervention.
- Allows therapeutic intervention over MRCP.

Ancillary tests
- Assessment of bile for crystals.
- Cytology for biliary/pancreatic strictures.
- Manometry for sphincter of Oddi dysfunction.

Oesophageal pH measurement

Indications
Assessment of suspected or established gastro-oesophageal reflux disease:
- In a patient with atypical symptoms, e.g. asthma, non-cardiac chest pain.
- Poorly controlled reflux disease.
- Prior to antireflux procedure.

Preparation
Acid suppression therapy stopped 7 days prior to procedure and patient fasted for 4h.

Procedure
A fine catheter is passed transnasally with the use of a local anaesthetic spray so that the tip of the pH catheter is placed 5cm above manometrically determined lower oesophageal sphincter. This is linked to a data recorder and is carried for a 24h period. The patient keeps a symptom diary. The computer-generated report is produced which gives the following information.

Measurements
- Percentage of time pH <4.
- Number of reflux episodes.
- Number of episodes longer than 5min.
- Duration of longest reflux episode.
- Correlation between symptoms and reflux episodes.

Interpretation
Values that lie outside the normal values shown below indicate significant reflux but are subject to interpretation:
- Reflux time upright <6.3%.
- Reflux time supine <1.2%.
- Total reflux time <4.2%.
- Number of episodes of reflux <50%.
- Reflux episodes longer than 5min <3.
- Longest episode of reflux <9.2min.

Pitfalls
The values need to be taken together with clinical information to form a full picture; investigation is not indicated for well-defined reflux responding to appropriate therapy.

GI manometry

Indications
- Determine the position of lower oesophageal sphincter in 24h pH monitoring.
- Prior to antireflux procedure.
- Assessment of motility disorder giving rise to dysphagia or non-cardiac chest pain.

Patient preparation
As per 24h monitoring.

Procedure
A multi-lumen catheter with several perfusion ports at various lengths along the catheter is placed transnasally to beyond 40cm past the lower oesophageal sphincter. The catheter is pulled back once the low oesophageal sphincter is identified and pressure measurements are taken throughout the length of the oesophagus with dry and wet swallows.

The following measurements are taken
- Upper and lower sphincter and body basal pressure.
- Peak pressure.
- Duration, frequency and pattern of contraction.

Results
- Achalasia—non-relaxing hypertonic lower oesophageal sphincter with atonic body.
- Nutcracker oesophagus—high amplitude prolonged body contraction but with normal peristalsis.
- Diffuse oesophageal spasm—prolonged body contractions simultaneously throughout the body.
- Non-specific motor disorder—a mixture of normal body contractions with incomplete propagation.

Pitfalls
Should not be used as initial test for atypical chest pain or other oesophageal symptoms because of low specificity.

Anorectal manometry
The methodology is similar to oesophageal manometry.

Indications
- Faecal incontinence.
- Chronic constipation.
- Pre-operatively for anorectal surgery.

Sphincter of Oddi manometry
A manometry catheter is used during ERCP.

Indications
Biliary type abdominal pain with abnormal LFTs ± dilated common bile duct. If sphincter of Oddi pressure is high, sphincterotomy may be beneficial.

Endoscopic ultrasound

Indications
- Pre-operative staging for cancer (oesophageal, gastric, pancreatic, ampullary, bile duct, colorectal and bronchial).
- Assessment of submucosal lesions and prior to endoscopic resection.
- Assessment of patient with suspected common bile duct stones.
- Assessment of chronic pancreatitis.
- Assessment of anal sphincter/faecal incontinence.

Preparation
As per OGD (no preparation for last indication). This is a relatively new technique and requests should be discussed before it is carried out.

Procedure
Intubation as per OGD. The tip of the endoscope has an ultrasound transducer which provides a cross-sectional (360°) or transectional (100°) scanning field. The endoscope is passed distally and then withdrawn as ultrasound images are assessed.

Therapeutic interventions include
- Fine needle aspiration.
- Cyst aspiration.
- Coeliac axis block.
- Stent placement.

Results
The exact place of endoscopic ultrasound is being assessed with other imaging modalities and it may replace other procedures although its role is likely to be complimentary. By providing information for better local staging, it will alter patient management.

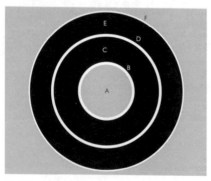

Fig. 7.1 A, lumen; B, mucosa; C, muscularis mucosa; D, submucosa; E, muscularis propria; F, serosa.

Chapter 8

Respiratory medicine

Airway hyperresponsiveness test or histamine/methacholine challenge test

Clinical indications
Suspected asthma.

Patient preparation
1. Explain procedure to patient.
2. Obtain informed consent.
3. Warn that wheezing and shortness of breath may occur and that a bronchodilator may be given.
4. Baseline FEV_1 measured.
5. Patient breathes in a nebulised aerosol of histamine (or methacholine) of increasing concentrations. This stimulates bronchoconstriction in a dose-dependent manner.
6. The FEV_1 is measured after each dose.
7. Patient must remain in department for 30min following the procedure to observe any delayed reactions.

Possible results
The % fall in FEV from baseline is plotted against the dose of inhaled histamine on a logarithmic scale. A dose–response curve is constructed and the provocation concentration (PC) of inhaled histamine required to reduce the FEV_1 by 20% (PC_{20}) can be derived by linear extrapolation. This figure has been arbitrarily chosen to assess degrees of bronchial reactivity for ease of comparison and safety.

Interpretation
Asthma suggested by PC_{20} <8mg/mL.

A direct relationship exists between the severity of asthma and requirement for medication and the PC_{20} value as an index of bronchial hyperresponsiveness.

Non-asthmatic subjects almost always have a PC_{20} >8mg/mL.

Advantages over other tests
- Easy to do.
- Cheap.
- Non-invasive.
- Quick.
- Reproducible.
- Safe: bronchoconstriction may be reversed by inhaled β-adrenergic agonist.

Contraindications
- Documented cholinergic hypersensitivity, e.g. cholinergic urticaria or angio-oedema or both.
- Allergy to histamine/methacholine.
- Unstable cardiac status, e.g. recent MI, arrhythmia or heart failure.
- Pregnancy.
- Severe baseline obstruction with FEV_1 <1.5.

Ancillary tests
PEFR chart: diurnal variation.

Pitfalls
- Bronchial hyperresponsiveness in asthma is not a static phenomenon and may vary widely from day to day.
- May change quite markedly without any change in symptoms (and vice versa).
- Represents only one component contributing to the symptomatology of asthma:
  - Others include airway oedema and mucus hypersecretion.

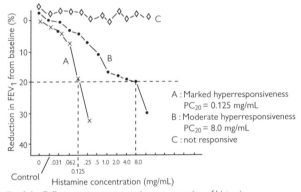

A : Marked hyperresponsiveness
PC$_{20}$ = 0.125 mg/mL
B : Moderate hyperresponsiveness
PC$_{20}$ = 8.0 mg/mL
C : not responsive

Fig. 8.1 Differing responses to varying concentration of histamine.

Pratter MR, Irwin S. (1984) The clinical value of pharmacologic bronchoprovocation challenge. *Chest* **85**, 260–265; Lotvall J, Inman M, O'Byrne P. (1998) Measurement of airway hyperresponsiveness: new considerations. *Thorax* **53**, 419–424; Smith CM, Anderson SD. (1989) Inhalation provocation tests using nonisotonic aerosols. *J Allergy Clin Immunol* **84**, 781–790.

357

Arterial blood gas sampling

Clinical indications
- Breathlessness (acute or chronic).
- Cardiorespiratory failure.
- Metabolic disturbance.
- Poisoning with drugs.
- Acute asthma with O$_2$ saturation <92% (on air).
- *OHCM p353.*

Patient preparation
Informed consent (verbal usually satisfactory).

Common sites Radial/brachial/femoral arteries.

Contraindications to radial
- Absent ulnar circulation.
- AV fistula for dialysis.
- Fractured wrist.
- Poor peripheral circulation.

Contraindications to brachial
- AV fistula.
- Fractured elbow.
- Poor peripheral circulation.

Contraindications to femoral
- Presence of graft/extensive vascular disease.

Procedure
1. Identify pulse.
2. Clean skin with alcohol swab.
3. Confirm position of maximum pulsation with non-dominant hand.
4. Local anaesthetic reduces pain.
5. Insert 23G needle attached to heparinised syringe.
6. If using low-resistance syringe this will fill automatically, otherwise aspirate gently.
7. Remove needle and apply firm gentle pressure with cotton wool ball for 5min.
8. Label hazardous specimens.
9. Expel air bubbles from sample.

Possible results
- Hypoxia with normal CO_2.
- Hypoxia with ↑ CO_2.
- Normoxia with ↓ CO_2.
- Metabolic acidosis *vs.* compensation.

📖OHCM pp154, 684.

Interpretation
Must be aware of the patient's inspired oxygen concentration (FIO_2) at time of sampling.

Advantages over other tests
- Easy, quick, cheap.
- No real alternative for assessing CO_2 or acid-base balance.
- Greater precision in upper ranges of SAO_2 curve.

Ancillary tests
- Pulse oximetry: gives indication of oxygenation status but not CO_2 levels.
- Arterialised blood sampling.

Complications
- Haematoma.
- Nerve damage.
- Inadvertant venous sampling.

Pitfalls
- If sample is to be analysed in a laboratory with >5min transit time it should be kept in melting ice to slow the metabolic activity of the cells.
- Avoid arterial puncture if possible in patients on anticoagulant therapy, with bleeding disorders or who have received thrombolytics in previous 24h.

- Failure to note FIO_2 will lead to difficulty in interpretation and potential therapeutic errors.

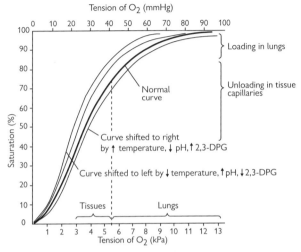

Fig. 8.2 Dissociation curve for oxyhaemoglobin.

Carruthers DM, Harrison BD. (1995) Arterial blood gas analysis or oxygen saturation in the assessment of acute asthma? *Thorax* **50**, 186–188; Syabbalo N. (1997) Measurement and interpretation of arterial blood gases. *Br J Clin Pract* **51**, 173–176.

Diagnostic pleural aspiration

359

Clinical indications
Pleural effusion either detected clinically or with imaging, e.g. CXR, USS, CT chest.

Patient preparation
1. Informed consent (verbal usually acceptable).
2. Patient sitting with arms forward supported on table/pillows.
3. Posterior or axillary approach if effusion large (otherwise be guided by USS).
4. Clean skin with iodine solution.
5. Infiltrate area one rib space below upper level of dullness to percussion with local anaesthetic (1 or 5% lignocaine).
6. Insert 19G needle attached to 50mL syringe. *Note:* Ensure needle enters immediately above rib to avoid the neurovascular bundle.
7. Aspirate fluid. If no fluid then try adjusting angle of needle.
8. Remove needle and apply plaster.

9. Post-aspiration CXR.

Possible results
- Pleural fluid is normally straw coloured.
- Pleural fluid analysed for protein, glucose, LDH, microbiology, cytology and pH.
- If heavily bloodstained suspect malignancy, pulmonary infarction or trauma. A traumatic tap will become progressively less bloodstained.
- If pus present: empyema.
- If creamy opalescent fluid: chylothorax (lymphoma, trauma to thoracic duct, yellow nail syndrome, lymphangioleiomyomatosis) or pseudochylothorax, e.g. in TB or RA.

Interpretation

Cytology	+ve in ~60% especially carcinoma of lung/breast Increased diagnostic rate with repeated sampling
Protein	Exudate >30g/L protein Transudate <30g/L protein
pH	<7.0: empyema, oesophageal rupture >7.0 and <7.3: collagen disorders, TB, malignancy, empyema
Glucose	↑ in RA, TB, malignancy, infection
Microbiology	Organisms, ZN stain
Eosinophilia	>10% in benign asbestos effusions, parasitic, hydropneumothorax
Neutrophilia	>1.0 × 10^9/L in acute inflammation, e.g. pneumonia, infarction
Lymphocytosis	Chronic effusions, e.g. TB, malignancy or RA
Amylase	↑↑↑ in pancreatitis ↑ in oesophageal rupture (salivary amylase) ↑ in malignancy
ANF	>1:160 virtually diagnostic of SLE
LDH	↑ in infection
RhF	+ve in RA
Complement	↓ in RA, SLE, malignancy, infection

Advantages over other tests
- Quick and easy.
- Cheap.
- Relatively non-invasive.
- Provides cytological, microbiological and biochemical data.

Ancillary tests
- Thoracoscopy.
- Pleural needle biopsy.

Pitfalls
- Traumatic tap.

Light RW. (1997) Diagnostic principles in pleural disease. *Eur Respir J* **10**, 476–481.

- Difficult to locate effusion if loculated: use USS/CT chest to guide aspiration attempt.

Complications
- Haemorrhage.
- Pneumothorax.
- Large volumes (>1000mL) should not be aspirated at one time due to risk of inducing pulmonary oedema.

Epworth test/Epworth sleepiness scale (ESS)

Clinical indications
Screening tool for obstructive sleep apnoea. Measures general level of daytime sleepiness.

Patient preparation
1. Ask patient to fill in questionnaire.
2. Subject rates on a scale of 0–3 the chances that, as part of his usual life in recent times, he would doze in each of 8 different situations.

Use the following scale to choose that most appropriate number for each situation:

0 = Would NEVER doze
1 = SLIGHT chance of dozing
2 = MODERATE chance of dozing
3 = HIGH chance of dozing

Situation
- Sitting and reading.
- Watching TV.
- Sitting inactive in a public place (e.g. theatre or a meeting).
- As a passenger in a car for an hour without a break.
- Lying down to rest in the afternoon when circumstances permit.
- Sitting and talking to someone.
- Sitting quietly after lunch without alcohol.
- In a car, while stopped for a few minutes in the traffic.

361

Possible results
ESS score is the sum of eight item scores and can range from 0 to 24.

Interpretation
Clinically normal score ≤10. Each ESS item gives an estimate of sleep propensity in one of eight specific situations whereas the total ESS score

Johns MW. (1993) Daytime sleepiness, snoring, and obstructive sleep apnea. *Chest* **103**, 30–36; Bennett LS. (1999) Adult obstructive sleep apnoea syndrome. *J Roy Coll Physicians Lond* **33**, 439–444.

gives a measure of more general average sleep propensity. Does not measure 'subjective' sleepiness.

Advantages over other tests
- Cheap.
- Easily administered.

Ancillary tests
- Polysomnography/Visi-Lab studies.
- Stanford sleepiness scale.
- Multiple sleep latency test.
- Maintenance of wakefulness test.

Pitfalls
Limited by patient's ability to read and comprehend the questionnaire and answer questions honestly.

Exercise testing

Clinical indications
- To confirm that reduced exercise tolerance exists.
- To determine the degree of impairment and disability.
- To investigate which system appears responsible for the reduction.
- To evaluate treatment results.
- To plan rehabilitation.

Patient preparation
1. Evaluate patient's medical history for contraindications to test.
2. Warn patient of cardiovascular complications*.
3. Obtain written consent.
4. Patient to wear comfortable clothes and shoes.
5. Monitoring: ECG, O_2 saturation, BP.
6. Exercise: treadmill/bike/free run on flat surface.
7. Steady state 5–12min walking test (usually 6min) or stepped stress test.
8. During a maximal exercise test the patient should be able to achieve 85–90% of predicted maximum heart rate.

Contraindications to test
- Unstable myocardium (recent MI, unstable angina, arrhythmias, severe valvular heart disease, congestive heart failure).
- Acute asthma.
- Acute febrile illness.
- Uncontrolled diabetes.
- Systemic hypertension (systolic >200mmHg, diastolic >120mmHg).

Possible results
Cardiac response: ECG, BP, cardiac output and stroke volume response.
Ventilatory response: ventilatory limitation (reduced breathing reserve), pattern of response, V_T, minute volume, respiratory rate.
Gas exchange: arterial blood gases, A-a gradient, P_aCO_2.
Ventilatory (anaerobic) threshold: normal or ↓.
VO_2 max (maximum oxygen uptake) normal or ↓.

*Mortality = 1 per 10000 tests

Interpretation

Useful in making the distinction between exertional dyspnoea secondary to lung disease or fatigue secondary to cardiac dysfunction. In patients known to have asthma, exercise test is +ve in 75% of cases with a single treadmill run and 97% if the test is repeated in −ve responders. A fall of 10% or more from baseline in PEFR or FEV_1 suggests exercise-induced asthma.

Advantages over other tests

Best assessment of exercise capacity. Adds to diagnostic accuracy quantitatively (measurement of work capacity, maximum VO_2 and sustained work capacity) and qualitatively (identification of the cause of exercise limitation).

Ancillary tests

- Static lung function tests.
- For asthma: histamine/methacholine inhalation challenges PEFR diary.

Pitfalls

- Dependent on patient effort and compliance.
- Not suitable for patients with severe objective measurement of respiratory impairment.

Complications

▶Bronchospasm: usually easily reversed with an inhaled adrenergic agent.
▶Cardiac arrhythmias/arrest: appropriate equipment and drugs should be available in the exercise testing area. Personnel should be trained in basic and advanced cardiopulmonary resuscitation.

Hughes JMB, Pride NB, eds. (1999) *Lung Function Tests. Physiological Principles and Clinical Applications*, WB Saunders Philadelphia pp, 133–148; König P. (1989) Exercise challenge: indications and techniques. *Allergy Proc* **10**, 345–348; Sue DY. (1994) Exercise testing in the evaluation of impairment and disability. *Clin Chest Med* **15**, 369–387.

Fibreoptic bronchoscopy/video bronchoscopy

Clinical indications

- Any patient with persistent/substantial haemoptysis.
- Suspected lung neoplasm:
  - For histology.
  - To assist with staging.
- Infection:
  - To identify organism.
  - To determine course of recurrence/persistence.
- Diffuse parenchymal lung disease (DPLD) to obtain transbronchial biopsies (useful in diagnosis of sarcoidosis, extrinsic allergic alveolitis and lymphangitis carcinomatosa).

Pre-assessment
- CXR.
- FBC.
- Spirometry.
- Clotting.
- Pulse oximetry.
- ABGs on air if hypoxia suggested by oxygen saturation.

Patient preparation

Endoscopy suite
1. Patient informed and consented.
2. Frontal approach with patient lying on couch, trunk at 45°.
3. IV access obtained.
4. Basic monitoring: pulse oximeter and cardiac monitor.
5. Supplementary O_2 via single nasal cannula.
6. IV sedation: midazolam/alfentanil.
7. Topical lignocaine spray to nose and pharynx (30–50mg of 4 or 10%).
8. Bronchoscope lubricated with 2% lignocaine gel and passed via nostril or mouth guard.
9. Further boluses of lignocaine (4%) applied to cords and then bronchial tree (2%).

Possible results
- Direct inspection of nares, nasopharynx and oropharynx.
- Assess movement of vocal cords (ask patient to say 'eee').
- Direct inspection of bronchial tree down to subsegmental level.
- Able to take bronchial/transbronchial biopsies and brushings.
  Bronchoalveolar lavage (BAL): wedge tip of bronchoscope into a sub-segmental bronchus and instil 20mL sterile saline into the distal airway. Aspirate immediately aiming to obtain approximately 50% of instilled volume.

Interpretation		
Histology:	tumours/DPLD	biopsy
Cytology:	tumours	brush
Microbiology:	Gram stain	lavage
	ZN stain	
	Stain for *Pneumocystis carinii*	
	fungi	
	virus	

Some appearances diagnostic.
Screening: x-ray-guided biopsy of non-visible lesions.

Advantages over other tests
- Well tolerated.
- Quick, cheap.
- Provides histological and immunobiological confirmation (to back up CT/CXR diagnosis).
- Therapeutic: removal of retained secretions, mucus plugs, blood clots.

Ancillary tests
- Rigid bronchoscopy: under GA:

- Allows therapeutic interventions, e.g. laser therapy, cryotherapy, stent insertion, debulking of large tumours in the major airways and better control of haemorrhage.
- Preferable for removal of foreign body.

Side effects and complications
- Pneumothorax with transbronchial biopsies.
- Haemorrhage post-biopsy.
- Hypoxia.
- If performed on day case unit patient will not be able to drive home and will need a responsible adult in attendance overnight.

Pitfalls
- Only visualises proximal airways.
- Biopsies may be inadequate or from necrotic areas.
- Not easy to biopsy submucosal tumour.
- Needs good quality cytology preparation.

Flow volume loops/maximum expiratory flow-volume curve

Clinical indications
Patient in whom COPD/small airways disease or upper airway obstruction is suspected.

Patient preparation
- Advised to wear comfortable, loose clothing.

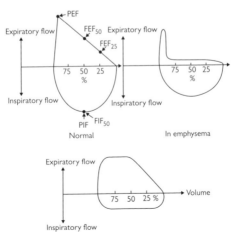

365

Fig. 8.3 Flow volume loops.

- Technician explains procedure to patient.
- Mouthpiece in position, patient breathes in maximally and then out as hard and fast as possible.
- 3 acceptable manoeuvres should be performed. Patients must perform the test with maximal effort each time and the results should be similar for each of the 3 attempts.

Interpretation

Particularly useful in recognising patients with narrowing of the central airway (larynx and trachea). Narrowing at this site has greatest effect on maximum expiratory flow and also on maximum inspiratory flow giving rise to a characteristic appearance. Also identifies patients with reduced elastic recoil (bullae, emphysema) or reduced airway lumen (asthma, chronic obstructive pulmonary disease, bronchiolitis).

Oscillation of flow gives a 'saw tooth' pattern. This usually signifies instability of the upper airway and has been observed in obstructive sleep apnoea, thermal injury to the airway, bulbar muscle weakness, extrapyramidal neuromuscular disorders, upper airway stenosis/tracheomalacia and snoring.

Advantages over other tests
- Allows early detection of small airway disease—more sensitive than FEV_1 alone.
- Reproducible.

Ancillary tests
- Spirometry.
- Transfer factor.

Pitfalls
- Dependent on patient understanding and maximal effort.
- Infection control necessary in patients with known or suspected transmissible disease (e.g. active pulmonary tuberculosis).

Peak flow charts

Clinical indications

Asthma
- Diagnosis.
- Assessment of severity.
- Assessment of treatment response to β_2 agonists.

Occupational asthma
- Diagnosis.

Patient preparation

Patients need to be equipped with a peak flow meter and peak flow and symptom diary and have a thorough understanding of how to use them.

Gelb AF, MacAnally BJ. (1973) Early detection of obstructive lung disease by analysis of maximal expiratory flow-volume curves. Chest **64**, 749–753.

Guidelines to patients should include:
1. Perform the test standing (if possible).
2. Hold the meter lightly and do not interfere with the movement of the marker.
3. Perform three tests each time and record the largest value.

Readings should be taken at various times throughout the day. Limiting the patient to two readings in each day may aid compliance. In occupational asthma 2-hourly peak flow readings are required during the day and evening.

Possible results
- Diurnal variability: as measured by the lowest PEFR value (usually on waking) and the highest PEFR value (usually in the afternoon/evening).
- Patient symptoms and PEFR can be examined together.

Interpretation
Diurnal variation is increased in patients with asthma compared to normals (amplitude >20%), i.e. peak flow falls significantly overnight and in the early morning.

Advantages over other tests
- Cheap.
- Saves time of respiratory physician and technician.
- Reproducible.
- Objective measure of response to treatment.

Ancillary tests for diagnosis of asthma
- Bronchoprovocation test.
- Exercise test.

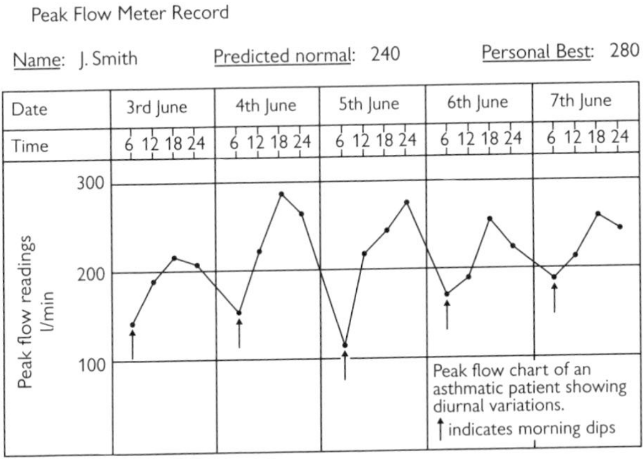

Peak Flow Meter Record

Name: J. Smith   Predicted normal: 240   Personal Best: 280

Peak flow chart of an asthmatic patient showing diurnal variations.
↑ indicates morning dips

Fig. 8.4

Normal Peak Expiratory Flow Rates

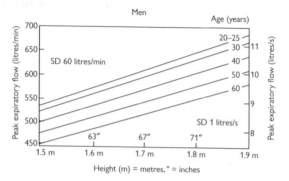

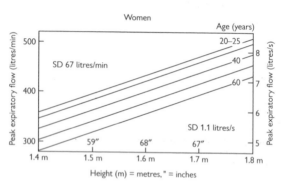

Fig. 8.5

Pitfalls

- Not all asthma exacerbations are associated with increased diurnal variability.
- Calculating diurnal variation can be complicated and tedious.
- Time of recording or recent use of β_2 agonist drugs may result in minor changes in peak flow, but can cause large errors in diurnal variability.
- Dependent on patient understanding, cooperation and accuracy.

Reddel H, Jenkins C, Woolcock A. (1999) Diurnal variability—time to change asthma guidelines? *BMJ* **319**, 45–47; Hetzel MR, Clark TJ. (1980) Comparison of normal and asthmatic circadian rhythms in peak expiratory flow rate. *Thorax* **35**, 732–738.

Pleural needle biopsy

Clinical indications

Pleural effusion of unknown aetiology especially if TB or malignancy suspected. *Note*: May be combined with diagnostic and/or therapeutic pleural aspiration. In which case, obtain diagnostic fluid sample first, then do needle biopsy, then follow with therapeutic aspiration.

Patient preparation
1. Informed written consent.
2. Patient sits with arms forward supported on table/pillows.
3. Posterior or mid-axillary approach.
4. Skin cleaned with iodine solution.
5. Lignocaine (1 or 5%) infiltrated in rib interspace: check pleural fluid aspirated.
6. Stab incision with narrow scalpel.
7. Insert closed Abrams needle (requires firm pressure to be applied until penetrates parietal pleura: take care not to apply too much force).
8. Attach 50mL syringe.
9. Twist open Abrams needle.
10. Aspirate fluid to ensure needle in pleural space.
11. Withdraw needle at angle to chest wall until side hole 'snags' parietal pleura.
12. Maintain lateral pressure and rotate to close hole thereby cutting biopsy. Remove needle and extract biopsy tissue.
13. Repeat with samples taken from 3, 6 and 9 o'clock (avoid the 12 o'clock position to avoid the neurovascular bundle).
14. May require suture to close.
15. Apply dressing.
16. Obtain CXR post-procedure.
17. Place samples in formalin for histological examination and saline for microbiological culture.

Possible results
- Slivers of white pleural tissue.
- Examine histology and culture for AFBs.

Interpretation
- Malignant mesothelioma may be diagnosed on histology, especially with addition of immunohistochemical methods looking at tumour cell markers.
- More sensitive than pleural fluid aspiration in diagnosing TB.
- Carcinoma cells may arise from direct spread from lung primary or represent secondary carcinoma. In either case, management is palliative.

369

Advantages over other tests
- Easy, quick, cheap; more reliable than diagnostic pleural aspiration.
- Less invasive than thoracoscopy for diagnosis of TB.

Ancillary tests
- Diagnostic pleural fluid aspiration.
- Thoracoscopy.

Complications
- Pneumothorax.
- Haemothorax.

Pitfalls
- Skeletal muscle biopsy: inadequate specimen.

Kirsh CM et al. (1995) A modified Abrams needle biopsy technique. *Chest* **108**, 982–986; Kirsh CM et al. (1997) The optimal number of pleural biopsy specimens for a diagnosis of tuberculous pleurisy. *Chest* **112**, 702–706; Prakash UB, Reiman HM. (1985) Comparison of needle biopsy with cytologic analysis for the evaluation of pleural effusion: analysis of 414 cases. *Mayo Clin Proc* **60**, 158–164.

Polysomnography

Clinical indications

Note: Symptoms alone do not help predict which patient with sleep disturbance has obstructive sleep apnoea (OSA).

- Patients with low probability sleep disorder, e.g. snores with no other features suggestive of OSA.
- Patients with high probability sleep disorder, e.g. typical symptoms and physiognomy. Need study for diagnosis and assessment of severity.
- Known OSA: assessing treatment response.
- Assessment of nocturnal hypoventilation syndromes, e.g. scoliosis.
- Patients with unexplained sleep–wake disorders.

Patient preparation

The patient is admitted to the sleep laboratory in the early evening. Monitoring is explained and attached, using some combination of the following:

Sleep	Electroencephalogram	
	Electro-oculogram	
	Electromyogram	
Oxygenation	Oxygen saturation probe (ear or finger)	
Breathing pattern	Airflow by:	Thermocouples
		Thermistor
		End tidal CO_2 pressure
	Thoracoabdominal movement by:	Inductance plethysmography
		Impedance
		Strain gauge
Miscellaneous	Snoring:	Microphone
	Leg movement by:	EMG
		Video
		Movement detector

Bennett LS. (1999) Adult obstructive sleep apnoea syndrome. *J Roy Coll Physicians Lond* **33**, 439–444; Douglas NJ. (1995) Sleep-related breathing disorder. 3. How to reach a diagnosis in patients who may have the sleep apnoea/hypopnoea syndrome. *Thorax* **50**, 883–886.

Possible results

Original diagnosis of OSA based on polysomnography—overnight recording of sleep, breathing patterns and oxygenation. It is relatively expensive and most centres use a combination of video to assess quality of sleep, identify transient arousals and paroxysmal leg movement disorder (PLMD) and oximetry (to detect desaturation) plus some form of measuring the breathing pattern to detect hypopnoea.

Interpretation

Obstructive sleep apnoea diagnosed in the context of multiple (typically >15/h) hypopnoeic/apnoeic events occurring throughout the night and resulting in desaturation.

Advantages over other tests

Demonstrates number of hypopnoeic (reduction in breathing) or apnoeic (absence of breathing) events occurring per hour. May be used to monitor effectiveness of treatment.

Ancillary tests

Epworth sleepiness score.

Pitfalls

- Expensive.
- Time-consuming.
- Most sleep study systems are poorly validated therefore need expert interpretation of results to consider false positives and negatives.
- Patients need to sleep for >3h/night and have rapid eye movement (REM) sleep.

Pulse oximetry

Clinical indications

- Any acutely unwell patient—avoids repeated blood gas measurements provided that hypercarbia is absent.
- Monitoring of long term oxygen therapy (LTOT)—but not suitable for initial assessment.
- Assessment of nocturnal FiO_2 and screening for sleep apnoea syndrome—identification of nocturnal desaturations.
- Exercise walk test.

Patient preparation

1. Clean probe site (ear or finger).
2. Ensure good contact of probe with warm well-perfused skin.
3. Avoid nail-varnished fingers.

Possible results

Oxygen saturations expressed as **%**.

Cross-sectional	Normal or low
Longitudinal	Stable/improve/deteriorate
Overnight	Normal/intermittent desaturations

Interpretation
- Respiratory failure unlikely if O_2 saturation >92% on air.
- Provides almost immediate arterial oxygen saturation data.
- Must know the inspired oxygen (FiO_2) concentration the patient is breathing.

Advantages over other tests
- Non-invasive.
- Easy, cheap.
- Instantaneous.
- Sensitive.
- Portable.

Ancillary tests
Arterial blood gas sampling.

Pitfalls
- Does not detect carbon dioxide levels.
- If carboxyhaemoglobin or methaemoglobin are present in the blood in elevated levels the pulse oximeter will give a falsely elevated reading for the arterial oxygen saturation.
- ↑ in jaundice.
- Erroneous information if patient poorly perfused.
- Excessive patient movement can give false readings.

Spirometry

Clinical indications
- To evaluate symptoms, signs or abnormal test results.
- Provide objective, quantifiable measures of lung function.
- Evaluate and monitor disease.
- Assess effects of environmental/occupational/drug exposures both adverse (e.g. amiodarone) and beneficial (e.g. bronchodilators).
- Pre-operative assessment.
- Employment/insurance assessment.
- Early detection of bronchiolitis obliterans in lung transplant patients.

Patient preparation
1. Explain what the test involves. Most respiratory technicians demonstrate technique to ensure maximal effort and cooperation of patient.
2. Patient must fully inhale before test.
3. Exhale into breathing tube. Must be maximal effort with no hesitation.
4. No cough/glottal closure in the first second.
5. Test must last at least 6s (up to 15s with obstruction).
6. No evidence of airflow leak/obstruction of mouthpiece.

Possible results

FEV$_1$:	Forced expiratory volume in 1 s.
	Test of mechanical function of the lungs.
	Depends on size and elastic properties of the lungs, calibre of the bronchial tree and collapsibility of airway walls.
FVC:	Forced vital capacity.

8 Respiratory medicine

Interpretation
At least three acceptable tracings should be obtained. Examine each tracing to ensure adequate effort made by patient, that it is reproducible, and that there are no artefacts.

FEV/FVC ratio:	Index of the presence/absence of airflow limitation. Young and middle aged healthy non-smokers rate ≥75%. Older normal patients ratio 70–75%.
FEV/FVC ↓:	Obstructive. Classify severity using FEV, expressed as % of predicted value, e.g. COPD, asthma.
FEV/FVC ↔ or ↑	Restrictive but need reduced TLC to confirm, e.g. lung fibrosis, chest wall problems, pulmonary effusion and oedema.

If used for monitoring purposes need adequate baseline study.

Advantages over other tests
- Cheap, quick.
- Bedside/outpatient test.
- Reproducible.

Ancillary tests
- Total lung capacity to confirm interstitial disease with restrictive spirometry.
- Pre- and post-bronchodilator studies: an increase of 15% in FEV_1 and 20% in FVC suggest reversibility.

Pitfalls
- Need standardisation of normal data for height, weight, age, sex and race.
- Level at which a result may be considered abnormal is contentious, usually accepted to be outside range of 80–120% of mean predicted.
- FEV may remain relatively normal in early stages of generalised lung disease.

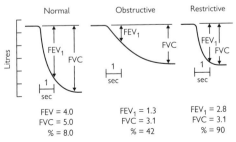

Normal	Obstructive	Restrictive
FEV = 4.0	FEV_1 = 1.3	FEV_1 = 2.8
FVC = 5.0	FVC = 3.1	FVC = 3.1
% = 8.0	% = 42	% = 90

Fig. 8.6 Examples of spirograms.

- FEV/FVC ratio is good guide to presence or significant airway narrowing but as disease progresses, both will fall and correlation with severity of disease is poor.
- Variability (noise) is greater in pulmonary function tests than in most other clinical laboratory tests because of the inconsistency of effort by patients.

See examples of spirograms 📖*OHCM p329.*

Crapo RO. (1994) Pulmonary-function testing. *NEJM* **331**, 25–30.

Sputum microscopy & culture/sputum cytology

Clinical indications
- Microbiology:
  - Productive cough with sputum.
  - Infective exacerbations of any chronic lung disease.
  - Pneumonia.

- Cytology:
  - Suspected lung cancer, especially in elderly/frail patients.

Patient preparation
- Explain need for the sputum sample.
- Provide suitable sputum pots.
- Early morning samples are best.
- Consider induced sputum—use ultrasonically nebulised hypertonic saline to facilitate sputum production in association with chest physiotherapy.

Possible results
Induced sputum results in successful sputum production in >70% of normal and asthmatic subjects who cannot produce sputum spontaneously.

Gram stain	Gram +ve or –ve organisms
ZN stain	AAFB
Microscopy	Differential cell count
	Eosinophils in asthma
Cytology	Malignant cells
	Small cell, squamous cell, adenocarcinoma cells

Interpretation
- Commensal organisms common.
- *Streptococcus pneumoniae* and *Haemophilus influenzae* likely pathogens in COPD.

Gibson PG *et al.* (1989) Cellular characteristics of sputum from patients with asthma and chronic bronchitis. *Thorax* **44**, 693–699; Parord ID *et al.* (1997) The use of induced sputum to investigate airway inflammation. *Thorax* **52**, 498–501.

- *Streptococcus pneumoniae* commonest organism in community-acquired 1° pneumonia.
- *Staphylococcus aureus* and *Pseudomonas* likely in bronchiectasis.
- Nosocomial infections:
  - *Staphylococcus aureus.*
  - *Pseudomonas.*
  - *Klebsiella.*
  - *Bacteroides.*
  - Gram −ve enterobacteria.
- Adenocarcinoma and small cell lung cancer diagnostic.
- Squamous cell carcinoma on cytology can reflect premalignant change.

Advantages over other tests
- Cheap, easy.
- Non-invasive.

Ancillary tests
- Bronchoscopy and bronchoalveolar lavage.
- Serum serology if atypical pneumonia suspected.
- PCR for drug-resistant TB.

Pitfalls
- Sputum may be diluted by saliva.
- Diagnosis of squamous cell carcinoma is not as robust as for small cell lung cancer or adenocarcinoma. Needs careful cross referencing to radiology and should be confirmed if possible with biopsies.
- Negative results should not preclude further investigations if malignancy suspected.

Static lung volumes/whole body plethysmography

375

Clinical indications
- Differentiate between obstructive and restrictive disease patterns.
- Identify and quantify trapped air (shown by ↑ RV/TLC ratio).
- Assess response to therapeutic interventions (e.g. drugs, radiation, transplantation).
- Identify presence and amount of unventilated lung.
- Assess chronic lung disease (e.g. sarcoidosis, rheumatoid lung).
- Pre-operative assessment.
- Assessment of pulmonary disability.

Patient preparation
1. Ask patient to wear comfortable clothes.
2. Place mouthpiece securely in mouth with lips tight around it.
3. Breathe in a relaxed manner through spirometer system (nose clips mandatory).

4. After total of 5 tidal breaths with consistent end-expiratory levels, patient asked to maximally inspire to total lung capacity followed by exhalation with encouragement to force out the last 5–15% of air.
5. A minimum of 2 attempts should be obtained.
6. More may be needed in the young and elderly to obtain reproducible results.

Most accurate results are obtained with whole body plethysmography.

Possible results

Total lung capacity
Volume of air in the lungs at the end of full inspiration.

Residual volume
Volume of air remaining in the lungs after maximal expiration.

Vital capacity
The amount of air expired (or inspired) between maximum inspiration and maximum expiration.

Functional residual capacity
The amount of air in the lungs at the end-tidal position.

Inspiratory capacity
The maximum amount of air that can be breathed into the lungs from the end-tidal position.

Tidal volume
The volume of air inspired and expired with each breath.

Inspiratory reserve volume
The volume between the peak inspiratory tidal position and maximum inspiration.

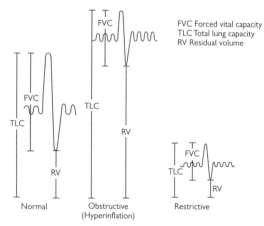

Fig. 8.7 Lung volumes: physiological and pathological.

Ries AL. (1989) Measurement of lung volumes. *Clin Chest Med* **10**, 177–186; Hughes JMB, Pride NB, eds. (1999) *Lung Function Tests. Physiological Principles and Clinical Applications*, WB Saunders, Philadelphia, pp4–16.

Causes of ↑ TLC:	Generalised airway obstruction, e.g. COPD
	Emphysema (including bullae)
	Bronchiectasis
	Asthma
	Other, e.g. Acromegaly
Causes of ↓ TLC	Intrapulmonary
	– pneumonectomy
	– collapsed lung
	– consolidation
	– oedema
	– fibrosis
	Extrapulmonary
	– pleural disease
	– effusion
	– thickening
	– pneumothorax
	– rib cage deformity
	– scoliosis
	– thoracoplasty
	– respiratory muscle weakness
Causes of ↑ RV:	Generalised airway obstruction
	Pulmonary vascular congestion, e.g. mitral stenosis, ASD
	Expiratory muscle weakness, e.g. spinal injury, myopathies
Causes of ↑ FRC:	Age, lung disease causing air trapping, e.g. asthma, emphysema, COPD
Causes of ↓ FRC:	Restrictive lung diseases, e.g. diffuse interstitial pulmonary disease of any aetiology, pneumonectomy

Interpretation

Only interpret if test is reproducible, i.e. if the 2 largest vital capacity values are within 5% or 100mL (whichever is the larger).

VC may remain within normal range in some pulmonary disease, e.g. emphysema.

↓ VC: restrictive pulmonary disease, neuromuscular disease, e.g. amyotrophic lateral sclerosis.

During the testing process, the patient is enclosed in a chamber equipped to measure either pressure, flow or volume changes. Because all the gas in the thorax is accounted for, this method is particularly useful in patients with trapped gas, e.g. bullous emphysema.

Advantages over other tests
Reproducible.

Pitfalls
- Patient cooperation essential: they must provide maximal effort and be capable of understanding instructions.
- Calibration should take place on a regular basis.
- Risk of disease transmission between patients and between patient and technician, therefore avoid if pulmonary TB suspected.

Sweat test

Clinical indications

Suspected cystic fibrosis (CF) in the context of
- Bronchiectasis/recurrent chest infections.
- Pancreatic insufficiency/diabetes mellitus.
- Family history.
- Fertility problems.

Patient preparation
1. Obtain informed consent: verbal usually sufficient but important to discuss reasons for test and possible implications. Perform two sweat tests simultaneously on each arm for greater accuracy.
2. Induce sweating by pilocarpine iontophoresis; a weak electrical current aids penetration of pilocarpine into skin. Stimulated in this way, the sweat glands of the forearm, previously washed and dried, secrete sweat.
3. Collect sweat on preweighed filter paper (>100mg), then measure eluted Na^+ and Cl^-.

Possible results
- 98–99% of children homozygous for CF have sweat Cl^- and Na^+ levels well >70 and 60mmol/L respectively.
- Sweat Na^+ concentrations tend to increase with age and show wide variability between individuals.
- Diagnostic accuracy is improved in borderline cases by a suppression test using fludrocortisone.

Interpretation
A +ve test is virtually diagnostic of cystic fibrosis. This should lead to counselling and genetic testing.

Equivocal results are defined as Na^+ or Cl^- concentrations between 50 and 70mmol/L.

The diagnosis should never rest on the sweat test alone and should be considered together with the clinical findings and laboratory evidence of pancreatic insufficiency.

Advantages over other tests
- Cheaper than genetic tests.
- Assesses functional deficit therefore capable of detecting patients who have rare variants of CF.

Ancillary tests
- Nasal potential difference.
- Pancreatic function tests (3-day faecal collection).
- Genetic studies.

Pitfalls
- A wide discrepancy between the results from each arm suggests a problem with technique.
- Accurate interpretation of sweat tests requires knowledge of the age-related changes in sweat Na^+ and Cl^- concentrations and should be done in a specialised centre.

False negatives
- Inexperience of operator.
- Low rates of sweating.
- Poor skin preparation.
- Poor iontophoretic contact with skin.
- Faulty chemical analysis.

False positives
- Evaporation of sweat secondary to inadequate sealing during collection.
- Untreated adrenal insufficiency.
- Nephrogenic diabetes insipidus.
- Hypothyroidism.
- Glycogen storage disease.
- Nephrotic syndrome.
- Severe malnutrition.
- AIDS (some reports of abnormal sweat electrolytes).
- Faulty chemical analysis.

Hall SK, Stableforth DE, Green A. (1990) Sweat sodium and chloride concentrations—essential criteria for the diagnosis of cystic fibrosis in adults. *Ann Clin Biochem* **27**, 318–320; Heeley AF, Watson D. (1983) Cystic fibrosis—its biochemical detection. *Clin Chem* **29**, 2011–2018; Green A, Dodds P, Pennock C. (1985) A study of sweat sodium and chloride; criteria for the diagnosis of cystic fibrosis. *Ann Clin Biochem* **22**, 171–176.

379

Medical thoracoscopy

Clinical indications
- Pleural effusions when pleural fluid analysis non-diagnostic.
- Pneumothorax.
- Staging of lung cancer.
- Diagnosis of malignant mesothelioma and other pleural abnormalities, e.g. neurinomas, lipomas, plastocytomas.
- Suspected empyema.

Pre-assessment
- CXR.
- FBC.

- Clotting.
- Spirometry.
- Pulse oximetry.
- ABGs on air if hypoxia suggested by oxygen saturation.

Patient preparation

Endoscopy suite
1. Patient informed and consented.
2. Intravenous access obtained.
3. Basic monitoring: pulse oximeter and cardiac monitor.
4. Supplementary oxygen given if necessary.
5. Intravenous sedation: midazolam
6. An absolute prerequisite for thoracoscopy is the presence of an adequate pleural space (i.e. at least 6–10cm diameter)
7. If pleural effusion: drain using 3-way tap. Replace with equal quantity atmospheric air.
8. If no effusion: create pneumothorax.
9. Insert needle connected to manometer into pleural space.
10. Introduce 400–1000mL air. Patient in lateral position with abdominal side upwards.
11. Skin incision 5th intercostal space, mid-axillary line 1.5–2cm.
12. Insert 5–10mm pleural trocar and cannula.
13. Introduce thoracoscope via trocar into pleural cavity.
14. After inspection remove trocar and insert drain.
15. CXR post-procedure.

Possible results

- Direct inspection of pleural surfaces.
- Biopsy of parietal and visceral pleura—histology/culture esp. AFBs.
- Pleural fluid $\longrightarrow$ MC&S
  $\longrightarrow$ cytology.
- Therapeutic options: pleurodesis, coagulation of blebs, resection of fibrinous loculations in empyemas.
- Drainage of large pleural effusions possible without risk of re-expansion pulmonary oedema due to rapid equalisation of pressures by entrance of air into pleural space.

Interpretation

Macroscopic appearance of pleura may be diagnostic, e.g. TB, RA, scleroderma, metastatic disease.

Advantages over other tests

- Better than blind pleural biopsy.
- Able to obtain diagnosis in 70–95% of cases.
- Especially good at diagnosing TB.
- Less invasive than thoracotomy.
- Less expensive than thoracotomy: does not require a theatre or anaesthetist.
- Done under sedation unlike VATS (video-assisted thoracic surgery) which requires a GA and selective one-lung ventilation.

Ancillary tests

Diagnosis of mesothelioma improved with use of immunohistochemical markers.

Pitfalls
Biopsies may be inadequate or non-representative.

Contraindications
- Obliterated pleural space.
- Small pneumothorax.
- Patient short of breath at rest unless secondary to pneumothorax or pleural effusion which can be treated during procedure.
- Disturbed haemostasis:
  - Platelets <40 × 10^9/L.
  - PTT >50% normal.
- Recent MI, arrhythmias, heart failure.

Complications
- Fever 24–36h post-procedure.
- Empyema (<1%).
- Wound infection.
- Subcutaneous emphysema.
- Air embolism.
- Bronchopleural fistula following lung biopsy.
- Seeding of metastases/mesothelioma along trocar wound. (Radiotherapy a few days post-thoracoscopy should be carried out to prevent this.)
- Haemorrhage.
- Arrhythmias.
- Mortality rate <0.01%.

Loddenkemper R. (1998) Thoracoscopy—state of the art. *Eur Resp J* **11**, 213–221; Colt HG. (1999) Thoracoscopy: window to the pleural space. *Chest* **116**, 1409–1415.

Transfer factor

Clinical indications
Test for abnormalities of pulmonary gas exchange.

Patient preparation
- Avoid smoking 6h prior and strenuous exercise 2h prior.
- Allow 15–30min for test.
- Usually measured by single breath inhalation technique.
- Patient breathes in air containing a known concentration of CO and holds breath for 10s.

Possible results
- Transfer factor (TLCO).
- Transfer coefficient (KCO).
- May need to correct for anaemia:
  - Result usually standardised to Hb 14.6g/dL.

- Effect of mild anaemia (Hb >10g/dL) slight but becomes progressively more marked at lower values.

Interpretation

↓ in DLCO
- Obstructive lung disease, e.g. COPD, emphysema.
- Diffuse interstitial lung disease, e.g. CFA, amiodarone lung.
- Pulmonary involvement in systemic disease e.g. SLE, RA, Wegener's.
- Cardiovascular disease e.g. pulmonary oedema, mitral stenosis, PE.
- Others: anaemia, cigarette smoking.

↑ in DLCO
- Diseases associated with polycythaemia.
- Pulmonary haemorrhage.
- Diseases associated with increased pulmonary blood such as from left to right intracardiac shunts.
- Exercise.
- Asthmatics (reasons not clear).

Advantages over other tests
- Quick.
- Relatively easy to perform.
- Reproducible.

Pitfalls
- Breath holding time may be difficult for some patients to achieve.
- Calculation of TLCO is based on assumption that ventilation and diffusion are homogeneous in the entire lung. With unequal distribution of ventilation and diffusion, the TLCO will be underestimated on the alveolar level.
- With extrapulmonary lung restriction and consequent inability to achieve full inspiration, KCO tends to be higher than normal.

Jansons H et al. (1998) Re-breathing vs single-breath TLCO in patients with unequal ventilation and diffusion. Resp Med **92**, 18–24.

Neurology

Lumbar puncture (LP)

Indications
- Meningitis.
- Encephalitis.
- Polyradiculitis, polyneuritis.
- Multiple sclerosis.
- Myelitis.
- Vasculitis.
- Suspected subarachnoid haemorrhage (SAH). Note: In general, a –ve CT does not exclude a SAH.
- Suspected malignancy with meningeal involvement.
- Assessment of CSF pressure:
  - High (e.g. idiopathic or 'benign' intracranial hypertension, BIH).
  - Low (e.g. 'low pressure' headache).
- Therapeutic trials, e.g.
  - BIH.
  - Normal pressure hydrocephalus, NPH (not particularly helpful).
- To seek specific antibodies/markers in CSF, e.g.
  - HIV.
  - Lyme (*Borrelia*).
  - Syphilis.
  - ACE (for neurosarcoid).
  - Tumour markers.

Preparation
- Decide exactly what investigations you want. If necessary, alert the appropriate laboratories and organise transport of samples. In particular, samples for xanthochromia and cytology should be rapidly taken to the laboratory to be spun down.
- If the patient is also due to have a neuroradiological investigation with contrast and LP is not urgent, delay LP until after scan as there may be diffuse meningeal enhancement after the LP.
- If the patient is extremely anxious, he may benefit from 5–10mg of oral diazepam prior to the LP.

Procedure
1. Explain to the patient what you are about to do.
2. Arrange all your equipment on a sterile tray, including assembled CSF manometer.
3. Position patient on his side, with back perpendicular to bed, at the edge of a firm bed. Place head on one pillow. Draw knees up and place one pillow between them.
4. Adjust height of bed so that you are comfortable.
5. Identify the bony landmarks. L3/L4 space is in line with the iliac crests, and is most commonly used. L2/L3 to L5/S1 are also. If you like, mark the target space with the imprint of your thumb nail. Take time over these first three stages.
6. The insertion of the needle should be a sterile procedure. Clean the skin over the lower back. Don sterile gloves and mask.
7. Insert a little (0.25–0.5mL) local anaesthetic—too much can obscure the bony landmarks.
8. Pass LP needle horizontally into the space, with tip angled at about 10–15° (toward the umbilicus), in the midline horizontal plane. At all times, stylet should be fully inserted and bevel of needle facing up.

9. Slight resistance should be felt as needle passes through ligamentum flavum and the dura, and then a 'give' as it enters the subarachnoid space.
10. Slowly withdraw the stylet. CSF drops should appear.
11. If CSF does not appear, reinsert the style and slightly rotate the needle—this sometimes frees it of obstructing nerve roots. A gentle cough from the patient can also help.
12. If the needle encounters bone, or the patient complains of pains shooting down the leg, check the position of the needle (is it in the midline? Is it angled correctly?) and then withdraw it entirely.
13. Insert a fresh needle, correcting for any error noted above.
14. If this second pass is unsuccessful, withdraw needle and inform patient. If he is happy for you to proceed, then attempt LP in another space, repeating all steps from 4 down. Use a fresh needle.
15. If you fail again, explain to patient and seek a more experienced operator to perform the LP. Multiple failed attempts are painful and discouraging (to both you and your patient).
16. If a more experienced operator fails, ask your friendly radiologist to do it under X-ray guidance, but give him the help he requests and precise instructions about the samples required.
17. When CSF collection is complete, gently pull out the needle and place a sterile dressing over the insertion site.
18. Allow the patient to mobilise shortly after the LP.

Measuring the CSF pressure

As soon as the CSF starts to flow, attach the pre-assembled manometer. Wait until the CSF stops rising. If the patient is very anxious, or uncomfortable, a falsely raised opening pressure may be recorded. Sometimes having the patient slightly relax his legs will help. Using the three way tap, let the CSF run into your first pre-labelled tube (do not waste the CSF!). Having collected all the CSF you require, if the opening pressure was elevated, note the closing pressure.

Collecting samples

- As always, tailor your investigations to the clinical picture. If you are just checking the CSF pressure, then no samples need necessarily be collected. If you suspect a subarachnoid haemorrhage, collect three samples in sequentially labelled bottles and send promptly to the laboratory for quantitative estimation of xanthochromia and haemoglobin breakdown products. If you are looking for evidence of malignant cells, then at least one sample should be send to the laboratory promptly for cytology.
- To avoid contamination, allow the microbiology lab to split samples rather than attempting this yourself.
- Collect at least 10 drops in each bottle. The microbiology and cytology laboratories in particular will thank you for greater volumes.
- As soon as the CSF is collected, a blood sample should be obtained (if necessary) for glucose and oligoclonal band detection.

Alternative positioning of patient

Sometimes there is a dry tap if the CSF pressure is too low to distend the lumbar cistern. This can sometimes be overcome by performing the LP with the patient sitting on a firm reversed chair, leaning forward to bend over its back. This manoeuvre maximises the separation of the vertebrae. Again the needle should be angled, slightly (10°) upward relative to the spine at that point. This position does not allow precise measurement of CSF pressure.

Which needle to use?
22G usually appropriate. Needles with larger bores tend to cause a greater CSF leak (and thus more headache). Some advocate even finer needles, but these make the collection of CSF take too long. 'Blunt' anaesthetists' needles probably also reduce the risk of post-LP headache.

Clinical record keeping
Record what you did in the notes after the procedure (e.g. if more than one pass was required; which space you used), the opening and closing CSF pressure, and what investigations you have requested. Note the appearance of the CSF (if normal, it will be clear and colourless). If the CSF appears bloody, record this and whether the final bottle collected is clearer than the first.

When *not* to attempt an LP
- Risk of herniation:
  - Space-occupying lesions.
  - Non-communicating hydrocephalus.
  - Cerebral oedema (if in doubt, cranial imaging should be performed first).
- Uncorrected bleeding diathesis/anticoagulant use.
- Caution) if previous lumbar spine surgery or known anatomical abnormalities.
- Local skin sepsis.

Complications and what to do about them

Headache
- Usually starts within 24h of LP.
- May last from a few hours to 2 weeks, but typically several days.
- Probably related to persistent CSF leak via the dural tear; therefore tends to have 'low pressure' characteristics (frontal, worse on sitting up, better on lying down). There may be mild meningism and nausea.
- Treatment has traditionally involved bedrest, analgesia and the encouragement of plenty of fluids.
- If nausea is a major problem, the patient may require IV fluids.
- Rarely, if the headache is severe and persistent, then an anaesthetist may place an autologous blood patch to 'plug' the dural tear. Surgical intervention is rarely required.

Low backache
- A variety of causes of post-LP backache exist; these may usually be treated conservatively.

Infection
- Very rare if sterile technique is used. Occasionally may occur if the needle passes through a region of infection. Meningitis typically develops within 12h; very rarely there may be an epidural abscesses or vertebral osteomyelitis. Treat with appropriate antibiotics and if necessary surgery.

Herniation
- Uncal or cerebellar herniation may occur, particularly in the presence of a posterior fossa mass. ►►*An LP should not be performed if there is suspicion of raised intracranial pressure without first obtaining cranial CT or MR imaging.*
- Should the CSF pressure be found to be very high (300mm of CSF), even after relaxing patient, and in the absence of idiopathic (benign) intracranial hypertension, manage as follows: nurse patient prone with no pillow, raise foot of bed, start infusion of 20% mannitol at 1g/kg over 20min, start neurological observation chart, arrange urgent CT of brain and notify neurosurgeons. ►►*Do not instill saline into the subarachnoid space.*

Haemorrhage
- A 'traumatic' tap may cause a little local bleeding, which is rarely of clinical significance. Patients with impaired clotting (remember warfarin) or platelet function are at risk of more extensive bleeding, and LP should not be attempted unless the coagulopathy is corrected. An arachnoiditis or a spinal subdural or epidural haemorrhage may develop.

CSF constituents: normal values
- White cells   0–4/mm^3
- Red blood cells   ideally none!
- Protein   0.15–0.45g/L
- Glucose   ~one-half to two-thirds of simultaneous blood glucose.
- Opening pressure   8–20cm CSF.

Note: If there is a traumatic 'bloody' tap, there may be hundreds or thousands of red blood cells/mm^3. If so, then white cells should be expected in the CSF, but in similar proportions to the peripheral blood.

OHCM p750.

Rules of thumb
1. **Pressure**:
   - ↑ by space-occupying lesions within the cranial vault, such as oedema, masses, chronic inflammation.
   - ↑ by increased central venous pressure, e.g. in the anxious patient with tensed abdominal muscles.
   - ↓ if the spinal subarachnoid space is obstructed, thus impeding CSF flow.
2. **Cells**:
   - Polymorphs (neutrophils): suggest acute bacterial infection.
   - Lymphocytes & monocytes: viral and chronic infections or tumours.
   - Eosinophils: tumours, parasites, foreign body reactions.
3. **Glucose**: ↓ by non-viral processes causing meningeal inflammation.
4. **Total protein**: ↑ by breakdown of the blood–brain barrier.
5. **Immunoglobulins** specific to the CSF, i.e. without matching Igs in a simultaneous blood sample: inflammation within the theca, e.g. MS, infection, tissue damage.

Condition	Glucose	Protein	Cells	Comments
Acute bacterial meningitis	↓	↑	often >300/mm³	polymorphs; lactate ↑
Acute viral meningitis	N	N or ↑	<300 mononuclear	culture, antigen detection may be possible
Fungal meningitis	↓	↑	<300 mononuclear	culture and antigen detection
Tuberculous meningitis	↓	↑	mixed pleocytosis	ZN stain organisms, culture
			<300	PCR
Herpes simplex encephalitis	N	mildly ↑	5–500 lympho	PCR
Guillain-Barre syndrome	N	↑	normal	
Subarachnoid haemorrhage*	N	may be ↑	erythrocytes	look for bilirubin pigments on spectro photometry; xanothochromia unreliable
Malignant meningitis	↓	↑	mononuclear	rapid cytospin and look for malignant cells
HIV	N	N or ↑	mononuclear pleocytosis	culture, antigen detection, antiviral antibodies
Neurosyphilis	N or ↓		<300	
— early		↑	lymphocytes	VDRL
— late		↑		Treponema pallidum immobilisation tests

*LP should be done >12h after onset of headache; the CSF should be spun down within 45min; decreasing numbers of RBCS in successive bottles *are* compatible with SAH.

Common patterns
These are shown in the table opposite.

Skull radiograph

Indications
Usually more modern imaging techniques are much more informative, but there are occasions when these may not be speedily available. However, the plain SXR has quite low specificity and sensitivity for detecting many abnormalities of neurological importance.

Used in (suspected) cases of
- Skull fracture.
- Pituitary fossa abnormalities.
- Tumours involving bone.
- Bone changes related to meningiomata.

Procedure
- Lateral view in the first instance.

Consider
- Occipitofrontal.
- Towne's (half axial).
- Basal (submentovertical).
- Specific views (e.g. orbits).

What to look for (*what you see will depend on the pathology*)
- Shape and symmetry of vault.
- Pituitary fossa.
- Position of calcified pineal (midline shift?).
- Bone density changes (e.g. tumour, meningioma, Paget's).
- Fractures.
- Evidence of neurosurgical procedures.
- Intracranial air.
- Post-nasal space.
- Craniocervical junction.

Indications for SXR after head injury

In an orientated patient
- History of loss of consciousness or amnesia.
- Suspected penetrating injury.
- CSF or blood loss from the nose or ear.
- Scalp laceration (to bone or >5cm long), bruise or swelling.
- Violent mechanism of injury.
- Persistent headache or swallowing.

Nel MR, Robinson N. (1997) Lumbar puncture and headache. Epidural blood patching can be used to treat headache. *BMJ* **316**, 1019; Peterman SB. (1996) Postmyelography headache: a review. *Radiology* **200**, 765–770; Thompson EJ. (1997) Cerebrospinal fluid, in *Neurological Investigations*, ed Hughes RAC, BMJ Publications, London; Broadley SA, & Fuller GN. (1997) Lumbar puncture needn't be a headache. *BMJ* **315**, 1324–1325.

In a child
- Fall from >60cm or on to a hard surface.
- Tense fontanelle.
- Suspected non-accidental injury.

In a patient with impaired consciousness
- All patients, unless CT is performed urgently (CT is the preferred imaging modality).

Indications for CT after head injury
- Uncertain level of consciousness in intubated and ventilated patients.
- Coma persisting after resuscitation.
- Deteriorating level of consciousness.
- Progressive neurological signs.
- Skull fracture with:
  - Confusion.
  - Seizure.
  - Neurological signs/symptoms.
- Open injury:
  - Depressed compound fracture of skull vault.
  - Fracture of skull base.
  - Penetrating injury.

Ultrasound

Ultrasound may be used in a variety of modes.

Mostly commonly used in neuroradiology
- B mode: gives 2-dimensional images.
- Doppler effect is used to assess alterations in the pattern (especially velocity) of flow in vessels.
- Duplex scanning combines B mode and Doppler.

Extracranial vessels

B mode
- Can image from clavicle (common carotid bifurcation), and internal and external carotids to angle of jaw.
- Can image proximal and distal subclavian, and vertebral arteries.
- Supraorbital artery (anterior circulation).
- Fibrofatty plaques and thrombus on plaques not very echogenic therefore missable.
- Fibrous plaques more echogenic.
- Calcification in plaque is highly echogenic.
- Can sometimes detect intraplaque haemorrhage or ulceration.

Note: Requires patient cooperation and considerable operator skill. High grade stenosis can appear as total occlusion.

Doppler mode
- Stenosis alters the normal pattern of velocities recorded.

Greenberg JO. (1995) *Neuroimaging*, McGraw-Hill, New York; Kuhn MJ. (1992) *Atlas of Neuroradiology*, Gower, New York.

Duplex
- Combination of anatomic and flow imaging more sensitive and specific for clinically significant stenoses.

Comment

Use of carotid ultrasound: most commonly in the assessment of patients with carotid territory ischaemic strokes or TIAs, who might be candidates for carotid endarterectomy. Recent work suggests that there is little value in performing such studies >2 years after a cerebral event. Irregular plaques are more pathogenic.

Intracranial vessels

Transcranial Doppler
- 2mHz to penetrate thinner bone.
- Flow velocity in anterior, middle, and post cerebral, ophthalmic and basilar arteries; carotid siphon.

What it shows
- Intracranial haemodynamics.
- Vasospasm in SAH.
- Monitoring of microemboli.
- This is an area of active research with new clinical indications being described frequently.

Tegeler CH. (1995) Ultrasound in cerebrovascular disease, pp 577–595 in *Neuroimaging*, ed Greenberg JO, McGraw-Hill, New York.

Angiography

Indications
- Strongly suspected or confirmed SAH.
- Suspected cerebral vasculitis.
- Delineation of other vascular abnormalities (e.g. arteriovenous malformations, AVM).
- Delineation of tumour blood supply (occasionally).

391

Procedure
1. Catheter passed via femoral artery to carotid or vertebral artery under image intensification.
2. Contrast is given.
3. In digital subtraction angiography, subtraction of pre-contrast from post-contrast images (pixel by pixel) is used to help remove signals from bone density.

Arch angiography (aortography)
- Visualises aorta, major neck vessels and sometimes circle of Willis.
- No venous imaging.

Selective intra-arterial angiography
- Later images show venous system.

Carotid artery
- AP, lateral and oblique views: anterior and middle cerebral and internal carotid arteries.

Vertebral artery
- Towne's and lateral views: vertebral, basilar, posterior cerebral arteries.

What can be demonstrated?
- Occlusion, stenosis, plaques.
- Aneurysms.
- Arteriovenous and other blood vessel abnormalities.
- Abnormal tumour circulation[*].
- Displacement or compression of vessels[*].
- Experimental role in acute stroke analysis.

Complications
- Sensitivity to the contrast medium.
- Cerebral ischaemia, e.g. secondary to dislodgement of embolic fragments by catheter tip or thrombus in the catheter lumen.
- The rate of transient or permanent neurological defect following angiography depends on the operator.

Osborne AG. (1999) *Diagnostic Cerebral Angiography*, 2nd edition, Lippincott, Williams & Wilkins, New York; Larsen DW, Teitelbaum GP. (2000) Radiological angiography, pp617–643 in *Neurology in Clinical Practice*, 3rd edition, eds Bradley WG *et al.*, Butterworth-Heinemann, Boston.

Although CT and MRI give finer spatial details, angiography is still useful, e.g. delineating blood supply of a tumour.

Myelography

Indications
- Largely superseded by CT and especially MRI.
- Still used in subjects in whom MRI is contraindicated (e.g. cardiac pacemaker, metallic implants, claustrophobia).
- Can screen whole spinal cord and cauda equina for compressive or expanding lesions.
- Can visualise roots.
- Spinal vasculature abnormalities.

Procedure
5–25mL of (usually water-soluble) radio-opaque contrast medium is injected via an LP needle in the usual location (occasionally cisternal puncture is used). By tipping the patient on a tilt table, the whole spinal subarachnoid space may be visualised.

Complications
- Those of LP.
- Spinal arachnoiditis (after months or years), now rare with water-soluble contrast.
- Acute deterioration if there is cord/root compression.
- Direct neurotoxicity (3 in 10,000):
  - Seizures, encephalopathy.
  - Usually resolves in 48h.

- Allergic reaction to contrast:
  - Give dexamethasone 4mg 12 and 2h prior to investigation if known allergy.

Note: Send CSF for usual investigations (p385).

📖OHCM p394.

Radionuclide scans

Gamma camera scanning
- Give potassium perchlorate (to stop choroid plexus and salivary gland uptake).
- Then 99m - technetium labelled sodium pertechnetate IV.
- Look at intracranial distribution with gamma camera from lateral, anterior, and posterior views.

What does it show?
- Areas of increased vascularity.
- Areas of BBB breakdown.

However it has been superseded by CT and MRI and is rarely available.

Positron emission tomography (PET)
Unstable positron-emitting isotopes (produced locally by a cyclotron or linear accelerator) are incorporated into biologically active compounds. The distribution of isotope shortly after IV administration is plotted. A range of compounds may be labelled, such as ligands for specific neurotransmitter receptors. Commonly, PET is used to determine regional cerebral blood flow.

Single photon emission computed tomography (SPECT)
- Stable radioactive isotopes are incorporated into biologically active compounds.
- Their distribution after IV administration is plotted.
- These images often lack fine spatial detail.

Although the range of ligands available is limited, SPECT has certain advantages over PET:
- Isotopes are stable and therefore a cyclotron or linear accelerator need not be on site.
- A labelled ligand can be given after a clinically important event, e.g. can give agent and scan within 20min of the occurrence of a seizure.

Uses of PET and SPECT
PET is not widely available as a clinical tool. With the advent of functional MRI (FMRI), the uses of PET in both clinical practice and in neuroscience research may well become more restricted. SPECT is more widely available in clinical centres.

Clinical/research applications of PET and SPECT have included

Determination of regional cerebral blood flow, glucose metabolism and oxygen utilisation
- Hypometabolism may be seen following a stroke. The affected area may exceed that with a demonstrable lesion on conventional CT or MR imaging.
- The epileptogenic focus may show interictal hypometabolism (ictal hypermetabolism may be demonstrated with SPECT).
- Regional hypometabolism may be seen in Alzheimer's, Parkinson's and related degenerative conditions.
- 'Pseudodementia' secondary to psychiatric disease such as depression (with normal SPECT scans) may sometimes be differentiated from dementia due to 'organic' neurological disease (with regional hypoperfusion), although psychiatric diseases may themselves be associated with regional hypoperfusion.

In vivo pharmacology (e.g. distribution of neurotransmitter receptors).

Cranial CT

Now widely available; it should be considered a basic neurological tool.

Look for
- Disturbances in the normal anatomy of the ventricular system.
- Skull base and vault.
- Width of cortical fissures/sulci.
- Midline shift.
- Areas of abnormal tissue density.
- Opacity or lucency of sinuses.
- Normal flow voids.

High density ('white') signal
- Fresh blood.
- Calcification:
  - Slow growing tumour.
  - AVM/aneurysm.
  - Hamartoma.
  - In pineal/choroid plexus/basal ganglia, may be normal.

Low density ('black') signal
- Infarction.
- Tumour.
- Abscess.
- Oedema.
- Encephalitis.
- Resolving haematoma.

Mixed density
- Tumour.
- Abscess.
- AVM.
- Contusion.
- Haemorrhagic infarct.

After administration of IV contrast medium, areas with a breakdown in the blood–brain barrier may 'enhance' (appear 'white'). This may reveal previously 'invisible' lesions (isodense with the surrounding tissue). Especially useful for tumour and infection.

Common patterns of enhancement include
- Ring enhancement of tumours and abscesses.
- Solid enhancement of meningiomas.
- Meningeal enhancement with meningeal disease involvement.

CT of spine
MRI is usually preferable but plain CT can give information about the discs and bony architecture. After myelography compressive lesions can be demonstrated.

📕OHCM p394.

Magnetic resonance imaging (MRI) *or* nuclear magnetic resonance (NMR) imaging

For most applications, MRI is superior to CT, but has more restricted availability.

Note: MRI is not safe in the presence of ferromagnetic materials (e.g. certain prostheses, metal filings in the eye).

Most common sequences are T1 and T2, but increasingly other sequences are being used clinically, such as FLAIR, proton density.

In general
- T1 CSF is hypointense ('black'); fat and mature blood clot white.
- T2 CSF is hyperintense ('white').

MRI with enhancement
Intravenously administered gadolinium leaks through areas of damaged blood--brain barrier to give a marked enhancement.
- Ischaemia.
- Infection.
- Tumour (may help differentiate from surrounding oedema).
- Active demyelination.

MR venography and angiography
MR may be used to obtain non-invasive images of blood vessels by using special MRI sequences and image reconstruction. While standard angiog-

T1	T2	Tissue or lesion
Good anatomical detail	Reveals most pathology better than T1	
Hypointense	Hyperintense	CSF
Hyperintense	Iso-intense	Fat, e.g. dermoid, lipoma, some metastases (melanoma), atheroma
Very hypointense	Very hyperintense	Cyst, hygroma
Hypointense	Hyperintense	Ischaemia, oedema, demyelination, many malignant tumours
Hyperintense	Moderately hyperintense	Subacute or chronic haemorrhage
Iso	Hypointense	Acute haemorrhage
Iso	Iso	Meningioma

raphy remains a 'gold standard' for many purposes, MR angiography has the advantage of being non-invasive and therefore 'safe'. MRA images flow rather than structure, and therefore may fail to 'pick up' low flow abnormalities such as cavernous angiomas.

Uses
- Assessment of patency of major arterial and venous vessels.
- Visualisation of large (~3mm diameter) aneurysms.

Functional MRI (FMRI)
A recent development allows certain (indirect) indices of neural activity (most commonly changes reflecting regional perfusion) to be imaged with sufficient temporal resolution to be useful for both research and clinical applications (although FMRI has been largely a research tool to date). As a conventional MRI machine, albeit with special software, is required, it is likely that FMRI will become a widely used clinical tool.

Clinical and research applications have included
- Demonstration of the language areas prior to epilepsy surgery.
- Demonstration of the functional anatomy of cognitive, sensory and motor processes.

📖OHCM p394.

Frackowiak RSJ et al. (2000) Functional neuroimaging, pp 665–675 in Neurology in Clinical Practice, 3rd Edition, eds Bradley WG et al., Butterworth-Heinemann, Boston.

Nerve conduction studies

Sensory nerve action potential (SNAP) and sensory conduction velocity

Procedure
Orthodromic conduction velocity: electrically stimulates distal sensory branches (e.g. index finger) and records the evoked sensory nerve action potential (SNAP) proximally (e.g. over median nerve at wrist). The distance between the two sites (D) and the latency (L) of the onset of the SNAP determine the sensory conduction velocity (D/L). The SNAP amplitude is also useful.

Antidromic conduction velocity: supramaximal electrical stimulation proximally; records distally (e.g. by a ring electrode on little finger). By varying the position of the stimulating electrode, the conduction velocity in various portions of the nerve may be ascertained.

Motor velocities are more commonly measured

Typical values	Latency	Amplitude
Median nerve (index finger to wrist)	2–3ms	9–40mV
Ulnar nerve (little finger to wrist)	2–2.6ms	6–30mV
Sural nerve (midcalf to below med. mall.)	2–4ms	5–40mV

med. mall, medial malleolus.

What does it mean?
- ↓ SNAP amplitude or SNAP absence altogether imply a lesion distal to the dorsal root ganglion.
- ↓ velocity/↑ latency—see table below.

Motor conduction velocity

Procedure
Supramaximally stimulate a peripheral nerve trunk at a proximal (p) and a more distal (d) site. Record the time to the onset of the evoked muscle response (CMAP) from each (Tp and Td), and the distance between them (D). The motor conduction velocity between p and d is therefore D/(Tp−Td).

Typical values
- Median nerve in forearm (to abductor pollicis brevis) >48m/s.
- Ulnar nerve in forearm (to abductor digiti minimi) >48m/s.
- Common peroneal nerve (to extensor digitorum brevis) >40m/s.

What does it mean?
See table below.

Distal motor latency
Latency from stimulation of most distal site on nerve to CMAP.

Typical values
- Median nerve (wrist to abductor pollicis brevis) <4.1m/s.
- Ulnar nerve (wrist to abductor digiti minimi) <3.8m/s.
- Radial nerve (spiral groove to brachioradialis) <5m/s.

Note: These latencies include time taken for impulses to pass along the most distal (unmyelinated) portion of the nerve, and for transmission at the neuromuscular junction (therefore they may not be used to calculate nerve conduction velocities). Compare with velocities elsewhere in the nerve being studied.

What does it mean?
↑ DML seen in:
- Conditions in which the very distal segment of a nerve is compromised (most commonly carpal tunnel syndrome).
- Early demyelinating neuropathy (e.g Guillain-Barré Syndrome).
- Chronic demyelinating neuropathy.

Compound motor action potential (CMAP)
The waveform, amplitude and area-under-the-curve of the CMAP reflect the number of depolarised muscle fibres (e.g. reduced in axonal neuropathy and denervated muscle) and the temporal dispersion of conduction velocities in the motor neurones to them (e.g. increased in demyelinating neuropathy).

	Conduction velocity	AP amplitude	AP dispersion
Axonal neuropathy	late stage: ↓ distally > proximally (loss of fastest conducting axons)	late stage: ↓	not seen
Demyelination	marked		greater dispersion, perhaps especially in acquired not inherited demyelination
Ganglionopathies	slowing proportional to loss of large fibres; often not marked	↓ proportional to loss of large fibres; often not marked	not seen

Note: limbs should be warm; look for asymmetries.
What are your laboratory's current values?

Late responses

F wave:
- If a motor nerve is stimulated, there are orthodromically directed action potentials that may cause a response in the muscle (CMAP). However, antidromically directed action potentials will also pass proximally towards the cell body. If these result in sufficient depolarisation of the axon hillock, then a second orthodromic volley will pass down the nerve. This may cause a second motor action potential (the F wave). Therefore the F wave (i) does not involve synapses (other than the neuro-

muscular junction of course) and (ii) depends on the integrity of the whole axon.
- It may be difficult to elicit.

Delay or absence of the F wave may reflect a lesion proximal to the site of stimulation, in parts of the nerve that may be inaccessible to electrodes, e.g. brachial plexopathy or thoracic outlet syndrome. May also be an early feature in GBD.

H wave:
- This is 'an electrical ankle jerk': submaximal stimulation of posterior tibial nerve in the popliteal fossa causes trans-synaptic activation of soleus, recorded as a CMAP.
- Amplitude may be ↓ by afferent or efferent problems, e.g. neuropathy or radiculopathy.

Repetitive stimulation
Procedure
- Stimulate a motor nerve with short trains of 2–4Hz while recording evoked CMAPs.

Normal response
- No change in CMAP potential.

In myasthenia gravis
- >10% decrement in CMAP amplitude after 1–2 of stimulation.
- After 10–30 of voluntary contraction of the muscle, the CMAP returns to normal.

In Lambert-Eaton myasthenic syndrome
After voluntary contraction, or after rapid stimulation (20–50Hz), the CMAP amplitude, often initially small, increases by 25% (suggestive) or 100% (diagnostic). At a slow (3Hz) rate of stimulation, there is a response decrement.

EMG

Procedure
- A concentric needle electrode is usually used.
- It is inserted into the muscle to be studied.
- The difference in potential between the inner part of the electrode and the outer core is amplified and displayed on an oscilloscope or computer screen.
- It is also 'displayed' as an auditory signal, and experienced electromyo- graphers as much listen to as watch the pattern of electrical activity.

Aminoff MJ, ed. (1992) *Electrodiagnosis in Clinical Neurology*, Churchill Livingstone, New York; sec- tions of *Neurology in Clinical Practice*, eds Bradley WG et al., Butterworth-Heinemann, Boston: EEG and EPs (pp473–496), EMG and NCS (pp497–519).

Normal muscle is 'silent' (electrically inactive) at rest (there is no 'spontaneous activity'), although there will be a brief burst of activity when the electrode is first inserted (the 'insertional activity').

The electrode can pick up electrical activity from muscle fibres within about 0.5mm of its tip, therefore muscle fibres from several motor units (each innervated by a different motor neurone) in this volume can contribute to the signal. However, with care, potentials from a single motor unit may be recorded when a cooperative subject tries to exert the muscle a little (the 'motor unit potential'). With increasing muscular effort, more muscle fibres are recruited, giving rise to the 'interference pattern'.

Various nerve and muscle problems cause characteristic alterations to these four patterns of activity
1. Insertional.
2. Spontaneous.
3. Motor unit potential.
4. Recruitment.
5. In addition, certain other patterns may be observed in certain diseases (myotonia).

1. Insertional activity
- Usually there is a brief burst of potentials which lasts <1.
- Insertional activity is normal in upper motor neurone (UMN) lesions and most non-inflammatory myopathies.
- It may be longer lasting in lower motor neurone (LMN) lesions, inflammatory myopathies and acid maltase deficiency.
- In myotonia, myotonic discharges occur (see below).

2. Spontaneous activity
- Normal muscles at rest are silent.
- This is also the case in UMN lesions, non-inflammatory myopathies (unless secondary denervation has set in) and myotonia.
- Fibrillation potentials and positive sharp waves are seen in LMN lesions and inflammatory myopathies. They occur in regular bursts of constant amplitude (unlike activity related to voluntary contraction).
- Fibrillation potentials are spontaneous APS in irritable, acutely denervated, muscle fibres. They are low amplitude brief negative potentials.
- Positive sharp waves are brief positive potentials, followed by a negative wave. Typically they can be seen for 2–3 weeks after denervation, but may persist.

3. Motor unit potentials (MUPS)
- If the electrode is positioned quite close to the fibres of a motor unit which is active during slight voluntary contraction, then a motor unit potential may be recorded. In normal muscle (and in UMN lesions), this waveform is triphasic, 5–10ms and has an amplitude of 0.5–1mV (larger muscles have larger motor units).
- In myopathies and muscular dystrophies, the motor units are smaller and polyphasic. They tend to be briefer but in some cases last longer than usual.
- In denervated and then reinnervated muscles (typically LMN lesions), the size of individual motor units increases (as the surviving motor neurones 'take over' the muscle fibres previously innervated by now absent other motor neurones). MUPs therefore are of greater amplitude and duration, and are polyphasic.

- In myotonia, myotonic discharges are seen.
Note: Up to 15–20% of MUPs in 'normal' muscle may be polyphasic.

4. Recruitment
- Normally, as the strength of voluntary contraction increases, increasing numbers of motor units are recruited, and these units tend to be larger (Heinneman's size principle). The potentials due to these active units overlap, and become difficult and finally impossible to tell apart— a full 'interference pattern', usually well below maximum voluntary contraction.
- In muscle diseases, a full interference pattern may be produced, but it is of low amplitude. In weak muscles, there may be 'early recruitment' (i.e. recruitment of many motor units at low levels of voluntary contraction).
- In denervated muscles, a full interference pattern may not be achieved, because of the decreased number of motor units.
- In UNM lesions, there is a lower frequency of 'normal' MUPs.

5. Other phenomena: myotonia
High frequency repetitive discharges occurring after voluntary movement or provoked by moving the electrode. The amplitude and the frequency wax and wane, giving the auditory signature likened to the sound of a Second World War dive bomber (or a motor cycle).

Note: Following the onset of a neuropathy, it may take at least 10–14 days for evidence of denervation to appear in the EMG, therefore a repeat study after this time is often useful.

Single fibre EMG
A recording electrode with a smaller recording surface than usually used samples a few muscle fibres from a single motor unit (supplied by a single motor neurone). The variability ('jitter') in the timing of action potentials from different muscles should be less than 20–25ms. Conduction block during voluntary contraction may also be shown. These techniques are used to investigate neuromuscular disorders and reinnervation in neuropathies.

EEG

The standard EEG is non-invasive. Electrodes are attached to the scalp with collodion adhesive. Stable recordings may be made for days. Usually they are arranged according to the international 10–20 system. This is a method for positioning electrodes over the scalp in an orderly and reproducible fashion. Additional electrodes can be applied to the scalp, depending on the region of interest.

Standard recording conditions
- **Rest.**
- **Hyperventilation** for 3–5min, can activate generalised epileptiform changes (and precipitate absence seizures):

- Can ↑ frequency of focal discharge.
- Can ↑ slow wave abnormalities.
- **Photic stimulation** (a strobe light at 30cm with a frequency of 1–50Hz); this can produce several patterns of activity:
  Photoparoxysmal response: bilateral spike or spike and wave discharges not time-locked to the visual stimulus, which may outlast the visual stimulus by hundreds of milliseconds. Generalised, but may have frontal or occipital predominance.
  - Commonly seen in idiopathic generalised epilepsies.
  High voltage occipital spikes, time-locked to the stimulus.
  - Weakly associated with epilepsy.
  Photomyogenic (photomyoclonic) responses: non-specific mostly frontal spikes due to muscle activity.
  - Associated with alcohol and some other drug-withdrawal states.
- **Sleep studies:**
  - Subject either stays awake the night before the recording or is given a small dose of choral prior to the recording (sometimes both).
  - Subjects tend to show the earlier stages of non-REM sleep.
  - These studies increase the yield of EEG abnormalities, including epileptiform ones.
  - By capture of 'natural sleep': certain seizure types are more common in sleep (e.g. juvenile myoclonic epilepsy).
  - Sleep deprivation itself increases the number of seizures and epileptiform changes.

📖 *Polysomnography* (p407).

The normal EEG

There are a wide range of normal EEG phenomena. Some of the common patterns in the awake adult are listed in the table below.

EEG abnormalities (not peri- or per-seizure)
- A variety of EEG abnormalities may be seen outside the peri- or per-seizure period.
- Abnormalities in the EEG are not restricted to the appearance of abnormal waveforms.
- The loss, or redistribution in the scalp location, of normal background activities is abnormal.

The classification of EEG abnormalities is complex. Below is a highly simplified guide
1. General excess of slow waves: commonly seen in:
   - Metabolic encephalopathy.
   - Encephalitis.
   - Post-ictal states.
2. Focal slow waves: commonly seen in:
   - Large cerebral lesions (e.g. tumour, haematoma).
   - Post-ictal states.
   - Migraineurs.
3. Localised intermittent rhythmic slow waves: may be seen in:
   - Idiopathic generalised and localisation related epilepsies.
4. Epileptiform abnormalities:

Activity	Frequency (Hz)	Amplitude (mV)	Scalp location	Behavioural state
alpha	8–12	20–60 eyes close	usually occipital	maximum relaxed, awake,
beta	>13	10–20	frontocentral slow wave sleep 1 and 2	wakeful, drowsy; REM and
theta	4–8	variable diffuse	frontocentral, temporal SWS (slow wave sleep)	minimally awake, drowsy,
delta	<4	variable	diffuse	awake; drowsy
mu	8–10	20–60	central	awake, suppressed in voluntary movements

The terms alpha, beta, theta and delta are often used to describe the background activity but are also used to describe the frequency of EEG activity.

Sharp activity may be a normal phenomenon.

- Spikes (if last <80ms) or sharp waves (80–200ms) may be associated with slow waves.
- Consistently focal spikes suggest epilepsy with a focal seizure onset.

Note: 2–4% of non-epileptics have occasional spikes or sharps.

5. Repetitive stereotyped 'periodic' complexes.

EEG patterns may show periodicity. These patterns may be epileptiform or not, and may be focal or generalised. They are an abnormal EEG feature, the interpretation of which depends on the clinical context.

Examples include
- Burst suppression: bursts of generalised high voltage mixed waveforms, alternating with generalised voltage suppression:
  - Coma.
  - Late stage status epilepticus (both convulsive and non-convulsive).
- Triphasic waves over one or both temporal lobes:
  - Common in herpes simplex encephalitis.
- Periodic lateralised epileptiform discharges (PLEDS) are localised sharp or slow wave complexes 0.2–1s long, every 1–5s.
  - Non-specific but suggest localised cerebral insult (stroke, haematoma, tumour).
  - Occasionally seen in migraine and focal epilepsies.
- BIPLEDS are bihemispheric PLEDs.
  - Suggest more widespread insults, e.g. anoxia, encephalitis.
- Bilateral or generalised high voltage complexes for 0.5–2s every 4–15s:
  - Characteristic of subacute sclerosing panencephalitis.
- Triangular waves:
  - Characteristic of Creutzfeldt-Jakob disease (CJD).
  - Not seen in VCJD may see a 'disorganised' EEG without repetitive complexes).
- Runs of broad triphasic waves (1.5–3Hz).
  - Severe metabolic encephalopathy (e.g. renal or hepatic failure).
- Periodic spikes or sharp waves; bi or multiphasic morphology (0.5–2Hz); usually generalised—suggest severe encephalopathy, e.g.
  - Herpes encephalitis.
  - CJD (in setting of rapid dementia and myoclonus).
  - Lithium intoxication.
  - Post-anoxic brain injury.
  - Tricyclic antidepressant overdose.

EEGs in epilepsy

Idiopathic (primary) generalised epilepsy (IGEs)
- Generalised, bilaterally synchronous epileptiform discharges with virtually normal background.
- Absence epilepsy: 3Hz spike and wave.
- Juvenile myoclonic epilepsy (JME): 6Hz multiple spike and wave.

Symptomatic (secondary) generalised epilepsy
- More variable.
- Interictal background activity: excess slow.

- Interictal epileptiform activity: irregular spikes or sharp and slow waves 1.5–4Hz. Usually generalised, but may show asymmetry or (multi) focal features.

Localisation-related partial epilepsy
- Interictal EEG is often normal, particularly if the focus is located deeply (especially common with frontal foci).
- There may be lateralised or localised spikes or sharp waves.

How to use the EEG

In suspected epilepsy
- Routine EEG with photic stimulation and hyperventilation gives about up to a 50% detection rate for interictal epileptiform abnormalities in a subject with epilepsy (higher 'yield' in primary generalised epilepsies than in localisation-related epilepsies).
- Sleep-deprived or choral-induced sleep recording: this may increase the yield of EEG abnormalities to up to 60–70%.
- Consider 24h or longer ambulatory EEG, ideally with audio/video monitoring. Most useful in helping to determine the nature of the seizure in a subject with frequent (e.g. daily) attacks.

In general, avoid reduction in antiepileptic drugs or drugs such as pentylenetrazole to induce seizures, except in exceptional circumstances, e.g. videotelemetry as part of workup for epilepsy surgery.

Note:
- No interictal spikes does not imply no epilepsy.
- Similarly, interictal spikes do not always imply epilepsy.
- A negative ictal EEG does not necessarily imply a non-epileptic ('pseudo') seizure, especially in simple partial and some brief complex partial seizures. Scalp electrodes may fail to record deep, especially frontal, activity.
- However, a tonic-clonic seizure with loss of consciousness should be associated with an epileptiform EEG during the ictus. This EEG activity may be obscured by muscle artefact, but post-ictal slowing may be seen (*see below*).
- The EEG may be slow after a tonic-clonic seizure for many tens of minutes.

405

Note: The diagnosis of epilepsy is mainly clinical!

In established epilepsy
- Classification (e.g. complex partial seizure (CPS) *vs.* absence).
- Assessment of frequency of seizures (e.g. ambulatory EEG to assess frequency of absence seizures).
- Reduction in interictal discharges in some syndromes (e.g. absence, photosensitive epilepsy) correlates with AED efficacy.

In focal cerebral dysfunction
Often not particularly helpful. Modern imaging studies usually provide more information.
- Small, deep or slow growing lesions often cause no effects.
- Asymmetric voltage attenuation may be caused by a subdural haematoma (or other fluid collection) overlying the cortex.
- Direct grey matter involvement may cause alteration/loss of normal EEG, or cause epileptiform discharges.
- Subcortical white matter changes can cause localised polymorphic slow waves.
- Deeper subcortical lesions tend to produce more widespread slow wave disturbances.

In CNS infections
- CJD and subacute sclerosing panencephalilits (SSPE) have relatively characteristic EEG associations.
- Meningitis and encephalitis cases may show diffuse background disturbances and polymorphic or bilateral intermittent slow wave abnormalities.
- Encephalitis usually causes more changes than meningitis.
- Focal changes may be seen over abscesses and in cases of herpes simplex encephalitis.

In dementia
- To exclude some conditions such as toxic encephalopathy, non convulsive status epilepticus (NCSE).
- A few dementing conditions have characteristic EEGs (CJD, SSPE).
- Slowing of background frequency occurs in Alzheimer's disease, but values may overlap with those of the normal aged, therefore not very helpful clinically.

In confusional states
- Helpful in diagnosing NCSE (absence and complex partial status).
- To exclude cerebral dysfunction.
- Not very useful in psychiatric diagnosis *per se*, but an abnormal EEG in a confusional state may help exclude psychogenic causes for an apparent reduction in level of consciousness.

In toxic-metabolic encephalopathies
- EEG always abnormal.
- Diffuse slowing in mild cases.
- Other abnormalities may develop in later stages.
- Specific patterns may be seen in certain aetiologies.
- Excess fast activity: barbiturate and benzodiazepine toxicity.
- Triphasic waves: hepatic and renal failure, anoxia, hypoglycaemia, hyperosmolality, lithium toxicity.
- Periodic spikes or sharp waves: anoxia, renal failure, lithium and tricyclic antidepressant toxicity.

In coma
- EEG, especially serial EEGs, provides an indication of degree of cerebral dysfunction.
- In general, any 'normal'-looking EEG, spontaneous variability, sleep–wake changes, and reaction to external stimuli are relatively good prognostic signs.

- An invariant, unreactive EEG is a poor prognostic sign; the pattern however is not uniform, it may include periodic spikes of sharp waves, episodic voltage attenuation, alpha coma, burst suppression.
- May give some diagnostic clues, e.g. localised abnormality—supratentorial mass lesion; persistent epileptiform discharges—status epilepticus.
- 'Alpha coma': monotonous unresponsive alpha with anterior distribution seen after cardio/respiratory arrest is a poor prognostic feature.
- Monotonous but partially reactive alpha may follow brainstem infarcts.

Invasive EEG techniques

These are generally restricted to specialist centres, most commonly used in the pre-surgical workup of patients.

Foramen ovale electrodes, corticography (usually done by laying strips of electrodes on the surface of the brain) and depth EEG (electrodes implanted into the parenchyma of the brain) may be used, depending on the region of interest. Sphenoidal electrodes are rarely used today, but can give useful EEG information about the medial temporal structures.

Sodium amytal (Wada) test

Sodium amytal is injected into the R or L internal carotid artery. It is a short-acting barbiturate, and temporarily causes hemispheric dysfunction on the injected side. If injected into the left in most right-handers, the ability to speak and continue to hold up the R arm is temporally impaired. If speech is preserved following R-sided injection, it suggests normal left-lateralisation for language function. More complex testing may also be undertaken during the period of hemispheric dysfunction, but it is usually used to determine language dominance prior to certain neurosurgical procedures.

Polysomnography

- This is the multimodal recording used in the analysis of sleep-related disorders.
- There is concurrent recording of EMG, EEG and EOG (electro-oculography—eye movements), often with audiovisual channels. Other physiological parameters may also be recorded, e.g. nasal air flow, chest expansion.

Sleep is classically divided into 4 stages (1–4), of progressively 'deeper' slow wave sleep (SWS), and a fifth stage of rapid eye movement (REM) sleep, characterised physiologically by bursts of rapid eye movements (saccades).

Stage	Behaviour	Main EEG pattern	Comments
1	drowsy	diffuse alpha →theta flat to medium	
2	light sleep	high theta	K complexes
3	medium sleep	delta	broad K complexes delta activation
4	deep sleep	continuous delta	none
REM	rapid eye movements		

There is progression through stages 1 to 4, and several episodes of REM during a typical night's sleep. Polysomnography can be important in understanding the pathophysiology of the insomnias, parasomnias and other sleep patterns.

Multiple sleep latency test

This is a diagnostic test for narcolepsy. Following a good night's sleep, normal subjects typically enter REM sleep with a latency of >>10min (usually ~90min). In narcolepsy the latency is <10min.

Sensory evoked potentials or responses (EPs or ERs)

While many techniques and protocols have been developed in research laboratories, there are only a few techniques in widespread clinical use. A stimulus is delivered to the periphery, thus activating a sensory system and evoking an electrical response over a more central, often cortical, area. Multiple surface electrode recordings time-locked to the peripheral stimulus are recorded and averaged, to help eliminate ongoing random background 'noise' from the sensory stimulus-evoked 'signal'. Deviations of this evoked potential or response (EP or ER) from the norm (especially in latency and waveform) suggest pathology in the sensory pathway tested.

Visual EPs

Pattern-evoked VEP

An alternating chequerboard pattern (temporal frequency 1–2Hz) is presented to each eye individually. The EP is recorded over the occipital (primary visual) cortex. Most commonly the first large positive wave, called P1 or P100 (as it typically occurs at about 100ms), is studied.

A delayed, smaller or dispersed VEP indicates disease in the retino-geniculo-striate pathway (if severe refractive errors or cataracts have been excluded), but most commonly affecting the optic nerve (a uniocular deficit implies a lesion anterior to the optic chiasm) or at the chiasm.

Flash-evoked VEP

In subjects with very poor vision or fixation, and in the very young, a bright flash may be used as the stimulus. This gives less reproducible results, particularly in the P100 latency.

Common uses
The VEP is used in general to document intrinsic, inflammatory or compressive lesions of the optic nerve (or chiasm).
1. Suspected optic or retrobulbar neuritis.
2. In a patient with suspected MS, evidence of a VEP abnormality in an asymptomatic eye would suggest a previous episode of an optic neuritis.
3. Evaluation of hysterical blindness (may need to use a strobe light stimulus if patient non-cooperative).
4. Evaluation of optic nerve function in compressive lesions such as dysthyroid eye disease, optic nerve glioma.
5. Follow up after surgery to decompress the optic nerve or chiasm.
6. Assessment of poor visual acuity in patients unable to cooperate with usual testing. Vary the size of the chequerboard squares; subjects with poor acuity will only have a VEP to the coarser patterns.

Somatosensory EPs
- Stimulation site over a peripheral nerve, eg. ulnar or median at wrist, common peroneal at knee, posterior tibial at ankle.
- Record over Erb's point (above the medial end of the clavicle), C7 or C2 vertebra, parietal cortex for arm stimulation; L1, C7, C2 or vertex for leg stimulation.
- Calculate absolute and interpeak latencies.
- Need to show with nerve conduction studies (NCS) that distal parts of the somatosensory pathways are conducting normally.
- Assesses dorsal column not anterolateral (spinothalamic) tract pathways:
  - E.g. stimulate median nerve at wrist, prolonged latency to Erb's point; suggests brachial plexus (or more distal) lesion.
  - Prolonged Erb's point to C2 latency suggests spinal cord lesion.

Uses
- Diagnosis of plexopathies.
- Evaluation of subclinical myelopathy in possible MS.
- Evaluation of hysterical sensory loss.
- Per-operative monitoring (e.g. during scoliosis surgery).

Brainstem auditory evoked potentials (BAEPs, BAERs, BSAEPs)
- Stimulus: rarefaction clicks of 50 or 100ms duration, presented monoaurally at 10Hz at 60–70DB above threshold (masking noise to other ear).
- Record over mastoid and vertex of skull.
- Classic waveform has seven peaks, said to be generated by sequential auditory nuclei:

I	VIIIth nerve (must be present to interpret subsequent waves)
II	Cochlear nucleus (may be absent in normals)
III	Superior olive
IV	Lateral lemniscus (may be absent in normals)
V	Interior colliculus (should be 50% or more of wave I's amplitude)
VI	Medial geniculate (too variable for regular clinical use)
VII	Auditory thalamocortical radiation (too variable for regular clinical use)

Latency I to V (central conduction time) should be no more than 4.75ms. The difference between left and right central conduction times should be <0.4ms.

Uses

- Hearing assessment, especially in children.
- Evaluation in suspected MS and other myelinopathies (e.g. adrenoleukodystrophy; MRI more important now).
- Evaluation and detection of posterior fossa lesions (eg. acoustic neuromas; MRI more important now).
- Evaluation of brainstem function (e.g. tumour, CVAs).
- Evaluation of brainstem function in coma and brain death.
- Per-operative, e.g. acoustic neuroma excision.

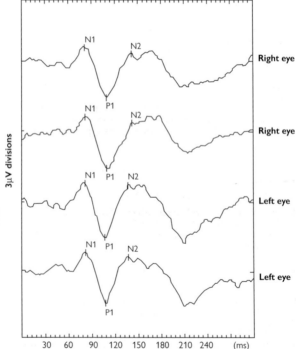

Fig. 9.1 Visual evoked potential (to checkerboard stimulus).

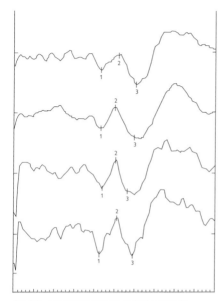

Fig. 9.2 Leg somatosensory evoked potentials.

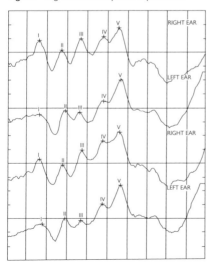

Fig. 9.3 Brainstem auditory evoked potentials.

Transcranial magnetic stimulation (TMS)

- Brief, high-current pulse produced in a circular or figure-of-eight-shaped coil held over the scalp.
- This induces a magnetic field with flux perpendicular to the coil.
- This in turn produces an electric field perpendicular to the magnetic field.
- The result is excitation or inhibition of the subjacent cortex (depending on stimulus parameters).

Measurement of central motor conduction time

- TMS over the motor cortex indirectly (presumably via synaptic activation of corticospinal neurones) causes a volley of activity in the corticospinal tracts. The latency of the EMG in, say, the abductor digiti minimi may be measured.
- May be used in cervical myelopathy and MS to show increased latency of EMG in hand muscles evoked by TMS over the motor cortex. If the EMG latency to more distal stimulation (e.g. at C7 over the spinal cord and in the ulnar nerve) is normal, then an increased central motor conduction time may be inferred.
- Latency may also be increased in other neurogenerative conditions.

Psychogenic limb weakness

Some authorities have used TMS to evoke muscle activity in 'paralysed' limbs in patients with psychogenic paralysis. This needs to be done in the context of an 'holistic' approach to the patient, aimed at dealing with any psychological pathology.

Potential clinical applications

There have been many TMS studies; some that may prove useful as clinical tests, e.g.

- Determination of lateralisation of language function by repetitive TMS (rTMS) prior to surgery for epilepsy.
- Assessment of cortical excitability in certain epilepsy syndromes.
- Assessment of decreased intracortical inhibition in dystonia.

Neurological investigation of sphincter disturbance

EMG

- Of pelvic floor muscles may be helpful in faecal incontinence, stress urinary incontinence and cauda equina syndrome.
- Pelvic floor and sphincter muscle EMGs may reflect pudendal nerve damage.
- Anal sphincter EMG abnormalities may reflect damage to Onuf's nucleus, e.g. in multi-system atrophy. It is characteristically unaffected in motor neurone disease.

MRI

- In suspected sacral spinal cord, conus medullaris and equina equina lesions.

Fowler CJ. (2000) Neurourology, pp 743–757 in *Neurology in Clinical Practice*, 3rd edition, eds Bradley WG et al., Butterworth-Heinemann, Boston.

Urodynamics

Flowmetry
- Measurement of rate and amount of urine flow over time.
- Allows calculation of parameters such as time to maximal flow, maximum and mean flow rate, volume voided.
- Post-micturition ultrasound can determine residual volume.

Cystometry (needs urinary catheterisation)
- Measurement of intravesicular pressure during filling (usually at 50mL/min) or emptying. Typically bladder filling sensation starts at about 100mL, and the bladder is full at 400–600 mL (with no more than a 15cm of water rise in pressure). Detrusor instability may cause sharp rises in the pressure during filling.
- During voiding, flow rate should be >15mL/min (♂) or >20mL/min (♀) with pressures of <50cmH$_2$O (♂) or 30 cmH$_2$O (♀).

Edrophonium (Tensilon) test

Procedure
- Explain the test to patient.
- Select weak and/or fatiguable muscles to be assessed.
- Attach ECG monitor.
- Draw up 0.6mg atropine (for use if extreme bradycardia develops), 10mg of edrophonium in 5mL normal saline (A), 5mL normal saline (B) and, saline flush.
- Administer 1mL of test solution (A or B, ideally patient and administrating physician should be blinded to the nature of the solution).
- If no adverse reaction, administer remaining 4mL.
- Repeat with other solution (B or A).

Note: If the diagnosis of MG is clinically obvious, and the patient has responded to pyridostigmine given empirically, there is little point in stopping this and performing an edrophonium test.

413

Interpretation
- In myasthenia gravis, there should be a response within 30–60s, which should wear off in 2–4min.
- There may be a response in LEMS, polymyositis and motor neurone disease (MND).

Biopsies

- Always liaise with those taking the biopsy and those processing it!
- A biopsy should be undertaken to answer specific questions, in the light of a differential diagnosis formulated following history, examination and other investigations.

Skeletal muscle

Indications
- Primary muscle disease, e.g. metabolic myopathy, polymyositis, muscular dystrophy.
- Neurogenic atrophy.
- Mitochondrial cytopathies (even in the absence of clinical muscle involvement).
- Multi-organ disease, e.g. vasculitides.

Which muscle to biopsy?
- An involved but not endstage muscle.
- One that has not been used for EMG recording or had an injection for >1 month.
- Quadriceps and deltoid often used.

Open or needle biopsy?

Open biopsy:
- Larger specimen.
- Can fix specimen at *in situ* length.
- Especially for inflammatory myopathy and in vasculitis.

Needle biopsy:
- Smaller scar.
- Multiple biopsies possible.
- But:
  - Smaller biopsies.
  - Difficulties in orientating the sample.

What may be done to the tissue?
- Routine histology.
- Examination of small blood vessels.
- Histochemistry.
- Electron microscopy.
- Tests of muscle metabolism.
- Mitochondrial DNA studies.

Nerve

Indications
- Distinction between segmental demyelination and axonal degeneration (if not already determined).
- Certain neuropathies with characteristic histological features, e.g. due to amyloid deposition, sarcoid, vasculitis, neoplastic involvement.
- Certain myelinopathies (e.g. leukodystrophies) with PNS and CNS involvement.

Which nerve to biopsy?
- The cutaneous branch of the sural nerve at the ankle (usually).
- Superficial peroneal (sometimes).
- Superficial radial (occasionally).
- Occasionally small motor nerve twigs are obtained in muscle biopsy.
- Overlying skin may be co-biopsied.

What is done?
- 2–3cm of full-thickness nerve or fascicle.

What may be done to the tissue?
- Routine light microscopy (morphometry, structural survey; amyloidosis).
- Frozen section light microscopy (immunochemistry).
- Electron microscopy (ultrastructure).
- Teased out single fibres (to examine sequential myelin internodes).

Brain/meningeal biopsy

Indications
- Diagnosis and management of suspected primary and some metastatic brain tumours.
- Differential diagnosis of other mass lesions (inflammatory and infective).
- Differentiation of radiation necrosis and tumour regrowth.
- Differentiation of neoplastic and non-neoplastic cysts (and their drainage).
- Diagnostic biopsy of a suspected infectious lesion that has not responded to a trial of therapy.
- Diagnosis of cerebral vasculitis or vasculopathy.

What is done?
- High quality cranial CT/MRI, possibly with contrast, to delineate lesion.
- If no discrete lesion, generally an area of non-dominant, non-eloquent cerebrum is taken.
- Stereotactic needle biopsy with image guidance:
  - Deep, small, lesions in 'eloquent' areas.
  - Multiple biopsies along needle track (useful in heterogeneous lesions such as some gliomas).
- And/or open biopsy:
  - Accessible lesions.
  - When resection considered during procedure.
- Intra-operative evaluation of frozen samples:
  - E.g. can a biopsy be made?
  - E.g. is the sample adequate?

Note: Caution in suspected CJD!!

Skin
- Some storage diseases:
  - Lafora body.
  - Batten's disease.
- Mitochondrial cytopathies.

Bone marrow
- Niemann-Pick type C.
- Haematological and other malignancies.

Rectal and appendicectomy
- Most neuronal storage diseases affect the autonomic nervous system, so evidence can be sought in neurones of the gut's intrinsic plexi.
- Amyloid in rectal biopsy.

Tonsillar biopsy
- Research tool in VCJD.

Oligoclonal bands (OCBs)

- Electrophoresis of serum and CSF separates protein components by size and charge.
- OCBs may be present in serum and CSF. Bands in the CSF not seen in the serum suggest intrathecal specific synthesis of immunoglobulins.
- This pattern is seen in most (95%) cases of established MS but may also occur in other conditions such as chronic meningitis, neurosyphilis, SSPE and neurosarcoid (although uncommonly).

Thompson EJ. (1997) Cerebrospinal fluid, pp 443–466 in *Neurological Investigations*, ed Hughes RAC, BMJ Publications, London.

Diagnostic & prognostic antibodies and other markers in blood & urine

Multi-system disorders
PNS and CNS are affected in many multi-system disorders; markers in blood and other fluids and tissues for these are therefore commonly requested in neurology patients.

Vasculitides, e.g.
- Extractable nuclear antigens in SLE.
- ANCA in Wegener's.
- Rheumatoid factor in RA.

Enteropathies, e.g.
- Gliadin and endomysial antibodies in coeliac disease.

Systemic infections, e.g.
- Serology for many diseases e.g. *Borrelia* in Lyme disease; HIV.
- PCR for TB.

Disorders of coagulation: thrombophilia screen currently commonly includes
- Protein S and C levels.
- Antithrombin III levels.
- Screening for the Leiden mutation in factor V.
- Lupus anticoagulant.

Tumour markers, e.g.
- CEA for gut neoplasia.
- Serum and urinary paraproteins in haematological disorders like myeloma.

Sarcoid
- ACE and ACE genotype.

Endocrinopathies, e.g.
- TSH, FT4 and FT3, thyroid autoantibodies in thyroid dysfunction.

Other metabolic disorders, e.g.
- Wilson's disease: blood copper and caeruloplasmin; some authorities also request 24h urinary copper excretion. *Note:* Slit lamp examination performed by an experienced ophthalmologist reveals Kayser-Fleischer rings in most cases of Wilson's disease with neurological involvement.
- Phaeochromocytoma: catecholamine metabolites in three 24h urine collections.

Disease-specific markers
- Anti-acetylcholine receptor antibodies in MG.

Paraneoplastic antibodies

Certain neurological syndromes are 'paraneoplastic', i.e. due to remote but non-metastatic effects of non-nervous system cancers. These paraneoplastic syndromes are rare, but important to recognise. In perhaps 50% of cases, the neurological symptoms may predate those of the cancer. This is an area of intensive research. Antibody tests include:

Antibody	Neurological presentation	Possible underlying cancer
Hu	encephalomyelitis sensory neuronopathy cerebellar degeneration	small cell lung cancer (SCLC)
Yo	cerebellar degeneration	breast ovary
Ri	ataxic myoclonus/opsoclonus	breast ovary SCLC
Tr cerebellar degeneration		Hodgkin's
Anti-voltage-gated calcium channel (VGCC) antibodies	LEMS	SCLC
Anti-amphyphisin	stiff person syndrome	breast SCLC
CV2	limbic encephalitis cerebellar degeneration optic neuritis sensory neuropathy LEMS	SCLC uterine sarcoma thymoma
Anti-recoverin	cancer-associated retinopathy	SCLC

Note: There is no one-to-one relationship between the cancer, the antibody and the paraneoplastic syndrome.

417

Genetic tests

The list of diseases for which we have specific genetic tests grows each month. Individual single gene neurological diseases are rare, but there are a lot of them, so about 0.1% of the population has one!

When might a neurologist refer to a clinical geneticist?
- Genetic counselling of an index patient and his family.
- Cytogenetic or molecular diagnosis.
- Long-term follow up of family:
  - Notification of advances.
  - Counselling family members as they become adult.
  - Coordinating care with paediatric and adult neurologists.

Cytogenetics: when to do it
- Female with an X-linked disorder.
- Unexplained mental retardation.
- Unexplained major CNS malformation.
- The coexistence of two genetic diseases in a patient.

What is done?
- Conventional karyotype.
- Fluorescent *in situ* hybridisation (FISH) for suspected submicroscopic chromosomal aberrations:
  - E.g. a p13.3 deletion may cause lissencephaly.

Molecular genetics: when to do it
- Confirming a clinical diagnosis.
- Identify carriers in the family.

What is done?
An ever-increasing range of diseases may be tested for. Some of these tests may be routinely available at your local clinical genetics lab; others at regional, national or even supranational centres. Other tests may be available on a 'research' basis. It is clear, however, that tests for genetic 'lesions' or risk factors will become increasingly available. Rather than give an, at best, partial list of readily available tests, we give a few examples below of the kinds of tests that are available. The astute reader will spot that different mutations within a given gene can give rise to different clinical phenotypes. Indeed, recent work has shown that the same mutation in some genes can give rise to more than one phenotype: we clearly have a great deal yet to learn about the genetics of neurological diseases!

Detection of deletions
- E.g. in mitochondrial (mt)DNA in MELAS and MERFF.
- E.g. of dystrophin gene in Duchenne and Becker muscular dystrophies.

Detection of DNA rearrangement
- E.g. PMP22 gene duplication in some case of Charcot Marie Tooth disease type 1 (or hereditary motor-sensory neuropathy type 1, (HMSN1); deletions within this gene cause hereditary neuropathy with liability to pressure palsies (HNPP).

Detection of trinucleotide repeats
- Found in >10 neurological diseases.

- So far, there in no overlap in the number of repeats in controls and affected patients (except rarely in Huntingdon's, in the region of 33 to 36 repeats).
- Anticipation (more severe phenotype and earlier onset) often reflects in increased number of repeats in the most recent generations (especially myotonic dystrophy).

Disease	Gene	Triplet repeats	Transmission
Fragile X	FMR1	CGG	X-linked
Myotonic dystrophy	DM	CTG	AD
Friedreich's ataxia	FRDA	GAA	AR
Spinobulbar muscular atrophy	androgen receptor	CAG	X-linked
Huntingdon's disease	IT15	CAG	AD
Spinocerebellar atrophy			
SCA 1	SCA I	CAG	AD
SCA 2	SCA 2	CAG	AD
SCA 3	SCA 3	CAG	AD
SCA 6	SCA 6	CAG	AD
Dentorubropalli-doluysian atrophy	DRPLA	CAG	AD

Note: SCA 6 is a CAG triplet expansion in the CACNL1A4 calcium channel gene. Other (non triplet repeat) mutations in the gene cause other conditions: episodic ataxia type 2 and familial hemiplegic migraine.

A variety of more time-consuming methods may be needed to look at, for example, single base mutations

These involve fragmenting the DNA of the gene into manageable pieces, then amplifying these so that there are multiple copies. Subsequently, various methods may be used to detect fragments with abnormal sequences, even if only differing at a single base from 'wild type'. There are several such techniques, constantly being refined, and many are restricted to research laboratories.

- However, molecular genetics is proceeding at a tremendous pace, both in terms of the number of conditions with identified genetic lesions, and the laboratory techniques for analysis.
- High speed DNA sequencing will facilitate sequencing large pieces of DNA.
- Progress is being made on the analysis of polygenic diseases.
- E.g. point mutations in the MPZ gene, which encodes for P0, a component of the myelin sheath, have been found in some families with Charcot Marie Tooth disease type 1B.

Genetic risk factors

Another area of clinical genetics which is likely to become more important is the detection of genetic 'risk factors' for diseases. Certain allelic variants, whilst not 'causing' a disease in the traditional sense, may predispose an individual to exhibiting a certain clinical phenotype, or alter the age at which it might become apparent.

- E.g. there are three allelic variants in the apolipoprotein E (APOE4) gene, e2, e3, e4. Homozygosity for e4 is likely to be a risk factor for developing Alzheimer's disease, and for developing it at an earlier age. However, the majority of e4 homozygotes do not develop the condition (therefore it is not 'causative').

Detection of the presence of abnormal protein or altered levels of normal protein

Immunocytochemistry and immunoblotting (western blots) on tissue samples from the patient allow direct visualisation of the presence of abnormal protein, or absence or reduced levels of normal protein, in a variety of conditions. (These techniques are not genetic in the strictest sense, but are often useful in 'genetic' conditions.)

- E.g. Duchenne and Becker muscular dystrophies have absent or reduced levels of dystrophin in muscle biopsy samples.

Useful website

Online Mendelian Inheritance in Man (OMIM) is a continually updated catalogue of 'genetic' diseases in man, giving data about the genotype, mode of inheritance and the clinical phenotype of thousands of disorders (not just neurological).

🖰 http://www.ncbi.nim.nih.gov/Omim/

Young AB. (1998) Huntingdon's disease and other trinucleotide repeat disorders, pp 35–54 in *Scientific American Molecular Neurology*, ed Martin JB, Scientific American, New York.

Biochemical tests

Some basic principles

Many autosomal recessive and X-linked metabolic diseases are caused by reduced or absent activity of a specific enzyme, in turn due to a single gene defect. In some there is a tissue-specific deficit:

- E.g. McArdle's (glycogen storage disease V): demonstrates absence of phosphorylase activity in muscle biopsy (as only the myophosphorylase isozyme is affected).

In other conditions, notably the lipidoses, the enzyme is deficient in many tissues:

- E.g. in Niemann-Pick diseases A and B, sphingomyelinase is deficient in brain and spinal cord, but also in the gastrointestinal tract, liver, spleen and bone marrow. Abnormal lipid metabolism can therefore be demonstrated in relatively easily accessible tissue such as fibroblasts.

Not only may the absence or lower activity of an enzyme reduce the amount of the product of the reaction it catalyses, it may lead to the accumulation of precursors in the metabolic pathway:

$$A \xrightarrow{(1)} B \xrightarrow{(2)} C \xrightarrow{(3)} D$$

If enzyme (3) is reduced, A, B and C may accumulate, with lower levels of D than usual being produced:

- E.g. in acute intermittent porphyria, there is increased urinary excretion of δ haemaminolevulinic acid and porphobilinogen (intermediates in the heme synthetic pathway) during an acute attack.
- Decreased levels of porphobilinogen deaminase may be demonstrated in erythrocytes, leucocytes and cultured fibroblasts.

Ischaemic forearm exercise test (ischaemic lactate test)

Procedure
1. Rest patient supine for 30min.
2. Draw a baseline lactate sample from a catheter in an antecubital vein.
3. Inflate sphygmomanometer cuff on that arm to above arterial pressure.
4. Subject squeezes a rubber ball in that hand until exhaustion.
5. Rapidly deflate cuff.
6. Take further venous samples at 30, 60 and 240s.

Results
Normally the venous lactate will rise by 2, 3 or even 4-fold; if it fails to rise by 1.5-fold, then there is likely to be a glycogenolysis or glycolysis defect (or the patient has not exercised sufficiently!):

- E.g. in disorders of glycolysis and glycogenolysis the venous lactate fails to rise in the ischaemic forearm exercise test.

Neuro-otology

Pure tone audiometry
Measure threshold for air and bone conduction at frequencies from 250 to 8000Hz.

Typical patterns
- Conduction deafness BC > AC at all frequencies.
- Sensorineural deafness AC = BC at all frequencies, but increasing deafness as frequency rises.

(AC = air conduction; BC = bone conduction)

More specialised tests
- Tone decay.
- Loudness discomfort.
- Speech audiometry.
- Acoustic impedance.

Caloric testing

Procedure
1. Inspect eardrum; if intact, proceed.
2. Place patient supine with neck flexed 30° (on pillow).
3. Irrigate external auditory meatus with 30°C water (ice water if testing for brain death).
4. Observe for (or record*) nystagmus.
5. Repeat after 5min with 44°C water.

What should happen
1. Cold water induces convection of fluid in ipsilateral lateral semicircular canal (LSCC).
2. There is less output from ipsilateral LSCC.
3. Imbalance of signals from the two LSCCs results in eye drift towards the irrigated ear.
4. Fast phase contraversive movements correct for eye drift (hence nystamus with fast phase away from irrigated ear).
5. This nystagmus starts in about 20s and persists for 1min.
6. Warm water reverses the nystagmus.

Common pathological responses

Canal paresis
1. Reduced duration of nystagmus following irrigation on one side (with cold or warm water).
2. Suggests ipsilateral peripheral or central lesion.

Directional preponderance
1. Prolonged nystagmus in one direction.
2. Suggests central lesion on side of preponderence or contralateral peripheral lesion.

Combination of clinical examination, audiometry and caloric testing of the vestibulo-ocular reflex will help localise a lesion (peripheral *vs.* central; L *vs.* R).

Brainstem auditory evoked responses
📖p409.

*There are various techniques for recording eye movements. Although quite crude, electronystography has the advantage that it requires no instrumentation of the eyeball directly, allows recordings in the dark or with closed eyes (thus abolishing visual fixation and other responses that can interfere with the vestibulo-ocular reflex) and is relatively cheap.

Troost BT, Arguello LC. (2000) Neuro-otology, in *Neurology in Clinical Practice*, 3rd edition, eds Bradley WG et al., Butterworth-Heinemann, Boston.

Renal medicine

Estimation of renal function

Serum creatinine

Creatinine is the non-enzymatic breakdown product of creatine and phosphocreatine (almost exclusively found in skeletal muscle). Daily production is constant in an individual. It is excreted mainly by filtration at the glomerulus, but is also secreted to a certain extent (up to 15%) by the tubules. Because of the secretory component, serum creatinine overestimates GFR, particularly at low GFR. Because of the reciprocal relationship between clearance and serum creatinine, serum creatinine does not rise outside the normal range until there has been a substantial fall in GFR, particularly in patients with low muscle mass (Fig. 10.1). However, in an individual patient, a progressive increase in serum creatinine over time, even within the normal range, implies declining GFR. Wide variation between individuals based on muscle mass, sex and age make serum creatinine an imperfect screening test for renal failure.

Drugs, e.g. cimetidine, trimethoprim and pyrimethamine, can block the secretory component. Ingestion of cooked meat and severe exercise causes a rapid, temporary rise in serum creatinine.

A variety of formulae have been devised to incorporate age, sex and weight differences to improve the ability of serum creatinine to predict GFR.

> The most popular formula is that of Cockcroft and Gault:
>
> GFR = [140−age (y)] × weight (kg)/serum creatinine (μmol/L)] × 1.23 (♂)
> GFR = [140−age (y)] × weight (kg)/serum creatinine (μmol/L)] × 1.04 (♀)

Serum urea

Urea is synthesised predominantly in the liver (by-product of protein catabolism). Production is increased by high protein intake, catabolic states, breakdown of blood in the gut lumen in GI bleeding and tetracycline, and may ↓ in liver disease. Urea is freely filtered at the glomerulus with variable reabsorption, which is influenced by extracellular volume status. Intravascular volume depletion, diuretics, CCF, GI bleeding, tetracyclines and renal failure cause elevated levels. Disproportionate rise in serum urea compared to creatinine occurs in hypovolaemia and GI bleeding. Reduced levels are seen in chronic liver disease and alcohol abuse.

24h creatinine clearance

The patient is instructed to completely empty their bladder soon after awakening in the morning, discard the urine and subsequently start the clock on the 24h collection period. During this time all urine voided is collected in the container provided. At the end of 24h the patient empties the bladder one last time, and the urine is saved. The time of the final urine specimen should vary by no more than 10min of the time of starting the collection the previous morning. The container is handed in and a blood sample to estimate serum creatinine is taken. In some centres the result obtained is normalised to the person's body surface area if the height and weight are known and is expressed as mL/min per $1.73m^2$.

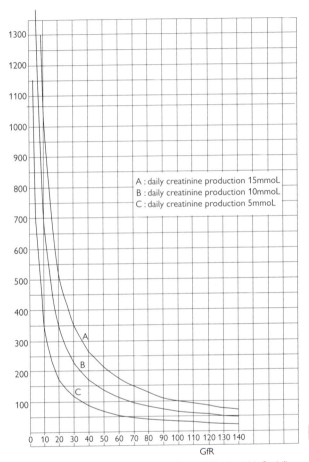

Fig. 10.1 Creatinine production is dependent on muscle mass which varies widely. Graph illustrates the theoretical relationship between GFR and plasma creatinine, ignoring effects of tubular secretion of creatinine, which results in overestimation of GFR from plasma creatinine or measurement of creatinine clearance. Note that in a patient with low muscle mass, serum creatinine does not rise outside the normal range until the GFR has fallen <30mL/min, whereas a patient with higher muscle mass will reach the same level of creatinine at a GFR of 90mL/min.

> The creatinine clearance is calculated as follows
>
> **Urine flow rate (mL/min)=**
> Urine volume (mL)/time of collection (min)
>
> **Creatinine clearance =**
> {Urine creatinine [mmol/L]/[plasma creatinine [mmol/L]} × urine flow rate [mL/min]

Since creatinine is excreted predominantly by filtration at the glomerulus, and partly due to secretion by the tubules, the above formula overestimates GFR. The secretory component can be completely blocked by cimetidine (400mg qds starting the night before commencing urine collection and continued till completion) to produce values closer to the true GFR.

The most common source of error is an incomplete collection of urine or incomplete bladder emptying. In spite of its inadequacies, creatinine clearance based on 24h urine collections and cimetidine-enhanced clearance studies are cheap, easily repeatable, and widely available and can be done in an outpatient setting. It will not replace more accurate estimates of GFR, but precise measurements are rarely needed in clinical practice.

Cystatin C
Cystatin C, a 13kDa protein of the cystatin superfamily of cysteine protease inhibitors, is produced by all nucleated cells at a relatively constant rate. It can be assayed using efficient, enzyme-linked immunoassays. Preliminary studies suggest serum cystatin C may be a more sensitive and specific marker than creatinine for assessing impaired excretory renal function. Minor reductions in GFR cause cystatin C levels to rise above normal when serum creatinine is still within normal range.

Measurement of glomerular filtration rate
Indications
- When accurate measurement of renal function is needed, as in clinical research, to calculate dose of chemotherapy agents which have renal excretion and in patients with abnormal muscle mass, e.g. paraplegics with bilateral lower limb muscle wasting.
- The 'gold standard' for measurement of GFR is measurement of inulin clearance: inulin is freely filtered, not protein bound, and not reabsorbed or secreted. However, measurement of inulin is difficult.

Radionuclide studies
Radionuclide studies are contraindicated during pregnancy and women of childbearing age need to have a negative pregnancy test before proceeding with the test.

A variety of radioisotope markers are available for estimating GFR. An ideal marker should be safe, not extensively protein bound, be freely filtered but not secreted or reabsorbed by the tubule and should be excreted only by the kidney. Inulin is the gold standard as it satisfies all the above requirements. However since its administration and measurement is cumbersome it is available only as a research tool.

- The commonly used markers are ^{51}Cr EDTA, ^{99m}Tc DTPA and ^{125}I iothalamate. Iothalamate is also available without radiolabelling and can be measured by fluorimetry.
- These substances are injected intravenously (SC in ^{125}I iothalamate) and after allowing for equilibration, plasma levels are measured at pre-determined intervals. Plasma clearance and hence renal elimination is calculated from the rate of fall of the substance from circulation.
- ^{51}Cr EDTA has been the most extensively studied marker and is widely available. Extensively used in Europe as a single injection technique followed by plasma sampling at 0, 90, 120, 150 and 240min. ^{51}Cr EDTA is reliable even at low levels of renal function. Studies in humans suggest renal clearance estimated by this method is ~10% lower than that of inulin.
- ^{125}I iothalamate is only slightly protein bound and studies suggest clearance values similar to that of inulin. Unlike other markers it can also be administered SC, and this allows for slow equilibration with

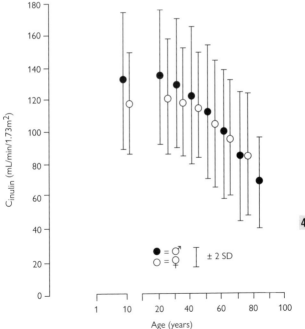

Fig. 10.2 Glomerular filtration rate, measured by inulin clearance, in normal individuals according to age.

stable plasma concentrations. It is considered safe, but potential problems of thyroid uptake necessitate pre-treatment with oral iodine.

- ^{99m}Tc DTPA is also widely available. There is some evidence that renal clearance can be estimated with a gamma camera placed over the patient, without the need for plasma sampling. Also anatomical correlation to renal function, like information on relative contribution from each kidney, can be obtained. ^{99m}Tc has a very short half-life, and radiation exposure is minimized. Protein binding can result in diminished renal clearance.

Assessment of proteinuria

Proteinuria may result from ↑ glomerular permeability or tubular disease, causing ↓ reabsorption of filtered protein or ↑ excretion of tubular enzymes. Severity of proteinuria is best measured by absolute protein excretion over 24h, rather than protein concentration (influenced by urine dilution). Although dipstick tests are useful, they can be misleading, with false +ve (concentrated urine) and false −ve (dilute urine) results.

Indications for quantitation of proteinuria

Diagnosis of nephrotic syndrome

Nephrotic syndrome is defined as triad of **oedema**, **hypoalbuminaemia** and **proteinuria** >3g/24h. In a patient with oedema and hypoalbuminaemia it is worthwhile obtaining a 24h urine protein, to confirm that these are indeed due to renal disease. It is worthwhile measuring creatinine clearance on same sample, and measurement of 24h urinary Na^+ excretion may also help in planning management.

Prognosis of progressive renal disease

Proteinuria is one of the most potent risk markers for progressive loss of renal function in renal disease, e.g. diabetic nephropathy, chronic glomerulonephritis and reflux nephropathy. In addition, treatments that reduce proteinuria (e.g. antihypertensive drugs, particularly ACE inhibitors) ↓ rate of progression. Because reduction of proteinuria is an important therapeutic aim, regular assessment of the severity of proteinuria is important in monitoring the effects of treatment.

Diagnosis of early diabetic nephropathy

Diabetic nephropathy is most treatable in its early stages—characterised by an ↑ in GFR, ↑ albumin excretion, and then by hypertension. 'Microalbuminuria' is the term for pathologically increased albumin excretion below the limit of detection of standard tests for proteinuria.

Quantitation of proteinuria

'Gold standard' is 24h urine collection for measurement of *total protein* or *albumin*. Protein measurement is cheap but does not differentiate between the various proteins present in urine. Proteinuria >300mg/24h is usually defined as pathological, but patients with early diabetic nephropathy have total protein excretions below this limit. Only when proteinuria >1g/24h is there a high suspicion of underlying renal disease. Albumin measurement is more expensive but justified when the detection of 'microalbuminuria' would alter management—either in the diagnosis of diabetic nephropathy or in the early detection of other forms of glomerular disease. An alternative is to measure the urine protein:creatinine ratio or albumin:creatinine ratio on a 'spot' urine sample—ideally an early morning urine sample (because protein excretion ↑ with activity—*see below*). Because creatinine is produced at a fairly constant rate throughout the day and night, its concentration depends purely on daily production rate and on urine dilution.

Assuming an average creatinine production of 10mmol/day (ignoring inter-individual variation due to variation in muscle mass), a protein:creatinine ratio of *n* mg/mmol allows estimation of the daily protein excretion as **10 × *n* mg/24h**.

Diagnosis of postural proteinuria
Protein excretion ↑ with activity and upright posture. In some individuals increase is exaggerated, resulting in +ve dipstick tests for proteinuria and even ↑ 24h urine protein excretion. This 'postural proteinuria' has a nearly completely benign prognosis. In patients with proteinuria who have no other evidence of renal disease it is worth quantitating proteinuria separately in urine collected while the patient has been recumbent overnight and in a daytime specimen. This can either be done by measuring protein:creatinine (or albumin:creatinine ratio for even greater accuracy) on both an early morning urine and one taken after period of activity, or a 24h urine divided into 'night-time' and 'daytime' aliquots. Normal protein excretion during the night with increased protein excretion during the day indicates postural proteinuria.

Assessment of tubular proteinuria
Occasionally of value to detect the relatively low grade proteinuria that results from tubular disease, e.g. Dent's disease (rare genetic disorder caused by mutation in a tubular chloride channel), which causes calcium stone formation and tubular proteinuria. Other examples include screening for generalised tubular dysfunction and for drug toxicity, e.g during treatment with platinum derivatives. Tubular proteinuria is best diagnosed by measurement of specific proteins whose presence in the urine result from tubular disease, e.g. retinol binding protein (RBP), N-acetyl-β-D-glucosaminidase (NAG) or α1-microglobulin, either in 24h urine specimens or as ratios between the protein concentration and creatinine concentration.

Assessment of selectivity of proteinuria
The more severe the damage to glomerular permeability, the larger the protein molecules which pass through the glomerulus in glomerular disease. Measurement of the ratio of clearance of transferrin or albumin (a small molecule) to immunoglobulin G (a large molecule) can therefore be used as a measure of selectivity, and is calculated as follows:

> Albumin/IgG clearance = {(urine [IgG] × serum [albumin])/(serum IgG × urine [albumin])} × 100%

Transferrin/IgG clearance is calculated similarly.

A ratio of <0.16 indicates highly selective proteinuria.

In children, minimal change nephropathy causes selective proteinuria, whereas non-selective proteinuria raises the possibility of an alternative type of renal disease and might led to a recommendation of renal biopsy to avoid steroid treatment when this would be unlikely to be of benefit. Measurement of selectivity in adults is of very limited use.

Detection and quantitation of urinary light chains (Bence Jones protein)
Measurement of urinary light chains requires specific immunoassays for light chains and is performed on 24h urine samples as part of the regular assessment of disease activity in multiple myeloma. These tests are probably a less reliable marker of disease activity in the presence of renal impairment.

Assessment of renal tubular function

There are two main types of renal tubular diseases: those due to a single defect, usually genetic, in solute secretion or reabsorption, and those due to generalised tubular damage.

Screening tests for generalised tubular dysfunction test for
- Renal glycosuria (dipstick or lab test for glucose in urine plus normal plasma glucose).
- Hypophosphataemia (can be followed by estimation of phosphate reabsorption, see below).
- Low molecular weight proteinuria (due to failure of tubular reabsorption plus increased release of proteins derived from tubular cells).
- Normal anion gap metabolic acidosis—serum bicarbonate, plus sodium potassium and chloride to permit calculation of the anion gap (followed by tests to confirm renal tubular acidosis, see below).
- Aminoaciduria—detected by amino acid electrophoresis on a random urine sample.
- Hypouricaemia—plasma urate may be low due to decreased tubular reabsorption. (This can be followed by measurement of fractional urate excretion, see below.)

Assessment of phosphate reabsorption
Occasionally useful in the differential diagnosis of hypophosphataemia, e.g. in confirming the diagnosis of X-linked hypophosphataemic rickets.

Procedure
- The patient is asked to fast overnight.
- The overnight urine is discarded.
- The next urine sample is obtained, together with a blood sample.
- Both are analysed for phosphate and creatinine.

Fractional phosphate excretion is calculated as:

$$FE_{PO4} = C_P/C_{Cr} = [\text{serum creatinine} \times \text{urine phosphate}]/[\text{urine creatinine} \times \text{serum phosphate}]$$
—this is the fraction of filtered phosphate which appears in the urine

Fractional tubular reabsorption of phosphate (TRP) is calculated as $1-FE_{PO4}$

TmP/GFR, the tubular maximum for phosphate reabsorption can be read off a nomogram[1], or can be calculated as follows:

If TRP<0.86, TmP/GFR = TRP × plasma phosphate

If TRP>0.86, TmP/GFR = {0.3 x TRP/[1 − (0.8 x TRP)]} × plasma phosphate

Interpretation

The adult reference range for TmP/GFR is 0.80–1.35mmol/L. Higher values of normal are seen in infancy and childhood[2]. Low values are seen in X-linked hypophosphataemic rickets and in osteogenic osteomalacia, both of which are thought to be due to overproduction or failure of inactivation of an as yet unidentified phosphaturic hormone, phosphatonin. TmP/GFR is raised in hypoparathyroidism and reduced in hyperparathyroidism and by PTH-related peptide secretion.

Reduced phosphate reabsorption may also be seen in hypercalciuric stone formers, but it remains difficult to be certain whether this is the primary disorder, causing increased production of $1,25-(OH)_2$ vitamin D, or secondary to tubular damage as a result of renal stones.

Reduced phosphate reabsorption is also seen in a number of primary and secondary disorders of renal tubular function.

Assessment of tubular urate handling

The relative contributions of production rate, glomerular filtration, presecretory reabsorption, secretion and post-secretory reabsorption to control of plasma urate concentration cannot be dissected out without complex tests involving selective pharmacological blockade of some of these processes. However, it is possible to determine whether an abnormal plasma urate concentration is due to abnormal production or abnormal renal handling.

24h urinary urate production is increased in overproduction but normal in patients whose hyperuricaemia is due to decreased excretion. (*Note*: it is not decreased, because in underexcretion the steady state is maintained at the expense of a raised plasma level.) If 24h urinary urate is raised, the collection should be repeated on a low purine diet.

Fractional excretion of urate is calculated as:

{(urinary [urate] × plasma [creatinine])/(plasma [urate] × urinary [creatinine])} × 100%

Normal values are dependent on age and sex but in adults are of the order of 10%. High fractional excretion is a cause of hypouricaemia in SIADH and several other conditions; low fractional excretion occurs in primary gout but also in a familial syndrome of hypouricaemia with early- onset gout and progressive renal failure.

Walton RJ & Bijvoet OLM. (1975) Nomogram for derivation of renal threshold phosphate concentration *Lancet* **ii**, 309–310; 2 Payne RB. Renal tubular reabsorption of phosphate (TmP/GFR): indications and interpretation (1998) *Ann Clin Biochem* **35**, 201–206

Assessment of acid-base balance

Plasma HCO_3^- and Cl^- are the two major anions in extracellular fluid. The major reason for measuring them is to assess acid-base status. Changes in serum $[HCO_3^-]$ concentration reflect changes in acid-base balance, with a ↓ in $[HCO_3^-]$ reflecting metabolic acidosis and an ↑ reflecting alkalosis. Plasma Cl^- is helpful in assessing the cause of acidosis or alkalosis.

▶There is *no* justification at all for performing an arterial puncture to measure arterial pH as part of the assessment of metabolic acidosis or alkalosis—it can be adequately assessed from serum $[HCO_3^-]$. Arterial samples are needed when it is unclear whether the acid-base disturbance is respiratory or metabolic in origin, or in mixed disturbances.

Plasma bicarbonate
The most reliable way to interpret plasma HCO_3^- is to use the acid-base diagram (Fig. 10.4), which allows assessment of how much the change in $[HCO_3^-]$ concentration is due to changes in CO_2 excretion via the lungs and how much to changes in $[H^+]$ or HCO_3^- wasting. In the absence of significant respiratory disease it can often safely be assumed that any change is due to metabolic causes, in which case low plasma HCO_3^- indicates increased H^+ production (or, occasionally, increased HCO_3^- loss) and vice versa. If arterial blood gases are obtained, the 'standard bicarbonate' is a calculated value which indicates what the plasma HCO_3^- would be if CO_2 excretion were normal, and is thus a way of allowing assessment of whether there is a metabolic component to an abnormal HCO_3^- concentration or whether it is solely due to the respiratory disturbance.

Remember that the kidneys compensate for respiratory disease and the lungs for metabolic disease: for instance, metabolic acidosis causes hyperventilation, resulting in lower PCO_2 and lessening the acidosis seen. However, overcompensation does not occur.

Plasma chloride
Many laboratories omit plasma Cl^- assays from 'routine' serum chemistry measurements, but this measurement is helpful if a systemic acid-base disturbance is suspected. As a useful oversimplification, low bicarbonate with high chloride can be seen as accumulation of hydrochloric acid, which can only result from altered renal handling of acid, as in renal tubular acidosis. If HCO_3^- is low with a normal or low Cl^-, some other acid must be accumulating. More precision in deciding the cause of metabolic acidosis can be obtained by calculating the anion gap.

The anion gap
The anion gap is the difference between the sum of the concentrations of the positively charged ions routinely measured in plasma and the negatively charged ions:

Anion gap = {[Na$^+$] + [K$^+$]} − {[Cl$^-$] + [HCO$_3^-$]}

Obviously, the total positive charges in plasma must be balanced by the same number of negative charges. The normal anion gap is caused by the fact that there are more unmeasured anions in plasma (mostly albumin, but including lactate, sulphate and others) than cations (including calcium and magnesium). The concentrations of all of these unmeasured ions can vary, so the normal range for the anion gap is wide; hypoalbuminaemia, for instance, reduces the anion gap by 2.5mEq per 1g/dL fall in serum albumin. The main use of calculation of the anion gap is in the differential diagnosis of metabolic acidosis.

A high anion gap acidosis is caused by an abnormally high concentration of an unmeasured anion, such as
- L-lactate (reflecting anaerobic metabolism or hepatic dysfunction).
- Salicylate (in aspirin poisoning).
- β-hydroxybutyrate (in diabetic ketoacidosis).
- Glycolate and oxalate (in methanol poisoning).
- Hippurate (in toluene poisoning, e.g. glue-sniffing).
- D-lactate (from gut bacterial fermentation in blind-loop syndrome).

A normal anion gap acidosis may be caused by loss of bicarbonate or failure of renal H$^+$ excretion, for instance
- Renal tubular acidosis.
- High ileostomy losses (bicarbonate wasting).
- Carbonic anhydrase inhibitors.
- Urinary diversions, e.g. ureterosigmoidostomy (Cl/HCO$_3^-$ exchange and NH$_4^+$ reabsorption in the colonic segment).

Beware: in North America the anion gap is usually calculated as [Na$^+$] − {[Cl$^-$] + [HCO$_3^-$]}, not including [K$^+$] in the measured cations. This results in a lower reference range for the anion gap. In addition, different laboratories use different assays for chloride. For these reasons, the local laboratory reference range for anion gap should be used.

In general, the anion gap is only useful when very high, confirming high concentrations of an unmeasured anion. If the diagnosis is not already obvious, this then justifies further investigation, including assay of plasma lactate concentration.

433

Assessment of urinary acidification

Indications
Unexplained hyperchloraemic metabolic acidosis.

Defects in the kidneys' ability to excrete acid in the urine may lead to permanent systemic acidosis, or to systemic acidosis at times of increased acid generation, depending on the severity of the defect. Acidification defects may occur as part of generalised tubular disease or as isolated, often genetically determined, alterations in function, most commonly of cell surface ion pumps.

Ammonium chloride loading test

This test is regarded as the 'gold standard' for the diagnosis of distal ('type 1') renal tubular acidosis, where there is impaired excretion of 'fixed acid' into the distal tubule.

Procedure
- The patient attends after an overnight fast, but is allowed to drink water.
- At the start of the test, a urine sample is sent to the laboratory for measurement of pH and a plasma or serum sample is sent for measurement of bicarbonate. Because pH changes rapidly in urine exposed to the air, the urine container should be filled to the top or the urine sent in a stoppered syringe, and sent to the laboratory without any delay.
- If the urine pH is <5.4, this indicates normal acidifying ability, and there is no need to continue with the test.
- If the venous blood bicarbonate is low, with a urine pH >5.4, the diagnosis of renal tubular acidosis is confirmed.
- If neither of these conditions is met, then proceed to give the patient ammonium chloride, 0.1g/kg body weight, PO. Ammonium chloride is

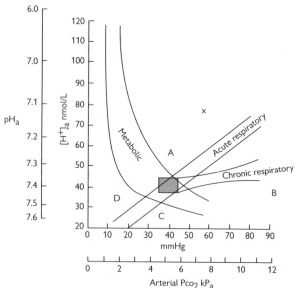

Fig. 10.4

given as capsules, is unpalatable, and frequently causes nausea and vomiting, but this can be reduced if the capsules are taken slowly, or with bread and honey. It is worth proceeding with the test even if the patient vomits, as acidosis is often achieved; no more ammonium chloride should be given.

- Urine samples are then collected hourly for the next 6–8h and sent, protected from the air (as above), for pH analysis in the laboratory. If any sample has a pH of ≤5.4 the test can be stopped, as this indicates normal acidifying ability of the distal tubule.
- At 3h after ingestion of ammonium chloride, a venous sample should be sent for plasma bicarbonate measurement to ensure that acidaemia has occurred.

Alternative tests of distal acidification

Rationale: the distal tubule reabsorbs sodium ions in exchange for hydrogen ions. Frusemide, by increasing delivery of sodium to the distal tubule, therefore causes a fall in urine pH. A fall in urine pH to <5.5 after frusemide confirms normal distal acidification ability, and may spare the patient the unpleasantness of the ammonium chloride test. The sensitivity of the test is increased in 'salt-avid' states produced by sodium restriction or fludrocortisone.

- The patient attends after a light breakfast without caffeine.
- Fludrocortisone 1mg is given, followed by frusemide 40mg an hour later.
- Drinking is discouraged unless the patient is very thirsty (very dilute urine can invalidate the test).
- Urine samples are collected for laboratory analysis of pH hourly, if possible, for 4–5h. A fall in urine pH to <5.5 excludes a distal acidification defect.

Bicarbonate infusion test

This is the 'gold standard' for the diagnosis of proximal ('type 2') renal tubular acidosis, which is characterised by impaired bicarbonate reabsorption. In this condition, urine pH may be <5.5 in untreated patients, because at steady state serum bicarbonate levels fall to the point at which filtered bicarbonate is reabsorbed, and distal acidification mechanisms are intact.

Procedure

- Sodium bicarbonate is infused IV at 0.5–1.0mmol/kg per hour. After 60min plasma bicarbonate is measured to confirm that this has risen to >20mmol/L. Urine pH is measured hourly and urine bicarbonate measured, to allow calculation of the fractional excretion of bicarbonate:

$$FEH_{CO3} = \{(\text{urine } [HCO_3] \times \text{plasma } [\text{creatinine}])/(\text{plasma } [HCO_3] \times \text{urine } [\text{creatinine}])\} \times 100\%$$

- Fractional excretion of bicarbonate is normally <15%.
- A level of >20% confirms type 2 renal tubular acidosis.

Plasma potassium

Although most of the body's potassium is intracellular, small changes in extracellular potassium concentration can have major changes in membrane excitability. Hypokalaemia causes increased excitability, causing atrial and ventricular cardiac arrhythmias; hyperkalaemia decreases excitability, causing a characteristic pattern of ECG changes and eventually causing asystole. Both hypokalaemia and hyperkalaemia can also be associated with skeletal muscle paralysis.

Plasma K^+ concentration is influenced both by distribution across cell membranes and by the balance between intake and excretion. Renal excretion is dependent on renal function, urine flow rate and aldosterone.

Pseudohyperkalaemia

Caused by excessive release of K^+ from cells after venepuncture, and should be considered when hyperkalaemia 'doesn't fit' with the clinical picture. The laboratory should report the presence of visible haemolysis (usually due to RBC trauma during difficult venepuncture), but pseudohyperkalaemia can also occur in the absence of visible haemolysis, as in:

- Haematological malignancies causing a high white cell or platelet count.
- Other causes of leucocytosis and thrombocytosis, e.g. leukaemoid reactions, rheumatoid arthritis.
- Familial pseudohyperkalaemia: rare disorder of RBC cation transport leading to an increased rate of release of K^+ from red cells at low temperatures.

Diagnosis can be confirmed by showing that plasma $[K^+]$ is normal in a heparinised sample analysed immediately, and then by demonstrating that delayed separation results in higher values being obtained. Pseudohyperkalaemia with a normal WBC and platelet count can be further investigated by measuring the rate of rise of plasma $[K^+]$ in samples incubated at 37°C and at 22°C, and studying the effects of drugs that affect cation exchange, e.g. thiazide diuretics and quinine. Artefactual hyperkalaemia can be caused by fist clenching plus a venous tourniquet during phlebotomy: plasma K^+ can rise by as much as 2mmol/L.

Hyperkalaemia due to redistribution across cell membranes

Hyperkalaemic periodic paralysis is an autosomal dominant genetic muscle disorder caused by mutations in the voltage-gated sodium channel. It presents in early infancy with attacks of paralysis associated with hyperkalaemia.

Other causes of release of potassium from tissues (including muscle) include

- Exercise.
- Acidosis (particularly inorganic acidosis).
- Muscle damage (rhabdomyolysis), e.g. crush injury, revascularisation of ischaemic limb, prolonged unconsciousness following drug intoxication.
- Burns.
- Tumour lysis, e.g. after initiation of chemotherapy for haematological malignancy.
- Drugs, e.g. digoxin, depolarising muscle relaxants, β-blockers.
- Malignant hyperthermia.

Hyperkalaemia due to altered external balance

- ↑ ingestion is seldom able to cause hyperkalaemia on its own, but can contribute to hyperkalaemia when combined with impaired excretion of a potassium load.
- ↓ excretion may be due to decreased glomerular filtration rate, ↓ urine flow rate, ↓ aldosterone production, drugs which inhibit renal tubular potassium excretion, or genetic defects in renal potassium excretion (pseudohypoaldosteronism, Liddle's syndrome).
- In most cases the cause is obvious.

Investigation of unexplained hyperkalaemia

- Serum creatinine, creatine kinase, bicarbonate.
- Urine K^+, creatinine, osmolality, allowing calculation of transtubular K^+ gradient (📖*Urine potassium & chloride measurements* (p438)): occasionally useful, for instance in confirming trimethoprim-induced inhibition of K^+ secretion.
- Tests for type IV renal tubular acidosis:
  - Normal synacthen test (to exclude Addison's disease).
  - 24h urinary aldosterone (low in type IV RTA).
  - Plasma renin and aldosterone response to upright posture and 40mg frusemide (subnormal levels of both suggest hyporeninaemic hypoaldosteronism).
  - Correction of hyperkalaemia with oral fludrocortisone 0.1mg/day.

Pseudohypokalaemia

Can be caused by delayed separation of samples kept at warm ambient temperatures, and is caused by continued uptake of K^+ into cells. This occurs more in heparinised samples than in those allowed to clot.

Hypokalaemia due to redistribution across cell membranes

- Alkalosis.
- Insulin treatment.
- β2-adrenergic stimulation (e.g. high dose nebulisers).
- B_{12} therapy of pernicious anaemia.
- Rapid cell division, e.g. acute leukaemia.
- Hypokalaemic periodic paralysis (precipitated by carbohydrate intake, rest after exercise):
  - Confirm diagnosis (under strict supervision) by infusing 2g/kg glucose and 0.1u/kg insulin; consider referral for mutation analysis of α1-subunit of calcium channel.
  - Consider thyrotoxic hypokalaemic periodic paralysis in non-familial patients, particularly of oriental background: check thyroid function tests.

Hypokalaemia due to increased renal loss
📖p125.

Urine potassium & chloride measurements

Measurement of urine potassium concentration is occasionally useful in the differential diagnosis of hyperkalaemia. The proportion of potassium filtered at the glomerulus which is excreted in the urine is extremely variable, and is modulated by the distal tubule in response to aldosterone, plasma potassium concentration, acid-base balance, urine flow rate, sodium status, and other factors. The final concentration of potassium in the urine also depends on urine dilution, controlled independently by factors (e.g. ADH) controlling water excretion.

Low urinary K^+ (<20mmol/L) with hypokalaemia is seen in
- Gastrointestinal potassium loss, e.g. diarrhoea, laxative abuse, villous adenoma, high ileostomy output, enterocutaneous fistula, ureterosigmoidostomy.
- Dietary deficiency.
- Skin losses, e.g. burns, severe eczema.

High urinary K^+ (>20mmol/L) with hypokalaemia and normal blood pressure is seen in
- Vomiting (K^+ is exchanged for hydrogen ions: acid-base preservation takes precedence)—note: urinary chloride will be low.
- Diuretic use, abuse and conditions which mimic diuretic use, e.g. Bartter's syndrome, Gitelman's syndrome.
- Tubular damage causing potassium wasting, e.g. renal tubular acidosis types 1 and 2.
- Diabetic ketoacidosis.

High urinary K^+ (>20mmol/L) with hypokalaemia and high blood pressure is seen in
- Hyperaldosteronism—adrenal adenomas, bilateral adrenal hyperplasia.
- Apparent mineralocorticoid excess.
- Liddle's syndrome.

Transtubular potassium gradient
This is a calculation that is promoted in the USA, but not widely used in the UK or Europe. The main purpose is to distinguish hyperkalaemia caused by decreased aldosterone action from hyperkalaemia due to effective volume depletion. The principle is that correcting for urine dilution, by using the ratio of plasma and urine osmolality, allows estimation of the urine potassium gradient in the cortical collecting duct, after the main site of potassium secretion (which is influenced by aldosterone) but before the main site of urine dilution or concentration (which is influenced by ADH). The index is only valid when the urine is concentrated, i.e. the urine osmolality exceeds the plasma osmolality, and when urine sodium concentration is >25mmol/L. It is calculated as follows:

$$\text{TTKG} = \{\text{urine } [K^+]/(\text{urine osmolality}/\text{plasma osmolality})\}/\text{plasma } [K+]$$

TTKG can vary widely in healthy subjects, but is commonly around 7–9
- Values <7 in a patient with hyperkalaemia suggest hypoaldosteronism.

- Values >7 in a hyperkalaemic patient suggest that aldosterone is acting normally, and that hyperkalaemia is due to low urine flow, limiting the rate at which potassium can be excreted.
- Values <7 in hypokalaemic patients suggest extrarenal potassium loss.
- Values >9 in hypokalaemic patients suggest renal potassium loss.

Urine chloride

This measurement is helpful in the differential diagnosis of otherwise unexplained normotensive hypokalaemia. Urine chloride is low if hypokalaemia is being caused by extrarenal sodium chloride or hydrogen chloride losses, as seen in diarrhoea or vomiting respectively: in these conditions potassium is exchanged in the distal tubule for sodium or hydrogen respectively, but chloride is conserved. Urine chloride is high when the cause of hypokalaemia is inappropriate loss of potassium chloride, as in diuretic use and in Bartter's syndrome (the genetic equivalent of being on permanent high dose loop diuretics) and Gitelman's syndrome (the genetic equivalent of being on permanent high dose thiazide diuretics). The distinction between the drug-induced and genetic causes can be very difficult to make, but temporary withdrawal from diuretics causes intense chloride retention and a very low urinary chloride concentration, which is never seen in Bartter's or Gitelman's syndromes. Repeated measurements of urine chloride are therefore helpful in this situation, together with screens for the presence of diuretics in the urine when urine chloride is high.

Urine sodium concentration

In health, serum electrolyte concentrations are kept constant because intake of electrolytes is balanced by excretion in the faeces and urine. Renal excretion is tightly regulated to achieve this balance. These basic principles imply that the urinary excretion of, for instance, sodium, is nearly totally dependent on dietary intake of sodium. Because this is very variable, there is no 'normal range' of urinary sodium, or any other urinary electrolyte. Measurements of urinary electrolytes therefore have to be interpreted with great caution.

24h urine sodium excretion is a good marker, at steady state, for dietary intake, and has been used in epidemiological studies of the relationship of salt intake to blood pressure. Dietary sodium intake varies from as little as 10mmol/day in the Amazon rainforest to >400mmol/day in Westerners living on processed foods. Current UK advice is to restrict sodium intake to around 100mmol/day.

In clinical practice there are several reasons for measuring sodium output, including

- Calcium stone formers. Sodium and calcium excretion are linked, and reduction of excessive salt intake results in a reduction in calcium excretion.

- Cystine stone formers. Similarly, cystine excretion is reduced by reduction of dietary salt intake.
- During antihypertensive and antiproteinuric treatment. Salt restriction amplifies the effects of ACE inhibitors in reducing not only systemic blood pressure but also protein excretion in renal disease, and may be more tolerable than diuretic treatment.

24h urine sodium is usually measured on a sample collected in a plain container. However, it can also be measured, by flame photometry, in a sample collected into an acid container, and this is useful if calcium and oxalate excretion are also being measured, for instance in stone formers.

Spot urine sodium concentration is of very limited value, because sodium excretion varies considerably through the day and because it is normally influenced by urine dilution and hence by recent water intake. However, there are two situations in which it may be of value:
- Acute renal failure. The normal response of the kidneys to underperfusion from hypovolaemia or hypotension is to retain salt avidly, urine sodium concentration dropping to <10mmol/L. If urinary sodium concentration is this low in acute renal failure, this indicates normal ability of the renal tubules to retain salt. Low urine sodium concentration is seen in 'pre-renal' renal failure; acute tubular necrosis results in loss of tubular salt reabsorption and a higher urine sodium concentration. The problem is that conditions other than underperfusion cause low urine sodium (e.g. contrast nephropathy, rhabdomyolysis) and a high urine sodium does not necessarily indicate acute tubular necrosis—indeed, it is seen in normal people. In any case, the measurement seldom has a useful impact on management, which both in pre-renal failure and in acute tubular necrosis is to restore renal perfusion by correcting hypovolaemia, hypotension and sepsis as quickly as possible.
- Syndrome of inappropriate ADH. This diagnosis cannot be made in a hypovolaemic patient, because hypovolaemia is a physiological stimulus to ADH secretion. For this reason, the diagnosis cannot be made if the urine sodium concentration is low (□p108).

Fractional excretion of sodium is calculated as

$$\{(\text{urine [sodium]} \times \text{plasma [creatinine]})/\text{plasma [sodium]} \times \text{urine [creatinine]})\} \times 100\%$$

This gives an index of avidity of sodium reabsorption independent of changes in overall renal function. An FE_{Na} of <1% is seen in pre-renal failure and >1% in acute tubular necrosis. However, this measurement is prone to the same criticisms as that of urine sodium excretion.

Sodium wasting and sodium retaining states
Sodium wasting is caused by diuretics, Bartter's syndrome, Gitelman's syndrome, and occasionally by renal tubular disease. It cannot be diagnosed by measurement of urine sodium excretion alone, as at steady state this equals sodium intake, but is diagnosed by finding clinical evidence of hypovolaemia without avid renal sodium retention.

Sodium retention is caused by diseases causing effective hypovolaemia (e.g. congestive cardiac failure), in which case the diagnosis is suggested by oedema and the clinical signs of the underlying disease. However, sodium retention can also cause hypertension without oedema, as in hyperaldosteronism, pseudohyperaldosteronism, chronic renal failure and inherited disorders of renal tubular sodium excretion (e.g. Liddle's syndrome). Again, measurement of sodium excretion alone is not helpful in the diagnosis of these conditions.

Urine dipstick testing

Urine analysis is useful for screening patients with potential renal disease and for serial assessment of patients with known renal pathology.

Many commercially available dipsticks rapidly test the urine for multiple chemical contents. The sticks use reagent strips, which change colour, following a chemical reaction with an active constituent depending on the presence (or absence) of a particular component.

Depending on the type of dipstick used, urine can be tested for
- pH.
- Specific gravity.
- Haemoglobin.
- Leucocyte esterases and nitrites.
- Glucose.
- Ketones.
- Protein.
- Urobilinogen.

The reagent strip is fully immersed in urine obtained by voiding or, if warranted, by urethral catheterisation, and the excess shaken off. The change in colour, if any, is read after the time specified by the manufacturer – usually 30s.

pH

Dipstick testing only gives a rough estimate of pH, because of the effects of storage and reaction on exposure to atmospheric air on urine pH *in vitro*. The dipstick contains a polyionic polymer bound with H^+, which is released on reaction with the cations in urine. Release of H^+ causes change in colour of a pH-sensitive dye. Normal pH varies between 4.5 and 8.0, depending on diet: vegetarians, in whom fixed acid ingestion is low, commonly have alkaline urine. Urine infection with urease-producing organisms also causes alkaline urine. Urine pH >5.5 in spite of metabolic acidosis is seen in renal tubular acidosis. Urine pH is important in some recurrent stone formers. For instance, uric acid solubility in urine is critically dependent on urine pH, and many uric acid stone formers are found to have normal 24h urinary urate but highly acidic and concentrated urine (e.g. as a result of high losses from an ileostomy). In patients with triple phosphate stones, alkaline urine is commonly seen due to infection with urea splitting organisms.

Specific gravity

Not accurate on dipstick testing. Non-ionic constituents including albumin, glucose and urea are also estimated. Normal values: between 1003 and 1030, vary with the patient's hydration status and hence urinary concentration. SG ↓ with age as the kidney loses its concentrating ability. Fixed SG of 1010 is seen in chronic renal failure.

Haemoglobin

Reagent strips use peroxidase-like activity of haemoglobin to induce a colour change in a dye linked to organic peroxide. Does not distinguish haemoglobinuria from erythrocyturia and myoglobin. False +ve results are obtained with myoglobin, contamination with menstrual blood and iodine. Positive dipsticks for blood with absence of RBC on microscopy suggest lysis of RBCs due to prolonged storage, myoglobinuria or haemoglobinuria. False −ve results are seen with high dose vitamin C and rifampicin.

Leucocyte esterases and nitrites

The esterase method relies on esterases released from lysed WBC. Esterases release pyrroles, which react with a diazonium salt on the dipstick resulting in a colour change. False +ve results seen in vaginal contamination. Presence of glucose, albumin, ketones, tetracyclines and cephalosporins in the urine can give false −ve results.

Most, but not all, uropathogenic bacteria convert nitrates to nitrites, which react with a diazonium compound resulting in a colour change. False −ve results are due to frequent bladder emptying, prolonged external storage and ascorbic acid. Some bacteria including *N. gonorrhoea* and *Mycobacterium* TB do not convert nitrates.

Sensitivity and specificity of the above tests vary, and are not useful for screening low-risk populations. However a −ve test is useful in excluding UTI in a patient with a high pre-test probability of infection.

Glucose

Most strips use the glucose oxidase/peroxidase method and can estimate levels as low as 50mg/dL. Ketones, salicylate and ascorbic acid can interfere with results. Estimates all reducing sugars including fructose and lactose. In the absence of concomitant hyperglycaemia, glycosuria is suggestive of proximal tubular disorders or, rarely, reduced renal threshold for glucose.

Ketones

Acetoacetic acid is detected by the nitroprusside test. Ascorbic acid results in false +ve result. Dipsticks do not detect beta hydroxybutyrate, which comprises the largest ketone fraction in blood.

Protein

Binding of proteins to the dye indicators is highly pH dependent and the indicators undergo a sequential colour change based on the concentration of protein in the sample. Albumin binds at a pH of 5–8 and has the highest affinity, so most commercially available dipsticks almost exclusively detect only albumin. Sticks with sensitivity as low as 250mg/L are available currently. Dipsticks are thus cheap, reliable and give rapid semiquantitative assessment of proteinuric renal disease. However, remember that these tests measure concentration of protein, rather than absolute excretion;

false negative tests are therefore possible in dilute urine caused by a high fluid intake, and false positive tests may be obtained in highly concentrated urine. At pH <5 or >8 results obtained by dipsticks are not accurate. Immunoglobulin light chains (Bence Jones proteins) do not result in positive dipstick tests for proteinuria even when present in high concentrations.

Urine culture

There are numerous situations in which accurate diagnosis of UTI is important. 'Sending an MSU' is not, however, quite as simple as it sounds and is not always the most appropriate test.

Obtaining a mid-stream urine sample
The aim is to obtain a sample of bladder urine, avoiding contamination by cells or organisms on perineal skin. Men should retract the foreskin prior to micturition; women should hold the labia well apart with the parted fingers of one hand to allow the urine to exit directly from the urethral meatus. The patient should be asked to begin to pass urine, and then, without stopping passing urine, pass a sterile container into the path of the urinary stream and collect a sample, before finishing passing urine normally. If a sterile foil container has been used to catch the specimen, the specimen is then transferred into a specimen container and sent to the laboratory.

Suprapubic aspiration of urine
In patients suspected of having bladder infection but in whom the results of culture of mid-stream urines are equivocal, it may be necessary to proceed to suprapubic aspiration (widely performed in paediatrics, but not in adults). After skin preparation a fine needle (e.g. a lumbar puncture needle) is introduced into the bladder by direct puncture just above the symphysis pubis, and urine aspirated. Ultrasound can be used to confirm that the bladder is full prior to the procedure.

'In–out' catheter urine specimens
Although bladder catheterisation carries a small (1–2%) risk of introducing new infection into the bladder, this risk is sometimes justified by the importance of obtaining urine direct from the bladder. A urethral catheter is passed into the bladder, the first few millilitres discarded, and sample collected.

Obtaining urine specimens from ileal conduits
Urine in ileal conduit bags is always contaminated by skin organisms, and the culture of 'bag urine' is not a useful way of diagnosing upper urinary tract infection in patients with conduits. In patients suspected of having ascending infection, a urine specimen should be obtained by passing a catheter as far into the conduit as it will go.

'Two glass test'

This is a test for urethritis, and is performed when a patient presents with dysuria or urethral discharge and a sexual history suggesting possible recent infection. Culture of a urethral swab or of the urethral discharge should also be obtained and sent for gonorrhoea testing (requires attendance at a sexual health clinic). Two urine samples are collected; the first 10mL passed and a mid-stream sample. Each is sent for culture; urethritis is diagnosed when the bacterial count is highest in the first sample. The first sample should also be sent for *Chlamydia* testing.

'Stamey-Mears test'

This test is performed for the diagnosis of prostatitis. A MSU sample is obtained, and then the patient is asked to stop passing urine. The prostate gland is massaged per rectum and 'expressed prostatic secretions' collected, followed by a final urine sample. In prostatitis, bacterial counts are higher in the expressed prostatic secretions or the post-massage urine sample than in the mid-stream sample.

Indwelling catheter urine specimens

Colonisation of the bladder is nearly inevitable within a fortnight of insertion of an indwelling urethral or suprapubic catheter. Unnecessary antibiotic treatment increases the selective pressure for the emergence of antibiotic-resistant organisms and must be reserved for symptomatic infection. There is no point in sending catheter specimens unless there is a suspicion of symptomatic infection at the time. 'Surveillance' samples sent to predict which antibiotics should be used if the patient becomes symptomatic at a later time are unjustified, because the colonising organisms may change over time. A fresh specimen of urine is obtained from the collection port into the collection pot. Samples should NOT be collected from the reservoir into which the catheter drains.

Localisation tests

- Occasionally it is justified to attempt to localise the site of infection to the bladder or to one or other kidney.
- The 'gold standard' is to obtain samples from each ureter and from the bladder during rigid cystoscopy under general anaesthesia.
- The 'Fairley test' requires passage of a urethral catheter followed by a bladder washout with a wide spectrum antibacterial and a fibrinolytic enzyme. Sequential samples of urine are then obtained. If infection is present in the upper tracts, this will not have been affected by the bladder washout, and organisms will be detected in the first specimen obtained after washout, whereas if infection was confined to the bladder, subsequent samples will be sterile.
- Infection may be confined to one or other kidney as a result of ureteric obstruction, or may be present within a renal cyst. In these situations, direct aspiration of urine under ultrasound control in the radiology department is necessary.

Microscopy and culture of urine

Once a sample has been obtained it is sent to a microbiology laboratory for microscopy and culture.

Microscopy is required to assess pyuria (WBCs in the urine) and contamination.

- Significant pyuria indicates inflammation within the urinary tract; if this persists despite negative urine cultures the patient has 'sterile pyuria', for which there are a number of causes, including infection with an organism which does not grow on conventional culture media, e.g. *Chlamydia*.
- Pyuria plus a positive culture confirm the diagnosis of urinary tract infection.
- The absence of pyuria makes a urinary tract infection less likely, but can occur in the early stages of infection or in the presence of a very high fluid intake.
- Contamination (in the female) is indicated by the presence of large numbers of squamous cells, which usually come from the vaginal wall; however squamous cells can occasionally come from the bladder.

Culture and sensitivity are necessary to decide what treatment is necessary and to differentiate contamination of the urine sample by organisms outside the bladder from true infection.

- A 'pure growth' of a single organism to $>10^5$ colony-forming units (cfu)/mL is the conventional criterion for urinary tract infection. However:
- Low counts of 10^2–10^4 cfu/mL can be associated with early infection, and should be taken seriously in the presence of suggestive symptoms in women.
- Low counts in men are likely to represent true infection, because contamination is uncommon.
- Genuine mixed growth may occur, in the presence of impaired urinary drainage or a foreign body within the urinary tract.

Urine microscopy

Urine microscopy is a useful, quick, reliable, cheap and underused investigation—the 'liquid renal biopsy'! Far more information can be obtained by careful microscopy than is usually obtained in the microbiology laboratory, where the priority is detection of significant urine infection.

Indications

- Suspected urinary tract infection (p443).
- Suspected acute glomerulonephritis.
- Suspected acute interstitial nephritis (requires staining for eosinophils).
- Unexplained acute or chronic renal failure.
- Haematuria (with or without proteinuria) on urine dipstick test.
- Suspected urinary tract malignancy.

Procedure

A freshly voided, clean catch, mid-stream, early morning specimen is ideal. The sample should be centrifuged and re-suspended in a small volume. Although bright field microscopy will allow identification of most formed elements in the urine sediment, phase contrast microscopy is useful for detection of red cell ghosts, 'glomerular' red cells and some other constituents. Staining of the urine sediment is not necessary for most purposes, but is useful for identification of eosinophils and malignant cells—this is usually performed in the cytology laboratory.

Haematuria

RBCs appear as non-nucleated biconcave disks. Even when urine is red in colour or dipsticks positive for blood it should be examined for the presence of red cells. The differential diagnosis of haematuria is broad, but it is broadly classified into glomerular (renal) and infrarenal causes. Transit of red cells through the renal tubules causes osmotic changes in their shape and size; 'dysmorphic' or 'crenated' red cells are best seen using phase contrast microscopy, and may be missed altogether if bright field microscopy is used. In experienced hands, detection of these glomerular red cells strongly suggests a glomerular origin for haematuria, although failure to detect these changes does not reliably indicate a lower urinary tract cause of bleeding—heavy haematuria in IgA nephropathy, for instance, can result in large numbers of normal red cells in the urine. Urine pH, concentration and storage can affect red cell morphology.

Leucocyturia

The presence of significant numbers of polymorphs (pyuria) in urine is highly suggestive of urinary tract infection (p443) but can also occur in glomerulonephritis, interstitial nephritis, and peri-ureteric inflammation, for instance in acute appendicitis. The presence of leucocyte casts is diagnostic of renal parenchymal infection ('acute pyelonephritis'). Eosinophiluria is associated with acute allergic interstitial nephritis and athero-embolic renal disease.

Other cells

Squamous epithelial cells are usually taken as indicative of vaginal contamination, but may also derive from the bladder and urethra. Occasionally malignant cells arising from the lower urinary tract are picked up on routine microscopy. Spermatozoa are also rarely seen.

Microorganisms

Identification of bacteriuria, in association with leucocyturia is very suggestive of infection. Organisms may be in chains or clusters and some are motile. Fungi including yeast and protozoans including *Trichomonas* can also be readily identified.

Casts

Casts are cylindrical bodies, which usually form in the distal tubule and collecting duct. They consist of cells or cell debris held together by Tamm-Horsfall protein. Staining and phase contrast microscopy improves identification and characterisation of casts, but results are operator dependent. Extreme shaking or agitation can disintegrate casts.

Hyaline casts appear translucent and homogeneous and are present in normal urine. Number may be increased in dehydration and proteinuria.

Cellular casts especially red cell casts, always indicate significant parenchymal renal disease. Red cell casts are strongly suggestive of acute glomerulonephritis, but may occur in interstitial nephritis and acute tubular necrosis as well.

White cell casts are seen in acute pyelonephritis and acute interstitial nephritis.

Granular casts are formed from cell debris and are seen in a wide variety of renal diseases.

Waxy broad casts form in atrophic renal tubules and are seen in chronic renal failure.

Crystals

A variety of crystals can be visualised and are of importance in stone formers. A freshly voided sample should be examined as storage and temperature changes can affect type and number of crystals found. A large number of calcium oxalate crystals are seen in hypercalciuria, hyperoxaluria and ethylene glycol poisoning. Presence of a single crystal of cystine is diagnostic of cystinuria as cystine is not a constituent of normal urine. Phosphate crystals can form in normal urine as it cools, and are of no pathological significance.

Investigations in patients with renal or bladder stones

Not all renal tract stones are formed because of abnormal urine chemistry. They may also be formed because of stasis, e.g. in calyceal or bladder diverticula. Infection ('struvite') stones are the result of chronic infection in the urinary tract with urease-producing organisms, which metabolise urea to form an alkaline urine in which struvite readily precipitates.

Indications

Although up to 75% of patients who present with renal stones eventually form a second stone, this may not be for 20 years. Most urologists therefore only refer patients for metabolic evaluation if there is a heightened suspicion of an underlying metabolic cause.

Situations in which evaluation is definitely indicated include
- Formation of stones in childhood or adolescence.
- Recurrent stone formation.
- Nephrocalcinosis (calcification in the renal parenchyma) as well as stone formation in the collecting systems.

447

Radiology

Intravenous urography will usually have been performed during the patient's presentation with stone disease, but the films should be reviewed to look for evidence of any cause of stasis within the collecting systems, and in particular for medullary sponge kidney. Radiolucent stones can be detected using ultrasound, intravenous urography or CT scanning, and can be made of cystine, uric acid or xanthine. 'Staghorn' calculi filling the collecting systems are most often struvite (infection) stones, but not always—calcium oxalate stones can grow to similar size and shape, particularly in hyperoxaluria.

Stone analysis

Depending on the facilities in the laboratory, this may be qualitative or semiquantitative. The purpose of analysis is to distinguish calcium stones from cystine, urate and struvite stones, to pick up the rare types of stone, and in addition to distinguish calcium oxalate from calcium phosphate stones. The result of stone analysis should be used to guide further investigation. Stones can be obtained for analysis either at surgery, including percutaneous nephrolithotomy, or by asking a patient to pass urine through a fine sieve.

'Spot' urine tests

Amino acid analysis on a random sample of urine shows increased excretion of cystine, ornithine, lysine and arginine in cystinuria, and this finding is sufficient to confirm a suspected diagnosis. However, measurement of 24h urinary cystine excretion is necessary for optimal management of this condition.

Random urine calcium:creatinine and oxalate:creatinine ratios are used in children to diagnose hypercalciuria and hyperoxaluria, but are not as reliable as 24h urine collections, which are preferred in adults.

24h urine collections

Collections must be made into an acidified container for measurement of calcium and oxalate, and into a plain container for measurement of urate (because acidification is necessary to prevent calcium binding to the plastic surface of the urine container and to prevent *in vitro* generation of oxalate, and because acidification precipitates uric acid crystals). Measurement of sodium and citrate excretion can be made on either type of collection.

Calcium excretion is not a good predictor of stone formation (calcium activity is less than concentration due to the presence in urine of anions that form soluble complexes with calcium). However, marked ↑ of urinary calcium is a risk factor for stone formation.

Oxalate excretion correlates well with the risk of recurrent calcium oxalate stone formation, even within the normal range. Marked hyperoxaluria may result from enteric hyperoxaluria (↑ colonic oxalate absorption resulting from small bowel resection, jejunoileal bypass or malabsorption), from excess dietary oxalate, or as a result of primary hyperoxaluria (one of several metabolic defects causing increased endogenous oxalate production).

Glycollate and L-glycerate should be measured in patients suspected of having primary hyperoxaluria to allow differentiation between type 1 and type 2 hyperoxaluria. This investigation is only available in a few laboratories.

Citrate excretion should be measured because citrate is a potent inhibitor of calcium stone formation; correction of hypocitraturia with, for instance, oral potassium citrate, reduces stone recurrence rate.

Sodium excretion (a good marker for dietary sodium intake) should be measured in calcium stone formers and in patients with cystinuria, because reduction of dietary sodium intake results in decreased excretion of calcium and cystine, respectively.

Cystine excretion should be measured in cystine stone formers. The aim of treatment is to maintain the cystine concentration well below the solubility limit for cystine (~1mmol/L at urine pH of 7). Worth asking the patient to split the urine collection into day-time and night-time aliquots to ensure that this target is met at night, when urine tends to become more concentrated, as well as during the day.

Urinary phosphate measurement of is of no proven value in the management even of calcium phosphate stone formers.

Tests of urinary calcium excretion
Tests performed after calcium restriction and following a high calcium test meal have been used widely in the USA to differentiate 'absorptive' from 'renal' hypercalciuria. These tests are necessary to define different phenotypes associated with hypercalciuria for research studies, but there is no evidence that management strategies based on them have any advantage over those based on simpler tests of urine chemistry.

Renal biopsy

Percutaneous renal biopsy is a valuable tool to establish diagnosis, suggest prognosis and guide therapy in renal diseases. It also has a major role in the management of a renal transplant recipient.

Definite indications (result likely to change management)
- Nephrotic syndrome (in adults).
- Steroid-unresponsive nephrotic syndrome in children.
- Acute nephritic syndrome.
- Rapidly progressive glomerulonephritis.
- Unexplained renal failure with normal-sized kidneys relative to body size and age.
- Renal involvement in multi-system disorders.
- Diagnosis of renal transplant dysfunction.

Relative indications (result may change management or help to define prognosis)
- Non-nephrotic range proteinuria with or without haematuria.
- Isolated haematuria.
- Unexplained chronic renal failure.
- Diabetic patient with renal dysfunction, particularly with features not typical of diabetic nephropathy.

▶▶Absolute contraindications
- Uncontrolled severe hypertension.
- Bleeding diathesis including platelets $<50 \times 10^9$/L, uncorrected familial bleeding/clotting disorders and patient on anticoagulation with prolonged clotting times.

449

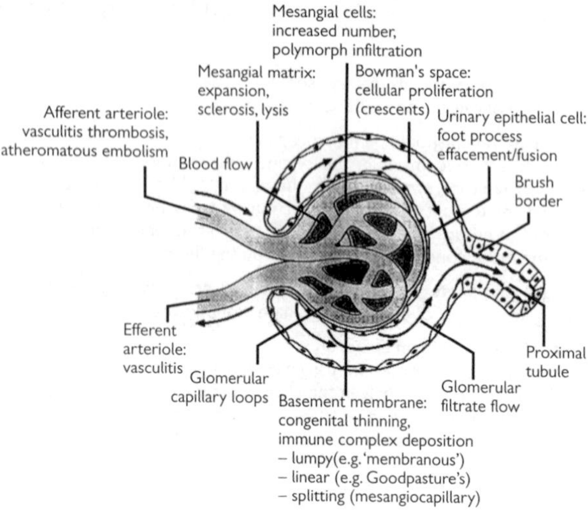
Mesangial cells:
increased number,
polymorph infiltration
Mesangial matrix:
expansion,
sclerosis, lysis
Bowman's space:
cellular proliferation
(crescents)
Afferent arteriole:
vasculitis thrombosis,
atheromatous embolism
Urinary epithelial cell:
foot process
effacement/fusion
Blood flow
Brush
border
Efferent
arteriole:
vasculitis
Glomerular
capillary loops
Proximal
tubule
Glomerular
filtrate flow
Basement membrane:
congenital thinning,
immune complex deposition
– lumpy(e.g.'membranous')
– linear (e.g. Goodpasture's)
– splitting (mesangiocapillary)

Fig. 10.3 The normal glomerulus and its repertoire of response to injury. Reprinted from Tomson CRV (1998) *Essential Medicine*, 2nd edition, p220, by permission of the publisher Churchill Livingstone.

Relative contraindications
- Single kidney.
- Kidney size small compared to patient's body size and age.
- Renal tumour/mass for fear of abdominal seeding.
- Uncooperative patient (can be done under sedation or under GA).
- Multiple renal cysts.

Complications
- Haematuria: microscopic haematuria almost universal. Macroscopic haematuria occurs in ~10% of patients. Severe macroscopic haematuria with need for transfusion 1–2%.
- Peri-renal haematoma: asymptomatic in 57–85% of patients. Symptomatic with need for transfusion in 1–2%.
- Renal arteriovenous fistula: usually asymptomatic with spontaneous resolution.
- Infection (very rare).
- Nephrectomy (<1:1000).
- Adjacent organ trauma.
- Death (<1:1000).

Procedure
1. Recent imaging of kidneys to document size and rule out obstruction is mandatory. A recent normal platelet count, clotting profile and informed consent is necessary.

2. The procedure is performed where proper ultrasound facilities are available and usually done under local anaesthesia. Sedation can be given to an uncooperative or tense patient.
3. An attending pathologist or technician at the time of sampling to comment on adequacy of tissue is very useful.
4. Biopsy with automated spring-loaded devices or a biopsy gun, under ultrasound visualisation is considered ideal but techniques vary based on availability of local expertise.
5. The patient lies supine and the kidney is identified with ultrasound.
6. The skin over the target area is prepared and anaesthetised with lignocaine.
7. A small cut in the skin is made using a scalpel. The kidney is localised with a fine bore 21G lumbar puncture needle and local anaesthetic infiltrated up to the level of the renal capsule. Either kidney can be biopsied: all parenchymal renal diseases are bilateral. After suitably protecting the ultrasound probe, the biopsy needle/gun is inserted along the anaesthetised track under ultrasound guidance to the level of the renal capsule, aiming to obtain a sample from the cortex of the lower pole. The patient is asked to hold their breath while the biopsy is taken.
8. The needle/gun is fired and subsequently withdrawn. The patient is then allowed to breathe normally.
9. Two cores of tissue are usually taken; this may require three or four 'passes' with the biopsy needle. If an attending pathologist or technician is present, they can comment on the adequacy of tissue by examining the core for glomeruli using a hand held magnifying glass or a simple microscope. If immunofluorescence is to be performed, part of one core is placed in saline; the remainder is placed in formalin.
10. Following the biopsy the patient is turned supine and strict bed rest enforced for a minimum of 6h. Vital signs are monitored every 15min for 2h, every 30min for 2h and hourly thereafter. If no complications are encountered at 6h the patient is allowed to mobilise. Most bleeding complications occur within the first 8h, but bleeding can start up to 72h after the biopsy. If macroscopic haematuria is present and does not resolve within the observation period, discharge should be delayed.

📖OHCM p249.

Renal imaging

Contrast nephropathy

Renal toxicity due to radiocontrast agents may cause or exacerbate renal impairment. Nephrotoxicity is due to a combination of local vasoconstriction and direct tubular injury. There is an increased risk in patients with pre-existing renal impairment, diabetes, myeloma, hypovolaemia or effective hypovolaemia (e.g. congestive cardiac failure), and concurrent administration of nephrotoxic medication including non-steroidal anti-inflammatory drugs and angiotensin converting enzyme inhibitors. Although usually reversible, contrast nephropathy can precipitate the need for dialysis in patients whose renal function is already seriously impaired. Non-ionic media, adequate hydration and acetylcysteine administered prior to the examination can reduce the risk in high-risk patients.

Details of the radiological investigation of the urinary tract appear on pp451, 515, 565, 567, 569.

Choice of investigation

Unexplained renal impairment

When a patient first presents with renal impairment it is important to decide whether this is acute—and therefore potentially reversible—or chronic. Although the history, examination and blood tests may give some clues, considerable doubt may remain.

All patients presenting with renal impairment should therefore undergo

- Ultrasound:
  - Hydronephrosis suggests obstructive nephropathy.
  - Small, smooth, kidneys with increased echogenicity and decreased corticomedullary differentiation suggest chronic parenchymal renal disease, e.g. chronic glomerulonephritis.
  - Irregular cortical scarring can be caused by reflux nephropathy, previous obstructive nephropathy (e.g. complicating renal stones) and renal infarction from vascular disease or embolism.
  - Renal asymmetry, particularly in a patient with known atherosclerosis elsewhere, suggests renal artery stenosis, although this can just as commonly be bilateral.
  - Renal enlargement can occur in acute tubular necrosis, renal vein thrombosis and renal infiltration, e.g. in haematological malignancy.
- Plain abdominal film (KUB—kidneys, ureters, bladder):
  - Nephrocalcinosis and urinary tract stones, particularly if outside the renal pelvis can be missed on ultrasound.

Further radiological investigations, including renal angiography and isotope scanning are sometimes helpful.

Suspected nephrolithiasis

IVU is the investigation of first choice: CT may be necessary, particularly for radiolucent stones.

Investigation of haematuria

In patients over 40, and possibly in some younger patients, it is important to exclude urinary tract malignancy. Ultrasound is the investigation of choice for the detection of renal cell carcinoma, but will miss some transitional cell carcinomas of the renal pelvis, which are best detected using IVU.

Investigation of suspected renal artery stenosis

In younger patients in whom fibromuscular dysplasia is suspected, conventional angiography should be performed. Atherosclerotic renal artery stenosis can be reasonably assessed by contrast CT angiography or by gadolinium-enhanced MR angiography.

Reflux nephropathy

Confirming this diagnosis can be important in counselling patients, as reflux nephropathy is often inherited as an autosomal dominant trait. Cortical scarring is best detected using a static DMSA renal scan. However, there are other causes of cortical scarring. The diagnosis is best confirmed by showing the combination of cortical scarring with underlying calyceal deformity on IVU. Demonstration of vesicoureteric reflux on direct or indirect micturating cystourethrography is useful in infants and small children, but reflux commonly resolves with growth, so these tests are seldom used in adults.

Obstructive uropathy

Although hydronephrosis demonstrated on IVU or ultrasound is usually sufficient to confirm obstruction, it is possible to have obstruction without much dilatation (e.g. complicating encasement by tumour). More commonly, there is uncertainty over whether dilatation of the collecting system and pelvis is due to previous obstruction, now resolved, or continuing obstruction. In these situations the options are diuretic MAG3 renography, insertion of nephrostomy, or retrograde insertion of ureteric stents. If doubt persists, a Whitaker test may be performed: this involves infusion of saline at a constant rate through a nephrostomy tube and measuring the relationship between pressure and flow down the ureter.

Renal transplant dysfunction

The differential diagnosis usually lies between obstruction, ureteric leak, rejection, acute tubular necrosis, nephrotoxicity and renal vein thrombosis. Depending on the centre, ultrasound with Doppler assessment of renal blood flow (giving resistance index) or isotope renography may be the investigation of first choice.

Renal bone disease

Parathyroid hormone

Indications
Diagnosis of primary, secondary or tertiary hyperparathyroidism.

Procedure
A heparinised sample is sent and separated within 4h of venepuncture. There are a variety of radioimmunoassays available, and fragments of parathyroid hormone (which accumulate in renal impairment) can cross-react in some of these.

Other markers of bone biochemistry

Serum calcium is often normal even in patients with significant renal disease, because a fall in serum calcium caused by reduced $1,25\text{-}(OH)_2$ vitamin D production results in an increase in parathyroid hormone secretion, returning serum calcium towards normal. Hypocalcaemia occurs after parathyroidectomy or after treatment with bisphosphonates. Hypercalcaemia occurs when the parathyroid hormone release loses sensitivity to serum calcium in tertiary hyperparathyroidism.

Serum phosphate is often increased in patients with renal impairment due to impaired renal excretion of phosphate.

Serum total alkaline phosphatase rises in severe hyperparathyroidism and in osteomalacia.

Serum bone alkaline phosphatase is a more sensitive marker of bone turnover, but quantitative measurement is not widely available. If total alkaline phosphatase is raised, alkaline phosphatase isoenzymes can be measured as an indicator of whether the increase is of bone origin.

Serum vitamin D metabolites are seldom measured in routine clinical management of patients with renal disease.

Serum aluminium and the desferrioxamine test
Patients with renal disease may be exposed to aluminium from contaminated water used for preparation of dialysate or by ingesting aluminium hydroxide as an antacid or, rarely nowadays, as a phosphate binder taken with meals. Because of the effects of aluminium on the brain, bone marrow and bones it is important to monitor patients at risk for evidence of aluminium accumulation.

Serum aluminium has to be taken into an aluminium-free glass tube. Serum aluminium levels reflect current exposure, and do not give any information about cumulative exposure. Serum aluminium levels may be increased by iron deficiency. Levels above 60µg/L (2.2µmol/L) are considered indicative of a dangerous level of exposure and should lead to a review of treatment.

The increment in serum aluminium 24 or 48h after IV desferrioxamine is a marker of aluminium 'load'. The original protocol requires the use of 40mg/kg desferrioxamine; a rise in serum aluminium of >200µg/L correlates well with the presence of aluminium-related bone disease on bone biopsy. Low dose protocols have also been described and validated.

Skeletal survey
Severe hyperparathyroidism causes erosion of the terminal phalanges, subperiosteal erosions, and in rare cases, brown tumours and pathological fractures. Severe osteomalacia causes loss of bone density and Looser zones (pseudo-fractures). These radiological signs are not commonly seen in modern renal patients because biochemical monitoring allows earlier detection of bone disease.

Transiliac bone biopsy
This is the 'gold standard' for the diagnosis of renal bone disease, but is not commonly used in clinical (as opposed to research) settings. However, it can be useful particularly for the confirmation of aluminium-related bone disease. For the maximum information to be gained from this invasive test, double tetracycline labelling should be performed.

Procedure
14 and 13 days before the procedure the patient takes a tetracycline antibiotic, e.g. oxytetracycline 250mg qds, and 4 and 3 days before the procedure a different tetracycline, e.g. demeclocycline 300mg bd. Under general anaesthetic a transiliac core of bone, including both cortical surfaces, is taken and placed in absolute alcohol. The sample should be sent to a laboratory specialising in the interpretation of bone biopsies in patients with metabolic bone disease.

Immunological tests in renal medicine

Immune-mediated diseases can affect the kidney in isolation or as part of a systemic disorder. Immunological tests commonly used to diagnose or monitor progress of renal disease are discussed here.

Complement

Indications

Acute nephritic syndrome, renal failure with skin ± neurological involvement and suspected SLE, endocarditis or cryoglobulinaemia. The normal complement system, its activation pathways and assay methods are discussed elsewhere (📖pXX). In relation to renal disease, hypocomplementaemia is important and relative deficiencies of various components can point to certain disorders.

	C3	C4
Post-streptococcal GN	Low	Normal
SLE	Low	Low
Cryoglobulinaemia	Low/normal	Very low
Membranoproliferative GN	Low	Low/normal
Subacute endocarditis	Normal/low	Low

GN, glomerulonephritis.

Successful treatment normalises complement levels in endocarditis, and in SLE except when SLE results from congenital complement deficiency.

C3 nephritic factor (C3Nef) is an IgG autoantibody that binds to and stabilises alternative pathway C3 convertase—C3bBb. This results in continuous activation of the alternative pathway with C3 depletion. It is detected by ELISA. C3Nef is classically associated with type 2 membrano-proliferative glomerulonephritis.

Immunoglobulins and serum electrophoresis for paraproteins

Indications

- Suspected myeloma or other clonal B cell disorders.
- Unexplained renal failure, with or without proteinuria, particularly in patients >50 years.
- Renal failure in association with hypercalcaemia.

Serum electrophoresis to identify a monoclonal immunoglobulin band is useful, but should always be combined with tests for urinary light chains

(Bence-Jones protein), as some types of myeloma cause light chain pro-teinuria **without** a monoclonal band in the serum.

Measurement of serum immunoglobulin concentrations is of value in patients with known myeloma, but is otherwise not useful in the assess-ment of patients with renal disease. Polyclonal hypergammaglobulinaemia is seen in chronic infections, connective tissue disorders (e.g. rheumatoid arthritis, Sjögren's syndrome), neoplasms and chronic liver disease. Measurement of serum IgA concentration is of **no value** in the diagnosis of IgA nephropathy.

Paraproteins are products of abnormal B cell clones and can be detected in serum as monoclonal bands on immunoglobulin electrophoresis or in urine as Bence-Jones proteins. Paraproteins may be whole immunoglobu-lins or heavy or light chains in isolation. Light chains are sufficiently small to be filtered at the glomerulus, are not reabsorbed and are not picked up on routine dipsticks. Bence-Jones proteins are light chains excreted in the urine. Bence-Jones proteins precipitate on heating to 45°C and redissolve on boiling but are now detected by electrophoretic techniques.

Paraproteins can cause a number of different renal lesions, including
- Myeloma cast nephropathy.
- Light chain nephropathy.
- AL amyloidosis.
- Fibrillary/immunotactoid glomerulopathy (although this appearance is more frequently not associated with a plasma cell dyscrasia).

Cryoglobulins
Cryoglobulins are immunoglobulins, which precipitate on cooling and redissolve on warming.

Cryoglobulinaemia should be suspected in
- Renal failure with otherwise unexplained hypocomplementaemia or positive rheumatoid factor.
- Renal failure in association with skin and neurological involvement.
- Unexplained proteinuria/renal failure in patients with clonal B cell dis-orders.

Meticulous attention to collection, transportation and assessment of the sample is required: a serum sample must be kept at 37°C and sent to the laboratory for analysis immediately, having warned the lab that the sample is on the way. False negative results are common due to improper han-dling of the specimen.

Once a cryoglobulin has been found, further electrophoresis and immunofixation allows identification of three distinct types:
- Type 1 has a single monoclonal immunoglobulin (IgG, IgA or IgM) and is associated with monoclonal B cell disorders.
- Type 2 has a monoclonal IgM directed against the Fc portion of IgG, and the cryoprotein therefore consists of monoclonal IgM with poly-clonal IgG. Tests for rheumatoid factor (i.e. anti-IgG antibodies) are positive. This may be associated with haematological malignancy, chronic hepatitis C infection or may be unexplained ('essential').
- Type 3 has polyclonal IgG and polyclonal IgM and occurs in chronic infections (e.g. bacterial endocarditis, viral hepatitis), autoimmune dis-

orders (e.g. rheumatoid arthritis, SLE) or may be unexplained ('essential').

Hypocomplementaemia, especially very low C4 levels due to classical complement pathway activation is characteristic and helpful in diagnosing active cryoglobulinaemic disorder. Renal disease can present as an acute nephritic disorder or as nephrotic syndrome and is usually seen in association with skin and systemic involvement.

Antineutrophil cytoplasmic antibody (ANCA)

These are autoantibodies directed against enzymes present in the cytoplasm of human neutrophils. They are present in nearly all patients with small vessel vasculitis (including Wegener's granulomatosis, microscopic polyangitis, renal limited crescentic GN and Churg-Strauss syndrome). However, a negative ANCA does not rule out vasculitis, and false positive tests occur, so the test is not a substitute for renal biopsy.

Indications
- Suspected rapidly progressive glomerulonephritis.
- Suspected pulmonary-renal syndrome.
- Unexplained multi-system disease with or without renal involvement.

The test requires a serum sample. Immunofluorescent techniques using alcohol-fixed human neutrophils are used as a screening test. In this test the staining pattern may be described as 'cytoplasmic, cANCA' or 'perinuclear, pANCA', depending on the distribution of fluorescence (reflecting binding of the autoantibody in the serum to cytoplasmic constituents). This test can be difficult to interpret in the presence of a strong antinuclear antibody.

Positive tests should be followed by an enzyme-linked immunoassay (ELISA) to confirm the specificity of the autoantibody. A positive cANCA is usually associated with autoantibodies against proteinase 3 (PR3), and positive pANCA with myeloperoxidase (MPO).

Presence of PR3 or MPO-specific ANCA has a sensitivity and specificity of greater than 90% for small vessel vasculitis. PR3-ANCA/cANCA is prevalent in Wegener's and MPO-ANCA/pANCA is seen more commonly in renal limited crescentic GN and microscopic polyangitis, but there is considerable overlap. ANCA titres usually but not always correlate with disease activity and can be used to monitor treatment and screen for relapse.

Non-specific ANCAs are occasionally detected in association with systemic infection and other autoimmune disorders and are of little diagnostic value.

Antiglomerular basement membrane antibody (anti-GBM antibody)

Indications
• Acute nephritic syndrome with or without lung haemorrhage.

Goodpasture's syndrome is caused by an autoantibody against a component of type IV collagen which is only found in the glomerular basement membrane and in the lung. It causes rapidly progressive glomerulonephritis and, particularly in smokers and patients with other pre-existing lung disease, pulmonary haemorrhage. The disease evolves rapidly, and the earlier that it is diagnosed and definitive treatment started (with plasma exchange, cyclophosphamide and corticosteroids), the better the outcome. Tests for circulating antiglomerular basement membrane are performed using an enzyme-linked immunosorbent assay (ELISA) using type IV collagen. A positive test in a patient suspected of having the disease is sufficient evidence to proceed to treatment pending confirmation by renal biopsy; a negative test is not sufficient to exclude the diagnosis.

Antinuclear antibodies
Autoantibodies against a wide range of nuclear antigens occur in SLE, Sjögren's syndrome, scleroderma and other 'connective tissue diseases'. These tests are described in detail elsewhere (📖p250). Some of these, particularly SLE and scleroderma, may involve the kidneys. It is unusual for renal disease to be the first manifestation of SLE, but monitoring of complement levels and anti-dsDNA titres are valuable in monitoring the progression of disease. Scleroderma may present with a scleroderma renal crisis, a syndrome of rapidly worsening renal function and severe hypertension that shares many characteristics with accelerated phase hypertension. In this setting, tests for the characteristic autoantigens (e.g. scl-70) can help confirm the diagnosis.

Chapter 11

Poisoning & overdose

General principles

Many poisoned patients recover without specific management other than supportive care. A minority have life-threatening toxicity. In assessing the poisoned patient it is important to ensure adequate airway, breathing and circulation, take an adequate history and undertake a full clinical examination. Tablets, bottles, syringes, aerosol containers and other items found with or near the patient should be retained, although it is usually best to analyse biological specimens (usually blood and/or urine) if analytical confirmation of exposure is required.

The role of blood or urine tests in toxicology
Close collaboration between analytical staff and clinicians is required if anything other than the simplest toxicological analysis is to be useful.

Toxicological analysis using blood or urine is used to confirm the diagnosis of poisoning when this is in doubt or for medicolegal purposes, to help the management, in the diagnosis of brain death, or to work out the time to restart chronic drug therapy. Few centres have full analytical toxicology services and a 'toxicology screen' rarely influences inpatient management, with the exception of paracetamol, salicylate, lithium, digoxin and iron poisoning, and on occasions a drugs of abuse screen. Toxicological analysis of blood plasma or serum is also of value if an extracorporeal method of elimination such as haemodialysis is being contemplated. Any toxicology 'screen' should be tailored to that patient's circumstances and the poisons commonly encountered in that country. In Western Europe and North America, most patients will have taken drugs, but pesticide poisoning, for example, is common in less developed countries.

Plasma paracetamol, salicylates, lithium, digoxin and iron measurements in blood are usually available on an urgent basis. For other patients, particularly those who present a complex clinical picture or who are unconscious, a 50mL sample of urine and a 10mL sample of heparinised blood should be collected on admission and stored at 4°C (→refrigerator). This can be analysed later if it is felt the result will influence your management, or is needed for medicolegal purposes (see below). Urine is useful for screening, especially for drugs of abuse, as it is often available in large volumes and often contains higher concentrations of poisons and their metabolites than blood. The samples should be obtained as soon as possible after admission, ideally before drug therapy is initiated. Urine samples usually provide qualitative results, e.g. detect the presence of amphetamines or benzodiazepines. Quantitative measurements in urine are of little use because some compounds, such as benzodiazepines, are extensively metabolised prior to excretion in urine.

Sample requirements

Plasma or serum is normally used for quantitative assays for drugs and drug metabolites and in general there are no marked significant differences in concentration between these fluids. Evacuated blood tubes and containers containing gel separators or softrubber stoppers are not recommended if a toxicological analysis is to be performed as plasticisers (phosphates and phthalates) used in many such tubes may interfere with chromatographic methods and volatile compounds such as carbon monoxide or ethanol may be lost.

EDTA tubes are preferred for carboxyhaemoglobin assays and for measurement of lead, and some other metals such as these are concentrated in red blood cells. A fluoride/oxalate tube should be used if ethanol, cocaine or benzodiazepines are being assayed, although special tubes containing 1% (W/V) fluoride are needed if enzymic hydrolysis of these and other compounds is to be completely prevented.

The use of disinfectant swabs containing alcohols should be avoided, as should heparin, which contains phenolic preservatives (chlorbutol, cresol) and preservatives containing mercury salts (see table opposite).

Samples of medicolegal importance
A toxicology screen is helpful if murder, assault or child abuse is suspected. Samples collected in such cases are often so important that they should be kept securely at −20°C or below, until investigation of the incident is concluded. Legal requirements mean that all specimens should be clearly labelled with the patient's family or last name and any forenames, the date and time of collection and the nature of the specimen, if this is not obvious. Strict chain of custody procedures should be implemented and the doctor or nurse taking the sample should seal the bag with a tamper-proof device and sign and date the seal. A chain of custody form must accompany the sample and should be signed and dated by every person taking possession of the sample. The sample should be secured in a locked container or refrigerator if left unattended before arrival at the laboratory.

Sample requirements for metals/trace elements analysis

Metal	Sample needed
Aluminium	10mL whole blood in plastic (not glass) tube – no anticoagulant/ beads*
Antimony	5mL heparinised whole blood; 20mL urine
Arsenic	5mL heparinised whole blood; 20mL urine
Bismuth	5mL heparinised whole blood
Cadmium	2mL EDTA whole blood*; 10mL urine*
Chromium	2mL heparinised whole blood*; 20mL urine*
Copper	2mL heparinised or clotted whole blood, or 1mL plasma; 10mL urine
Iron	5mL clotted blood or 2mL serum (avoid haemolysis)
Lead	2mL EDTA whole blood
Lithium	5mL clotted blood or 2mL serum (NOT lithium heparin tube!)
Manganese	1mL heparinised whole blood or 0.5mL plasma*
Mercury	5mL heparinised whole blood; 20mL urine
Selenium	2mL heparinised whole blood or 1mL plasma/serum
Thallium	5mL heparinised whole blood; 20mL urine
Zinc	2mL whole blood (not EDTA) or 1mL plasma/serum

* Send unused container from the same batch to check for possible contamination.

Methods used in analytical toxicology

A range of chromatographic and other methods such as radioligand immunoassays are available for toxicological analyses. Plasma concentrations associated with serious toxicity range from micrograms per litre (mg/L) in the case of drugs such as digoxin to grams per litre (g/L) in the case of ethanol. Specialised labs used a combination of solvent extraction and thin layer chromatography (TLC) together with gas-liquid chromatography (GLC) using either flame-ionisation or selective detectors such as nitrogen/phosphorus detectors or mass spectroscopy (MS) as the basis for a poison screen. It is unwise to use TLC without corroboration of results by another method, e.g. GLC, because the resolution power of TLC is limited and interpretation of chromatograms is subjective. A commercial kit for TLC (Toxi-lab, Marion Laboratories) is supplied with a compendium of colour plates but even so problems can arise in differentiation of compounds with similar mobility and colour reactions. The kit is aimed at the US market and some common UK drugs are not included.

Spectrophotometry is commonly used to measure salicylates, iron and carboxyhaemoglobin. However, UV spectrophotometry and spectrophotofluorimetry are often used as detectors for high-performance liquid chromatography (HPLC) and in immunoassays. Spectrophotometric methods and immunoassays often suffer from interference from metabolites or other drugs. Immunoassays have the advantage of long shelf life and simplicity, but all require confirmation with a chromatographic method if the results are to stand scrutiny. This is because immunoassays for small molecules are often not specific, e.g. some urine amphetamine immunoassays give positive results with proguanil, isoxuprine, labetalol, tranylcypromine and phenylethylamine. The Syva Emit antidepressant assay cross-reacts with phenothiazines after overdose. Chromatographic methods have the advantage of selectivity and sensitivity and ability to perform quantitative measurements, but are expensive. Generally, GLC is still used to measure basic drugs and HPLC is used to analyse specific compounds/groups of compounds.

Modern methods of assay for heavy metals vary enormously. Isotope dilution mass spectrometry is a reference method. Atomic absorption spectrophotometry, with either flame or electrothermal atomisation is used most widely. In the case of iron though, reliable kits based on the formation of a coloured complex are available.

There is wide variation in the units that various laboratories use to report results. This has caused confusion and errors in treatment and great care is needed to ensure that clinical interpretation is undertaken in full knowledge of the units used.

Flanagan RJ. (1995) The poisoned patient; the role of the laboratory. Br J Biomed Sci 52, 202–213; Baselt RC, Cravey RH. (1995) Disposition of Toxic Drugs and Chemicals in Man, 4th edition, Chemical Toxicology Institute, California.

Brainstem death testing & organ donation

Brain death cannot be diagnosed in the presence of drugs that mask CNS activity. There is a rule of thumb, based on the pharmacological principle that most drugs need five half-lives to be effectively eliminated from the circulation, to allow four half-lives of any drug to elapse before declaring death, or to allow at least 2–3 days for drug effects to wear off. Whether this is satisfactory for patients with organ failure and hence impaired drug elimination is unclear and often in such patients measurement of plasma concentrations of residual drugs is required to determine whether brainstem death tests are valid or whether a drug could be interfering with the results.

Selected donor organs from those who have died from poisoning by tricyclic antidepressants, benzodiazepines, barbiturates, insulin, carbon monoxide, cocaine, methanol and paracetamol have been used in transplantation. It is important to identify which organs act as reservoirs for drugs and either not consider such organs, e.g. a liver from a paracetamol-poisoned patient, or take prophylactic precautions like N-acetylcysteine administration in the case of donation of a heart from a paracetamol-poisoned patient.

Interpretation of arterial blood gases in poisoned patients

Interpretation of blood gas values is covered in OHCM pp154, 684. Essentially four patterns emerge, which may be mixed together.

Respiratory acidosis
Hypoventilation results in retention of carbon dioxide. This can occur after an overdose with any drugs that depress the central nervous system (CNS), e.g. tricyclic antidepressants, opioids and barbiturates.

Respiratory alkalosis
Hyperventilation with respiratory alkalosis is classically caused by aspirin (commonly measured as salicylates). It can also occur in response to hypoxia, drugs and CNS injury.

Metabolic alkalosis
Metabolic alkalosis is very uncommon in poisoning. Rarely it may result from excess administration of alkali, e.g. deliberate alkali ingestion.

463

Jones AL, Simpson KJ. (1998) Drug abusers and poisoned patients: a potential source of organs for transplantation? Q J Med **91**, 589–592.

Metabolic acidosis
This is the commonest metabolic abnormality in poisoning. If acidosis is particularly severe (e.g. pH<7.2), this should raise the question of poisoning by ethanol, methanol or ethylene glycol. Measuring the anion gap and osmolal gaps are helpful in further differentiation (*Ethylene glycol, ethanol & methanol* (p470)).

Amphetamines & derivatives (MDMA (ecstasy), MDEA (eve), MDA (adam))

The following investigations should be considered in patients presenting to hospital with acute amphetamine(s) intoxication.

Plasma urea and electrolytes and glucose
It is critical that at least one set of U&E are checked in every patient. Most are profoundly dehydrated and require vigorous rehydration. Some patients develop hyponatraemia, often after drinking excess water and antidiuretic hormone secretion may be responsible for this (OHCM p692). Hypoglycaemia may occur.

Dipstick test of urine for myoglobin and subsequent serum creatine kinase
A hyperthermic (serotonin-like) syndrome with autonomic instability and rigidity, can develop leading to rhabdomyolysis. Dipstick testing of urine is positive for blood as myoglobin is detected by the haemoglobin assay. This is an indication that serum CK should be then be measured. If found to be elevated, adequate rehydration is needed to avoid deposition in renal tubules and incipient renal failure.

Full blood count
Rarely, aplastic anaemia (OHCM p664) has been reported after ecstasy (MDMA) ingestion.

Clotting studies
Disseminated intravascular coagulation (OHCM p652) can occur, often in the context of hyperthermia. Once liver damage ensues the INR/PT (OHCM p648) will rise.

Temperature
Hyperpyrexia can lead to rhabdomyolysis, disseminated intravascular coagulation and hepatocellular necrosis. Risks relate to the time in hours spent above 39°C. A rectal thermometer is the most accurate measure of temperature.

Liver function tests
Acute liver injury can occur with a rise in aspartate aminotransferase (AST) or alanine aminotransferase (ALT), often of several thousands.

▶▶NB Don't miss a hidden paracetamol overdose—check paracetamol levels in blood, from the earliest sample you have on that patient!

ECG
Cardiac arrhythmias are common and deaths, which occur soon after ingestion, may be due to these. Arrhythmias are often supraventricular, though ventricular ones also occur.

Urine tests

Urine tests, e.g. EMIT dipstick system or by immunoassay in the laboratory, are sensitive and group specific for amphetamines and can confirm an amphetamine has been ingested if that is in doubt, e.g. agitated patient in A&E. *Note:* Amphetamine, MDMA, MDEA and MDA concentrations in blood do not correlate with clinical signs and are of no value in management.

Anticonvulsants

These can be assayed in blood by gas-liquid chromatographic (GLC) methods and in urine by thin layer chromatography (TLC) methods.

Carbamazepine toxicity

Plasma concentrations of carbamazepine and its active metabolite 10, 11-epoxide can be measured by high-performance liquid chromatography (HPLC) but do not correlate at all well with the degree of toxicity. Thus carbamazepine levels are seldom performed unless the diagnosis is in doubt or there is concern about a therapeutic excess. The therapeutic range is between 8 and 12mg/L (0.5–5.5 mg/L for the active metabolite, 10,11-epoxide). Toxicity has been seen with carbamazepine concentrations above 20mg/L (85mmol/L). Coma, fits, respiratory failure and conduction abnormalities have been seen with concentrations in excess of 40mg/L (170mmol/L).

An ECG should be performed in all but the most trivial carbamazepine overdosage (e.g. >4 tablets) and inspected for the following:
- First degree atrioventricular block.
- QRS prolongation.
- Loss of P waves.

The U&E should be checked as hyponatraemia and SIADH (□*OHCM* p638) have been reported. Hypoglycaemia has also been reported.

Lamotrigine toxicity

Plasma concentrations of lamotrigine can be measured for compliance purposes (therapeutic range 1–4mg/L; upper limit may be as high as 10mg/L) but are not of value in the overdose situation.

An ECG should be performed in all but the most trivial lamotrigine overdosage (e.g. more than four tablets) and should be inspected and reviewed for QRS prolongation.

Valproate toxicity

Plasma concentrations of sodium valproate can be measured by HPLC but do not correlate well with either with depth of coma or risk of seizures after overdose. Thus valproate concentrations are seldom performed unless the diagnosis is in doubt. The therapeutic range is 40–100mg/L. U&E and glucose should be measured as hypernatraemia, hypoglycaemia and hypocalcaemia have been reported after valproate overdosage.

Phenytoin toxicity

Most patients with acute phenytoin poisoning do not require measurement of the plasma phenytoin concentration. An urgent phenytoin measurement may be helpful however in severe phenytoin poisoning where charcoal haemoperfusion is contemplated, e.g. in the presence of deep coma, respiratory depression and/or arrhythmias, particularly if the diagnosis is in doubt. Charcoal haemoperfusion is considered if the plasma phenytoin concentration is rapidly rising towards or exceeds 100mg/L.

Patients with suspected chronic phenytoin toxicity as a result of therapeutic dosing should have their plasma phenytoin concentration measured. The 'therapeutic range' is 10–20mg/L. Routine measurements may be useful to monitor anticonvulsant therapy or to time re-institution of chronic therapy after overdose.

Benzodiazepines

Most patients who have taken an overdose with benzodiazepines just sleep off the drug without sequelae within 24h. However, more severe effects can occur when benzodiazepines are mixed with other drugs such as tricyclic antidepressants, especially in patients with pre-existing cardiovascular or respiratory disease. Pulse oximetry is useful for monitoring the adequacy of ventilation if significant CNS depression is present.

Generally, measuring benzodiazepine concentrations in blood or urine is not of value in the management of benzodiazepine overdose patients. Rarely a urine screen by EMIT (immunoassay) is undertaken to confirm ingestion. Liquid chromatography simultaneously assays diazepam and its polar metabolites, and postmortem blood concentrations of 5mg/L and 19mg/L have been found in fatalities.

Carbon monoxide

Carbon monoxide is the commonest cause of death by poisoning in the UK. Those particularly at risk include patients with pre-existing cardiac or respiratory disease.

COHb

A carboxyhaemoglobin concentration in blood confirms exposure and should be measured urgently in all patients with suspected carbon monoxide poisoning, including those with smoke inhalation. The space above the blood in the sample tube (headspace) should be minimised. Normally expected values for COHb are up to 5% in non-smokers and up to 10% in smokers. However, after acute exposure the blood HbCO concentration does not indicate the severity of poisoning because HbCO begins to dissociate from the moment of removal from the source of exposure, and the rate of dissociation is also dependent on factors such as oxygen administration in the ambulance. Thus the use of nomograms to 'back-extrapolate' to find the initial highest COHb is meaningless and pointless. Management of the patient is determined by the clinical condition and also on circumstantial evidence such as the intensity and duration of exposure, rather than a HbCO concentration *per se*, although a level of >40% has been used as one criterion to guide the use of hyperbaric oxygen. A patient should be administered high flow oxygen (e.g. 12L/min through a tightfitting, e.g. CPAP, mask) until the COHb is <5% and clinical signs of carbon monoxide poisoning such as impaired heel-toe walking and finger–nose incoordination have resolved.

Arterial blood gases
Any patient with suspected poisoning by carbon monoxide requires arterial blood gas analysis. Oxygen saturation monitors are misleading as they read carboxyhaemoglobin as oxyhaemoglobin (HbO) and the true oxygen saturation of the patient can only be determined by arterial blood gas analysis.

ECG
An ECG should be performed in anyone severely poisoned (e.g. drowsiness or any neurological abnormality, chest pain or breathlessness) or with pre-existing heart disease. ECG changes such as ST segment depression, T-wave abnormalities, ventricular tachycardia or fibrillation and arrest can occur. If ischaemia/infarction is seen on the ECG or suspected clinically, the patient should also have cardiac enzymes sent.

Cocaine

Cocaine is snorted into the nose or injected intravenously.

Blood pressure monitoring
Patients with cocaine intoxication should have frequent measurements of their blood pressure, as hypertension is a significant risk, and strokes or myocardial infarcts have been widely reported. A Dynamap or equivalent advice for repeated measurements is suitable.

ECG and cardiac enzymes
Cocaine-induced angina and myocardial infarction is common. ECG monitoring is advised for all but the most trivial exposure to cocaine. Appropriate cardiac enzyme activity, i.e. CK, AST, LDH, should also be performed in any patient with chest pain or ECG abnormalities. The predictive value of troponin T estimations in this condition has not been evaluated.

Urine or blood testing
Cocaine can be detected in urine by simple 'drugs of abuse' screening tests, e.g. EMIT testing. Gas chromatography-mass spectroscopy is more specific and can be carried out on blood or urine. Metabolites of cocaine (benzoylecgonine) can be detected in urine 2–3 days after exposure. Cocaine is unstable in blood and samples are best taken into 1% w/v fluoride oxalate tubes if medicolegal sequelae are a possibility. Nasal insufflation of 106mg of the drug to 6 volunteers produced mean peak plasma

concentrations of 0.22mg/L at 0.5h and 0.61mg/L for the metabolite ben-zoylecgonine at 3h. Smoking 50mg in 6 volunteers produced mean peak plasma concentrations of 0.2mg/L at 0.08h and 0.15mg/L for bezoylecgo-nine at 1.5h. Patients have survived plasma concentrations of 5.2mg/L but usually fatalities are associated with cocaine/benzoylecgonine concentra-tions in excess of 5mg/L, depending on the route of use. The IV route is the most dangerous.

Cyanide

Cyanide poisoning can occur by deliberate inhalation of gas, ingestion of salts or by exposure in industrial fires.

Arterial blood gas estimation
Such measurements are essential to determine the oxygen saturation and acid-base status of the patient.

Serum lactate
This is very helpful in confirming suspected toxicity. It is likely to exceed 7mmol/L in cases of significant exposure.

ECG
All patients should have an ECG. It should be examined for evidence of ischaemic damage, e.g. ST depression, ST elevation, T-wave inversion.

Cyanide assay
Blood cyanide concentrations are rarely of use in emergency management because they cannot be measured quickly enough. However, a sample should be taken before antidote administration for assay at a later stage. Cyanide concentrations of <0.2mg/L are 'normal'; 1.0–2.5mg/L causes obtundation and coma; and more than 2.5mg/L is potentially fatal.

▶▶NB Dicobalt edetate antidote should only be given if cyanide poisoning is certain, i.e. a proper history is available, otherwise you will kill your patient. Otherwise give oxygen, sodium thiosulphate and sodium nitrite and/or hydroxocobalamin; these are antidotes that can safely be given without certainty of cyanide ingestion. Excessive adminis-tration of sodium nitrite however can cause significant methaemog-lobinaemia.

Digoxin

Patients who are already taking digoxin and those with pre-existing car-diovascular disease are more susceptible to digoxin toxicity after over-dosage. Digoxin toxicity can also result from progressive renal impairment

Jones AL, Dargan Pl. (2001) Churchill's Pocketbook of Toxicology, Churchill-Livingstone, Edinburgh.

and hence reduced elimination of the drug or due to interactions with other drugs such as amiodarone, calcium channel blockers or quinine, as well as overdoses.

ECG

All patients with suspected digoxin poisoning should have a 12-lead ECG and all symptomatic patients should be attached to a cardiac monitor. Digoxin poisoning can cause virtually any type of cardiac arrhythmia. The combination of heart block with tachyarrhythmia is very common.

Plasma digoxin concentration

Absorption of digoxin often peaks at 4–6h after ingestion. Its half-life is in excess of 30h. Digitoxin is a structurally-related drug that has an even longer plasma half-life (6 days). A digoxin measurement is a useful, but not absolute, guide to toxicity as plasma digoxin concentrations correlate poorly with the severity of poisoning, particularly early in the course of acute poisoning. However it is desirable (though not essential) if anti-digoxin Fab antibody fragments are to be used, as it is useful in calculating the dose of fragments (*see below*), as well as confirming exposure. Plasma digoxin concentrations cannot be interpreted after administration of digoxin antibody fragments using normal assay procedures. Samples taken to investigate probable chronic digoxin intoxication should be taken at least 6h after dosing. They are not normally analysed urgently unless life-threatening features of toxicity are present and use of antibody fragments (Fab) is being considered. The therapeutic range for digoxin is 0.8–2.0mg/L.

Urea and electrolytes

It is important to ascertain if the patient has any renal impairment and plasma creatinine and urea are helpful, though of course do not exclude renal impairment completely. Hyperkalaemia is common in acute digoxin overdose and may be severe, e.g. >7mmol/L. If possible a magnesium level is helpful to exclude hypomagnesaemia, which contributes to risk of cardiotoxicity and is easily corrected.

Indications for Fab fragments and doses of Fab fragments
- Severe hyperkalaemia (>6.0mmol/L) resistant to treatment with insulin/dextrose infusion.
- Bradycardia or heart block associated with hypotension.
- Tachyarrhythmias associated with hypotension, especially ventricular arrhythmias.

Fab antibody fragment administration should be considered in less severe stages of poisoning in older patients and those with pre-existing cardiovascular disease.

The dose of Fab fragments to give can be calculated from either the dose of digoxin ingested or the plasma digoxin

Number of 40mg vials of Fab =

plasma digoxin concentration (ng/mL) × body weight × 0.0084

OR

ingested dose (mg) × 1.2

OR

best guess of 10–20 vials

📖 OHCM p828.

Ethylene glycol, ethanol or methanol poisoning

A history of ingestion or the presence of a metabolic acidosis raises suspicion of poisoning with these substances. Calculation of the anion gap and osmolal gaps is helpful in the assessment of such patients.

Anion gap

Calculating the anion gap =

$$([Na^+] + [K^+]) - ([Cl^-] + [HCO3^-])$$

The normal anion gap is 12 ± 2

Many toxins cause a high anion gap acidosis and these include
- Ethanol.
- Methanol (Note: the high anion gap is due to metabolites and may take several hours to develop).
- Ethylene glycol (Note: the high anion gap is due to the metabolites and may take 6–24h to develop).
- Metformin.
- Cyanide.
- Isoniazid.
- Salicylates (aspirin).

This list can be further reduced by measuring the osmolal gap.

Osmolal gap
This is the difference between the laboratory estimation of osmolality (Om) and calculated osmolality (Oc).

> *Calculating the osmolal gap =*
>
> $$Oc = 2([Na^+] + [K^+]) + [urea] + [glucose]$$
>
> The osmolal gap is normally <10

Toxic causes of a raised osmolal gap include
- Methanol.
- Ethylene glycol.
- Diethylene glycol.
- Isopropanol.
- Ethanol.

The acronym 'MEDIE' can be a helpful mnemonic.

Ethylene glycol and methanol plasma concentrations
Often the diagnosis of ethylene glycol or methanol poisoning can be difficult because assays for these substances are not widely available. If possible, their measurement can help manage severe intoxication. Other parameters may have to be used, i.e. anion gap, osmolal gap and arterial blood gas analysis. A normal osmolal gap does not exclude poisoning with ethylene glycol or methanol, but if the osmolal gaps and anion gaps are both normal and the patient is not symptomatic, then significant ingestion is unlikely to have occurred. In general, ethylene glycol or methanol measurements should not be carried out unless metabolic acidosis is present and there is an anion gap.

Ethylene glycol and methanol concentrations in blood are useful to confirm ingestion, and indicate when to stop antidotal treatment (with ethanol or 4-methylpyrazole) and/or haemodialysis (>500mg/L, *see below*). However, a low concentration may just mean that most of the parent compound has been metabolised. Formate (i.e. the methanol metabolite) levels can also be checked in patients who may have taken methanol.

Microscopy of urine for oxalate crystals
In suspected ethylene glycol poisoning, microscopy should be performed to look for oxalate crystals; however they are only present in 50% of cases, and often only many hours after ingestion. Treatment of a patient should not be delayed or dependent upon looking for crystals.

471

Plasma ethanol concentrations
Plasma ethanol concentrations are usually not needed in patients who are drunk unless there is doubt about the diagnosis, e.g. patients with a widening osmolar gap or the patient is so severely poisoned that haemodialysis is being considered for the ethanol poisoning. They are, however, essential to guide appropriate use of ethanol as an antidote in ethylene glycol or methanol poisoning (*see below*). Rarely, a plasma ethanol measurement will be needed in child protection cases and such sampling will need chain of custody and a specific (GLC) method by a specialist laboratory.

Antidotal therapy with ethanol

The dose of ethanol for treatment of ethylene glycol and methanol poisoning can be very difficult to predict because ethanol metabolism is variable and unpredictable. It is therefore important to frequently recheck the blood ethanol concentrations on patients receiving an ethanol infusion. The dose should be adjusted to achieve a blood ethanol concentration of 1–1.5g/L.

Indications for continued ethanol therapy are
- Methanol or ethylene glycol poisoning with blood concentrations >200mg/L.
- Metabolic acidosis with pH<7.3.
- Osmolal gap >10mOsmol/kg water.
- Formate concentration >10mg/L.
- Urinary oxalate crystals.
- Severe symptoms.

Indications for haemodialysis in methanol or ethylene glycol poisoning are

- Methanol or ethylene glycol concentration >500mg/L.
- Severe metabolic acidosis (pH<7.3) unresponsive to therapy, i.e. arterial blood gases are needed in all cases of high anion gap poisoning.
- Renal failure—hence it is essential to check plasma urea and electrolytes in all patients.
- Presence of visual problems in methanol poisoning.
- Formate concentration >500mg/L in methanol poisoning.

▶Haemodialysis should be continued until the methanol/ethylene glycol concentration is <200mg/L.

Iron

Serum iron concentrations

Serum iron concentrations should be measured urgently in all patients who may have ingested more than 30mg/kg of elemental iron, unless no symptoms have developed 6h or more after ingestion, and should be taken at 4h and a further one at 6–8h after ingestion. One 200mg tablet of ferrous sulphate contains 60mg elemental iron. If a sustained-release preparation of iron has been taken, an initial serum iron concentration should be taken. A blood sample taken later after ingestion may underestimate the iron as it may have already started distributing to tissues, i.e. in a late presenting patient a low concentration cannot be interpreted, but a high one indicates toxicity. If the antidote desferrioxamine is given before 4h have elapsed, it interferes with the colorimetric assay for iron and so a serum sample for iron should be taken off before it is given. If atomic absorption spectrophotometry is available for measurement of serum iron, there is no interference from desferrioxamine.

It is essential to interpret the serum iron concentration result in the context of the clinical state of the patient. If <55mmol/L (<300mg/dL), mild toxicity is expected. If above 90mmol/L (500mg/dL), severe toxicity is expected and treatment with desferrioxamine is necessary. Antidotal treatment is also indicated for patients with iron concentrations >55mmol/L if there is additional clinical evidence of toxicity, e.g. gastro-intestinal symptoms, leucocytosis or hyperglycaemia. Antidotal therapy with desferrioxamine is indicated without waiting for the serum iron concentration in patents with severe features (e.g. fitting, unconscious or hypotensive). Desferrioxamine is usually continued until the urine has returned to a normal colour, symptoms have abated and all radio-opacities of iron tablets on abdominal x-ray have disappeared. Urine free iron estimation is the best test of when to stop chelation therapy with desferrioxamine, but is not widely available.

Working out if the patient needs a serum iron level checked

If a patient has ingested <30mg/kg body weight of elemental iron (a 200mg ferrous sulphate tablet ≡ 60mg elemental iron) then no serum iron level is required. If in doubt a plain abdominal x-ray will usually indicate if lots of tablets are present. A serum concentration of <55mmol/L (<300mg/dL) also indicates low risk (see above).

Abdominal x-ray

This is required in patients who have ingested in excess of 30mg elemental iron/kg body weight. The AXR determines the need for gut decontamination either by gastric lavage or whole bowel irrigation with polyethylene glycol. Undissolved tablets appear radio-opaque but they disappear once dissolved, so the absence of radio-opacities does not exclude the possibility of toxicity.

Full blood count

This is needed in all cases of iron poisoning. A leucocytosis ($>15 \times 10^9$/L) is common with significant toxicity.

Blood glucose

Hyperglycaemia is common in serious poisoning.

Arterial blood gases

These should be checked in symptomatic or severely poisoned patients. Metabolic acidosis is common.

Total iron binding capacity

This has no role in the assessment of acute iron poisoning.

473

What to do if estimation of serum iron concentration is unavailable

If serum iron assay is not available, the presence of nausea, vomiting, leucocytosis ($>15 \times 10^9$/L) and hyperglycaemia (>8.3mmol/L) suggests significant ingestion and the need for treatment with desferrioxamine.

📖OHCM p828.

Lead poisoning

Blood lead concentrations

Blood lead concentrations are used to confirm the diagnosis and decide on whether chelation therapy is required. Samples are not 'urgent' (except in the case of suspected acute lead encephalopathy) and must be taken into an EDTA tube. 'Normal' concentrations are <100mg/L. Lead causes changes in red cell and urinary porphyrins, but these are not measured routinely. A plain AXR should be performed in all children, particularly if there is a history of pica, to exclude ingested paint or lead foreign bodies such as curtain pulls. Long bone x-rays in children may show lead lines.

There are two agents used for chelation therapy in lead poisoning: (1) intravenous EDTA (disodium calcium edetate) and (2) oral DMSA (2,3-dimercaptosuccinic acid). Before use, chelation therapy should be discussed with a poisons centre. In general patients with a blood lead concentration >450mg/L should be treated with chelation therapy and removal from further exposure. Children with encephalopathy or a blood lead concentration of >750mg/L require admission to hospital for urgent chelation therapy.

Other essential investigations

Patients should also have a full blood count and blood film (for basophilic stippling), urea and electrolytes, liver function tests and serum calcium measured.

Lithium

Blood lithium concentration

Lithium is available as sustained-release, non-sustained-release tablets and liquid. After ingestion of liquid preparations, plasma lithium concentrations peak at 30min. With sustained-release preparations peak concentrations occur at 4–5h. The plasma half-life is often in excess of 24h. Interpretation of plasma lithium concentrations depends on the clinical circumstances of exposure (see below). Do not take blood for lithium levels into a lithium heparin tube!

Acute overdose in lithium naïve patient

A single overdose in a lithium naïve patient is of low risk. However, onset of toxicity may be delayed for as much as 24h. Samples for lithium assay should be taken at 6h post-ingestion and measured urgently. Consider haemodialysis if plasma lithium concentration is >7.5mmol/L.

Chronic excess of lithium

Lithium toxicity can occur if the patient has been taking too high a dose, is dehydrated, or if an interaction with thiazide diuretics, NSAIDs, ACE inhibitors or tetracycline has occurred. Risk of toxicity is further enhanced by the presence of hypertension, diabetes, cardiac failure, renal failure or schizophrenia. Blood for plasma lithium assay should be taken at presentation. Consider haemodialysis if the plasma lithium exceeds 2.5mmol/L.

Acute on chronic lithium poisoning

A patient taking lithium chronically who takes an acute overdose is at risk of serious toxicity, because tissue binding of lithium is already high. The plasma lithium levels should be measured urgently at 6h post-ingestion. Lithium measurements should be repeated 6–12 hourly in symptomatic patients until clinical improvement occurs. Consider haemodialysis if plasma concentrations exceed 4mmol/L.

Indications for haemodialysis

Lithium is effectively removed by haemodialysis. It is indicated in all patients with severe lithium poisoning, i.e. coma, convulsions, respiratory failure or acute renal failure. Plasma lithium concentrations can also guide the need for haemodialysis. Each hour of dialysis will reduce the plasma lithium by 1mmol/L, but plasma lithium often rebounds after haemodialysis so the assay should be repeated at the end of dialysis and again 6–12h later.

Urea and electrolytes

Hyponatraemia is common in lithium toxicity. It is also important to check the serum potassium concentration and urea, as lithium is renally excreted and renal failure delays its elimination.

Methaemoglobinaemia

Oxidising agents convert haemoglobin to methaemoglobin and this renders it incapable of carrying oxygen. Common agents causing methaemoglobinaemia include: dapsone, sulphonamides, trimethoprim, chlorates, aniline dyes, nitrites, nitrates and local anaesthetic including lignocaine. The onset and duration of symptoms will depend on the agent. Nitrites cause breathlessness and flushing within minutes of exposure but dapsone may cause a methaemoglobinaemia several hours after ingestion but the methaemoglobinaemia may then persist for days.

Essential investigations

Patients with suspected methaemoglobinaemia should have the following
- Arterial blood gases.
- Full blood count (especially if dapsone has been taken due to haemolytic anaemia).
- Blood methaemoglobin concentration.

Methaemoglobin can produce a normal PO_2 in the presence of reduced oxygen saturation. Pulse oximetry measures both methaemoglobin and oxygenated haemoglobin, so can give false results.

Methaemoglobin estimation in blood

Measurement of blood methaemoglobin is required to confirm the diagnosis and assess the severity of poisoning. The measurement must be done urgently when administration of the antidote (methylene blue) is contemplated. Samples for methaemoglobin estimation need to be analysed as soon as possible after collection, as if left to stand around the methaemoglobin will be falsely low owing to a reduction by endogenous methaemoglobin reductase. The severity of symptoms correlates roughly with the measured methaemoglobin concentrations. Anaemia, cardiac or pulmonary disease will lead to more severe symptoms at a lower methaemoglobin level.

MetHb conc. (%)	Clinical effects
0–15	None
15–30	Mild: cyanosis, tiredness, headache, nausea
30–50	Moderate: marked cyanosis, tachycardia, dyspnoea
50–70	Severe: coma, fits, respiratory depression, metabolic acidosis, arrhythmias
>70%	Potentially fatal

If the patient has severe clinical features of toxicity or if the blood methaemoglobin concentration is >30% the patient should be given methylene blue. Methylene blue can be given at lower blood methaemoglobin concentrations in those who are symptomatic.

Opioids

Classic features of opioid poisoning
- Depressed respiration.
- Pin-point pupils.
- Coma.
- Signs of parenteral drug use, e.g. needlemarks.

Toxicity can be prolonged for 24–48h, particularly after ingestion of methadone, which has a long half-life. The life-saving measure is prompt administration of adequate doses of naloxone, before waiting for results of any investigations.

Adequacy of ventilation
Oxygen saturation monitoring and/or arterial blood gas analysis demonstrates the adequacy of ventilation in those whose respiration has been inhibited.

Drug screening
Qualitative screening of the urine (group-specific immunoassay) confirms recent use. This may not detect fentanyl derivatives, tramadol and other synthetic opioids.

Measuring opioids in blood with gas chromatography-mass spectroscopy
This is sometimes required for medicolegal purposes, particularly where a fatality or a child-care issue is involved. Plasma morphine levels as high as 0.3mg/L were observed in addicts taking IV doses of heroin (diamorphine)

of 150–200mg. Postmortem morphine levels in heroin overdose deaths vary depending on prior narcotic history but in general exceed 0.3mg/L. Following a single oral dose of 15mg of methadone, plasma concentrations peaked at 4h at 0.075mg/L and declined slowly ($t\frac{1}{2}$ = 15h) until 24h when the concentration was still 0.03mg/L. Plasma methadone concentrations in maintenance patients increases by approximately 0.26mg/L for every 1mg/kg increase in oral dose. Deaths are due largely to reduced tolerance and blood concentrations of 0.4–1.8mg/L have been found postmortem, though live patients with tolerance exceed these values. 8.75mg/70kg IV morphine given to adults produces mean serum concentrations of 0.44mg/L at 0.5min, with rapid decline to 0.02 mg/L by 2h. Average morphine concentrations in fatalities range from 0.2 to 2.3mg/L, depending on tolerance.

Paracetamol screening

Opioid tablets are frequently combined with paracetamol. All unconscious patients should therefore have a plasma paracetamol measured.

Organophosphorus insecticides

Measurement and interpretation of AChE

Measurement of red cell cholinesterase (AChE) is useful in confirmation of exposure to organophosphorus compounds such as insecticides or nerve warfare agents, where this is suspected, e.g. restlessness, tiredness, headache, nausea, vomiting, diarrhoea, sweating, hypersalivation, chest tightness, miosis, muscle weakness and fasciculation. In general, clinical features are more helpful than red cell cholinesterase measurements in determining the severity of intoxication and hence the prognosis. There is a wide degree of intersubject variation in cholinesterase activity and clinical effects (*see table below*).

Cholinesterase activity	Clinical effects
Approx. 50% of normal	Subclinical poisoning
20–50% of normal	Mild poisoning
<10% of normal	Severe poisoning

The need for treatment with cholinesterase reactivators such as pralidoxime is largely judged by the occurrence of convulsions, fasciculation, flaccid paralysis and coma. Such features rapidly reverse within 20–30min of pralidoxime administration, together with atropine. The need for further therapy is guided by clinical improvement, together with monitoring of cholinesterase activity. It may take 90–120 days for red blood cell cholinesterase to recover to normal values.

Other vital investigations

An ECG should be carried out in all organophosphorus poisoned patients, and urea and electrolytes and glucose should also be monitored. In those with respiratory embarrassment or muscular paralysis, frequent assessment of tidal volume/peak flow rates and oxygen saturations are essential in anticipating the need for intubation.

📖OHCM p829.

Paracetamol poisoning

Overview

▶▶Paracetamol is the commonest drug taken in overdose in the UK. Measurement of a plasma paracetamol concentration is essential for assessing the need for antidotal treatment within 16h of a paracetamol overdose and should be performed urgently in all patients with known or suspected paracetamol overdose. It can be measured by a variety of assay methods but HPLC is less susceptible to interference than some enzyme-based assays. It should also be done urgently in patients with undiagnosed coma, or where a history is unreliable. Routine measurement of paracetamol concentrations in awake patients who deny taking paracetamol is unnecessary. For most patients, only a single measurement of paracetamol concentration is indicated. It is important to err on the side of caution and to give the antidote N-acetylcysteine if the blood paracetamol concentration lies near or just below the treatment line (Fig. 11.1) as stated timing of the overdose may be inaccurate and other agents such as opioids may slow gastric emptying.

If N-acetylcysteine is given within 12h of the overdose, it provides complete protection against liver injury and renal failure. Beyond 12h after ingestion the protection is less complete and assessment of liver damage is required. Paracetamol poisoning can be deceptive, as there is a latent phase of many hours, where the patient remains well before liver damage develops.

INR/PT

The most sensitive marker of prognosis in paracetamol poisoning is the prothrombin time (PT) or INR. This often starts to increase within 24–36h of the overdose and peaks at 48–72h. Once the INR/PT starts to improve, this is a sign that hepatotoxicity is starting to improve and the patient will not go on to develop acute liver failure. Approximately half of patients with a PT of 36s at 36h post-ingestion will develop acute liver failure.

Plasma alanine and aspartate aminotransferases (ALT and AST)

These may begin to rise as early as 12h post-ingestion but usually peak at 72–96h. AST or ALT values in excess of 10,000iu/L are not unusual and a plasma ALT>5000iu/L is very suggestive of paracetamol poisoning (Fig. 11.2). Serum bilirubin may peak after the aminotransferase and this should not lead to concern for patients in whom the INR or PT have begun to fall. ▶▶Do not correct abnormalities in PT or INR with FFP or cryoprecipitate unless life-threatening bleeding is taking place, otherwise the most sensitive marker of how the patient is progressing will be lost.

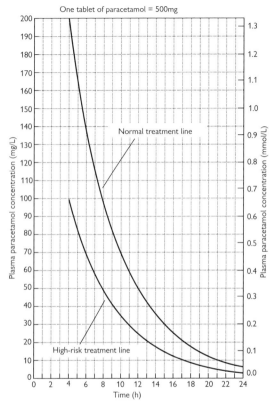

One tablet of paracetamol = 500mg

Fig. 11.1 *N*-acetylcysteine treatment graph. Patients whose plasma parac-etamol concentrations are above the **normal treatment line** should be treated with acetylcysteine by IVI (or, provided the overdose has been taken **within 10–12h**, with methionine by mouth). Patients on enzyme-inducing drugs (e.g. carbamazepine, phenobarbitone, phenytoin, rifampicin and alcohol) or who are malnourished (e.g. in anorexia, in alcoholism, or those who are HIV-posi-tive) should be treated if their plasma paracetamol concentrations are above the **high-risk treatment line**. *Note:* If paracetamol ingestion has been staggered (over some hours) serum levels may mislead: treat regardless, if significant amounts have been taken. Reproduced with permission from Dr Alun Hutchings and the *Oxford Handbook of Clinical Medicine*, 5th edition, Oxford University Press.

Other blood test abnormalities in paracetamol poisoning

Hypoglycaemia and metabolic acidosis are common. Early metabolic aci-dosis is often associated with very high plasma paracetamol concentra-tions, e.g. >400mg/L. Later, development of acidosis indicates incipient acute liver failure and the need to urgently check ABGs, liver function tests and INR/PT.

Pancreatitis with ↑ serum amylase has been reported. 5 cases of thrombocytopenia have been reported.

Renal failure can occur in the context of hepatic failure, but also in its absence (in 1 in 100 patients). It is treated with N-acteylcysteine and supportive measures, e.g. haemodialysis, if needed. Full recovery with supportive care is common.

Investigating the patient who has taken a paracetamol overdose <4h ago

Ingestion of >150mg/kg paracetamol or a paracetamol-containing product should be recognised as a hepatotoxic dose for most people. If ingestion of this amount or more has occurred within the last 1h, activated charcoal should be given orally (50g for an adult). Chronic alcohol ingestion (>14 units per week for ♀, >21 units per week for ♂), regular use of enzyme-inducing drugs (e.g. anticonvulsants) or the presence of eating disorders have been reported to reduce the ceiling of toxicity of paracetamol to 75mg/kg.

A plasma paracetamol should then be checked at 4h from the time of ingestion, to determine the need for N-acetylcysteine treatment from the treatment curve (Fig. 11.1). Very rarely, e.g. after ingestion of 4×500mg tablets by an adult, a confirmatory plasma paracetamol level is not needed, but in general it is cheap (approx £1) and safer to be certain by checking a blood concentration.

Investigating the patient who has taken a paracetamol overdose between 4 and 8h ago

A plasma paracetamol level should be checked as soon as possible to determine the need for N-acetylcysteine antidote treatment from the treatment curve (Fig. 11.1). ►►Use high-risk treatment line for patient with induced enzymes (e.g. anticonvulsants) or glutathione depletion (e.g. eating disorders).

Investigating the patient who has taken a paracetamol overdose between 8 and 24h ago

Start treatment with N-acetylcysteine straight away. Take blood for a paracetamol level, INR/PT, creatinine and plasma venous bicarbonate (if plasma venous bicarbonate is abnormal, check arterial blood gases). Checks results and refer to graph to determine whether treatment with N-acetylcysteine needs to be continued (i.e. is the plasma level above the treatment line?) or can be stopped (below the line). ►►Beyond 16h after ingestion the sensitivity of the assay for paracetamol may be too low to detect a treatable level—check and if in doubt, treat the patient with N-acetylcysteine! On completion of N-acetylcysteine, check blood INR/PT, creatinine and plasma venous bicarbonate (if abnormal check ABGs). If the patient is asymptomatic and the INR or creatinine is normal or falling discontinue the N-acetylcysteine. If the patient has symptoms (abdominal pain or vomiting) or the INR or creatinine is rising, continue maintenance N-acetylcysteine (50mg/kg in 500mL dextrose every 4h) until the INR improves. ►►Contact a poisons centre/liver unit.

11 Poisoning & overdose

Investigating the patient who has taken a paracetamol overdose >24h ago

It is too late for plasma paracetamol level estimation to be of any value. Start treatment with the antidote *N*-acetylcysteine straight away, unless a trivial amount has been taken. Take blood for baseline INR/PT, creatinine and venous bicarbonate (if abnormal check ABGs).

If the patient is asymptomatic and the lab tests normal, discharge the patient and advise to return if vomiting/abdominal pain develops. If the blood results are abnormal, phone a liver unit/poisons centre for advice.

Investigating the patient in whom the timing of overdose is unknown

Err on the side of treating the patient with the antidote *N*-acetylcysteine, checking an INR/PT, creatinine, plasma venous bicarbonate (ABGs if abnormal) at baseline and at the end of the first full course of treatment. If abnormal contact liver unit/poisons centre for further advice.

Investigating the patient who has taken a staggered overdose

Determine if the patient is in an at-risk group (i.e. enzyme induction or glutathione depletion) as discussed above. If the patient is not in an at-risk group but has ingested >150mg/kg body weight over 24h they should receive a full course of IV *N*-acetylcysteine. If they are in an 'at-risk' group and have ingested more than 75mg/kg body weight of paracetamol over 24h, they should receive a full course of *N*-acetylcysteine. There is no point measuring a plasma paracetamol level in this group of patients, unless the substance ingested is in doubt, and a 'not detected' result may

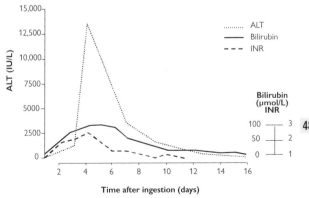

Fig. 11.2 Time course of liver function tests in paraetamol poisoning.

Dargan PI *et al.* (2001) Measuring plasma paracetamol concentrations in all patients with drug overdose or altered consciousness: does it change outcome? *J Emerg Med* **18**, 178–182.

be falsely reassuring. At admission and at the end of the course of N-acetylcystine a blood INR/PT, creatinine and venous bicarbonate should be checked. If abnormal at any stage, consult the poisons centre/liver unit.

📖 OHCM p830–831.

Salicylate (aspirin) poisoning

Features of severe poisoning
Ingestion of >150, 250 and 500mg/kg body weight of aspirin, respectively, produces mild, moderate and severe poisoning, respectively. Signs of serious salicylate poisoning include metabolic acidosis, renal failure and CNS effects such as agitation, confusion, coma and convulsions. Death may occur as a result of CNS depression and cardiovascular collapse.

▶▶The development of metabolic acidosis is a bad prognostic sign as it also indicates increased CSF transfer of salicylate.

Plasma salicylate concentration
Plasma salicylate should be measured urgently in all but the most trivial overdose, i.e. all those thought to have ingested >150mg/kg of aspirin or any amount of Oil of Wintergreen. It should be performed at 4h post-ingestion, because delayed absorption of the drug renders such levels uninterpretable before this time. As salicylates form concretions in the stomach, which delay absorption, it is recommended that a salicylate level is rechecked 3–4h after the first sample, to catch the peak salicylate concentration. There is no evidence for indiscriminate requesting of salicylate concentrations in every unconscious patient (unlike paracetamol) or in conscious patients who deny taking aspirin and who have no features suggesting salicylate toxicity. The plasma salicylate concentration is not an absolute guide to toxicity, as paracetamol levels are in paracetamol poisoning, but should be interpreted together with clinical features and acid-base status of the patient.

Urinary alkalinisation (📖 OHCM p830) is indicated for patients with salicylate concentrations of 600–800mg/L in adults and 450–700mg/L in children and the elderly. Metabolic alkalosis is not a contraindication to bicarbonate therapy as patients may have high base deficit in spite of an elevated serum pH.

Haemodialysis is very effective at salicylate removal and correction of acid-base and electrolyte abnormalities. It should be considered if the plasma salicylate levels are >700mg/L in children and >800mg/L in adults. Other indications for haemodialysis include resistant metabolic acidosis, severe CNS effects such as coma or convulsions, pulmonary oedema and acute renal failure.

Arterial blood gases
Acid-base problems are common in salicylate poisoning. Respiratory centre stimulation causes respiratory alkalosis. Uncoupled oxidative phos-

phorylation and interruption of glucose and fatty acid metabolism by salicylates often causes a concurrent metabolic acidosis. Serial ABGs are
needed in severe salicylate poisoning.

Theophylline

Acute theophylline poisoning can carry a high mortality and its management is best guided by the Shannon severity grading scheme[1], bearing in
mind that delayed effects tend to occur after sustained-release formula-
tions have been ingested. Most patients who die have grade 4 poisoning
(recurrent seizures, ventricular fibrillation, EMD arrest), sometimes grade
3 poisoning (non-repetitive seizure, sustained VT, mean arterial BP
<60mmHg and unresponsive to standard supportive therapy) toxicity with
plasma theophylline concentrations >100mg/L (770mmol/L). The adult
therapeutic range is 10–20mg/L.

Urea and electrolytes
It is vital to check the plasma K^+ concentration frequently, as
hypokalaemia is a life-threatening complication of theophylline overdose
and the serum K^+ concentration is a useful guide to severity. If
>2.5mmol/L the patient is less severely poisoned (grade 1) than if it falls
<2.5mmol/L (grade 2)[1]. Check blood glucose since hyperglycaemia is a
common complication.

Arterial blood gases
In potentially serious poisoning (e.g. ingestion of >20mg/kg body weight)
ABG analysis is helpful in optimising the acid-base status of the patient. An
initial phase of hyperventilation with respiratory alkalosis can be followed
by a further stage of metabolic acidosis.

Plasma theophylline concentrations
Measuring plasma theophylline concentrations confirms theophylline
ingestion where this is in doubt and is usually undertaken by HPLC. It is
also helpful in deciding when to employ charcoal haemoperfusion in seriously poisoned patients, particularly if plasma concentrations are
>100mg/L (770mmol/L) or are rapidly rising to approach this figure.
Charcoal haemoperfusion can be considered at lower concentration, e.g.
80mg/L, in the elderly or those with pre-existing ischaemic heart disease.
Charcoal haemoperfusion can also be decided on the basis of grade 3 or 4
severity grading alone, especially if administration of multiple doses of activated charcoal is not possible. However, for the vast majority of poisoned
patients, obtaining a plasma theophylline concentration does not guide
their management.

483

Therapeutic levels rarely exceed 20mg/L (155mmol/L). Theophylline peak
concentration in plasma may occur at 1–3h after ingestion of a standard-
release formulation. However, overdose is often with sustained-release
products and delayed absorption can result in delayed peak plasma concentration and toxicity, often 12–24h later.

Urine testing for myoglobinuria & measuring serum creatine kinase

Theophylline poisoning can be accompanied by rhabdomyolysis. Hence the urine should be dipsticked and if found positive for blood a serum CK should be obtained. This will then indicate that renal function should be closely monitored and the urine should undergo alkalinisation.

Tricyclic antidepressants

The main risks of overdose with these drugs are CVS and CNS toxicity.

ECG

An ECG should be performed in all but the most trivial cases of overdose.

ECG abnormalities are common in moderate–severe poisoning and include

- QRS prolongation: >110ms in adults predicts the risk of ventricular cardiac arrhythmias (and the need for IV sodium bicarbonate) and QRS >160ms predicts the risk of fits. In children a QRS >110ms is predictive of the risk of arrhythmias but *not* fits.
- Note: ECG criteria are not the only factors assessing risk of arrhythmias, fits and acidosis—electrolyte disturbances contribute. Supraventricular and potentially fatal ventricular arrhythmias can occur.

Cardiac monitoring

This is essential if ingestion of >10mg/kg body weight has taken place. It is seldom necessary beyond 24h after ingestion.

Arterial blood gas analyses

These should be done on all patients with marked symptoms and signs, particularly those with a reduced Glasgow coma score. It should also be performed on those with widened QRS or seizures, not least because such patients are receiving intravenous sodium bicarbonate therapy and a pH of 7.5 should not be exceeded.

Plasma concentrations

This is of no value as plasma concentrations of tricyclic antidepressants correlate poorly with clinical features of toxicity.

[1]Shannon M. (1993) Predictors of major toxicity after theophylline overdose. *Ann Intern Med* **119**, 1161–1167.

Table of conversion factors between mass & molar units

Drug	Clinical effects	Molar (SI) units	Conversion factor
Carbamazepine	mg/L	μmol/L	4.23
Digoxin	mg/L or ng/mL	nmol/L	1.28
Ethanol	g/L	mmol/L	1.28
Iron	mg/L	mmol/L	0.179
Lead	mg/L	mmol/L	0.0048
Paracetamol	mg/L	mmol/L	0.0066
Phenytoin	mg/L	mmol/L	3.96
Salicylate (aspirin)	mg/L	mmol/L	0.0072
Theophylline	mg/L	mmol/L	7.7

Rheumatology

Investigations

Investigations should be interpreted in the context of a careful history and physical examination.

Haematology

Full blood count: haemoglobin
Anaemia is common in rheumatic disease and may be:
- Microcytic (e.g. iron deficiency through blood loss resulting from treatment with analgesics or NSAIDs).
- Normocytic* (e.g. a manifestation of chronic disease).
- Macrocytic (e.g. folate deficiency, as may occur in RA).
*Note: ACD may be microcytic if longstanding.

White cell count may be increased or decreased
- Neutrophilia may accompany septic arthritis.
- Eosinophilia may occur in polyarteritis nodosa (PAN).
- Neutropenia is a feature of Felty's syndrome and of drug sensitivity.
- Leucopenia is a manifestation of SLE and of treatment with cytotoxic drugs (e.g. azathioprine).

Platelet numbers
- May be ↑, e.g. in RA (reactive phenomenon).
- ↓, as in SLE and as a side effect of treatment with D-penicillamine, gold or cytotoxic agents.

ESR and acute phase proteins
The ESR is an indirect measure of acute phase protein concentration; when ↑ it causes red cell rouleaux formation and results in a faster (higher) ESR. ESR and C-reactive protein (CRP) are both non-specific guides to inflammatory activity, e.g. in RA and SLE. Normally ESR is <20mm/h and CRP is <10mg/L.

A normal ESR generally excludes active inflammation. A falsely ↓ ESR can occur in sickle cell disease, anisocytosis, spherocytosis, polycythaemia and heart failure. A falsely ↑ ESR can result from prolonged blood storage or a measurement error. ESR and CRP levels may be inappropriately ↓ in some patients (e.g. seronegative arthritis and SLE, respectively) and are not infallible markers of inflammation.

Liver synthesis of acute phase proteins changes in response to inflammation. Some proteins increase whilst others decrease. Those whose levels fall are albumin, pre-albumin and transferrin.

An increased synthesis usually occurs rapidly (within hours) but varies in degree. Both C3 and caeruloplasmin increase only a little, whereas others such as fibrinogen and α1-antitrypsin increase two- to fourfold, and CRP and serum amyloid A (SAA) protein increase several hundredfold.

Biochemistry

Diagnostically useful plasma biochemistry includes
- Uric acid, which may be ↑ in gout.
- Urea and creatinine levels, which may ↑ when there is renal involvement.

- Alkaline phosphatase and other tests of liver function, which may be altered as a result of drug therapy with, for example, methotrexate.

Immunology

A number of markers of immune system function (e.g. antibodies, complement) that may be associated with specific diseases or disease groups can be measured. Autoantibodies and complement tests are discussed here because they are reliable and are commonly carried out (📖*Immunology investigations* p241).

Autoantibodies

Autoantibodies bind to a wide spectrum of antigens but their pathogenic relationship to disease has not been determined in most cases. The presence of autoantibodies may be used clinically:

- *To confirm a diagnosis*, e.g. rheumatoid factor (RF) may confirm a diagnosis of RA.
- *Point to a diagnosis*, e.g. antinuclear antibody (ANA) may indicate a diagnosis of SLE.
- *To forecast disease*, e.g. anticentromere antibodies are associated with the development of systemic sclerosis.
- *To indicate an exacerbation of disease*, e.g. anti-DNA is associated with an exacerbation of SLE.
- *To suggest early treatment*, e.g. coexistence of RF and reduced immunoglobulin G (IgG) galactosylation in RA is associated with severe disease later.

RFs are autoantibodies against antigenic determinants on the Fc fragment of IgG. They may be IgM, IgG or IgA.

RF tests are also positive in:

- Other rheumatic diseases.
- Viral infections (e.g. infectious mononucleosis).
- Chronic inflammatory disease (e.g. tuberculosis).
- Neoplasms or chemotherapy.
- 4% of healthy individuals—RFs may have a physiological role in immune regulation.

ANAs bind to cell nuclear components (DNA and RNA). Immuno-fluorescent cell staining is a useful screening test for them, and their specificity can be further defined by testing for the antibodies referred to below.

Antigen binding & disease associations of commonly measured autoantibodies

RA (correlation with severity)	IgG-Fc (rheumatoid factors)
SLE (correlates with activity)	DNA (double- and single-stranded) Extractable nuclear antigen (RNP)
SLE (highly specific)	SmRNP
Overlap syndromes	U1snRNP
Sjögren's syndrome, SLE	SS-A/Ro and SS-B/La
Systemic sclerosis	Scl-70 (topoisomerase 1) Centromere
Myositis	Jo1 (tRNA synthetase)
SLE associated with thrombotic events, thrombocytopenia and recurrent fetal loss	Phospholipids (i.e. anticardiolipin, lupus anticoagulant
Vasculitis	Neutrophil cytoplasmic antigen (A(anti)NCA); classified as **c** (cytoplasmic) and **p** (peripheral)
Wegener's granulomatosis	cANCA
PAN and other vasculitis syndromes	pANCA

RNP, ribonuclear protein; tRNA, transfer ribonucleic acid.

The pattern of ANA immunofluorescence is valuable diagnostically, but is not as specific as identification of a specific antigen–antibody reaction.

Five patterns of immunofluorescent are commonly recognised: homogeneous, peripheral, speckled, nucleolar and centromere.
- A *homogeneous* pattern (antibody to nuclear protein) and a *peripheral* pattern (antibody to DNA) are features of SLE.
- A *speckled* pattern (antibody to extractable nuclear antigens, e.g. ribonuclear protein) is seen in SLE, RA, systemic sclerosis and Sjögren's syndrome.
- A *nucleolar* pattern (antibody to nuclear RNA) is most common in systemic sclerosis.
- A *centromere* pattern is seen in limited cutaneous systemic sclerosis.

ANA testing may also be +ve, usually of low titre, in <20% of patients with chronic active hepatitis, infectious mononucleosis or lepromatous leprosy.

Complement

Total haemolytic complement, C3 and C4, are the factors usually measured to assess complement levels.

The main indication for these measurements is to diagnose SLE where immune complex activation of the classical pathway is thought to cause a reduction in these components. A genetic deficiency of the protein C2 is associated with SLE.

Arthrocentesis

Arthrocentesis or joint puncture is safe and easy to perform.

Indications
- To diagnose the cause of a joint effusion, particularly if there is a monoarthritis, which could be due to infection.
- To relieve pain by draining an effusion and injecting corticosteroids and/or local anaesthetic.

Complications
- Infection.
- Worsening symptoms.
- Induction of crystal synovitis due to joint trauma.
- Osteonecrosis as a result of repeated corticosteroid injection—it is recommended that only 3 injections are given into any one joint each year.

Synovial fluid examination

Synovial fluid obtained by joint aspiration is described in terms of its:
- Colour.
- Clarity.
- Viscosity.

Investigations when appropriate include
- White cell count.
- Gram stain, acid-fast methods and culture for bacteria (including *Mycobacterium tuberculosis*) and fungi (synovial fluid culture in suspected infectious arthritis should be accompanied by sputum, blood, urine and faecal cultures to detect a further source of infection).
- Crystal identification (using compensated polarised light microscopy to detect urate and calcium pyrophosphate).

491

Synovial biopsy may be necessary to detect *M. tuberculosis*, and EMU cultures are useful for suspected renal tuberculosis.

Diagnostic imaging

Diagnostic imaging is often necessary to allow an accurate diagnosis in rheumatology, and some techniques are more appropriate than others for certain disorders.

Plain radiographs

Radiographs are the first and usually only imaging test needed to investigate arthritis. They can demonstrate changes occurring in all components of the joint, and characteristic changes are seen, for example, in OA, RA and AS. Serial radiographs can be useful as they will document disease progression.

Ultrasonography

Ultrasound is a useful non-invasive technique especially for distinguishing synovial cysts (e.g. popliteal cyst) from solid tissue and in the examination of tendons (e.g. rotator cuff and biceps).

Computed tomography

Computed tomography (CT) is useful for visualising cross-sectional anatomy of calcified tissue (e.g. cortical and trabecular bone) and may be used to create a three-dimensional image.

Magnetic resonance imaging

Magnetic resonance imaging (MRI) is a valuable imaging tool. It works by detecting hydrogen ion mobility when tissues are subjected to pulsed radiowaves and a strong magnetic field causes them to emit a transient signal, which can be identified in space and time. The magnetic fields are known by their relaxation times, 'T1' and 'T2', which are characteristics of the tissues being measured and have to do with the rate at which energy is released by the magnetised tissue through which the pulse is passed.

MR imaging is especially useful for visualising organs in which there are contrasts of tissues (e.g. the spinal cord). Different tissues have specific hydrogen ion mobility in a magnetic field. Cortical bone contains virtually no mobile hydrogen ions and gives a very low signal intensity, whereas fat has a high signal intensity. Cortical bone is therefore better evaluated by radiographs or CT.

MRI of the musculoskeletal system has been most useful for viewing the spinal cord, intervertebral discs, hip joints and knee joints, and offers significant potential as it allows three-dimensional imaging and multiple plane examination.

Skeletal scintigraphy

The typical radionuclide scan uses ^{99m}technetium methylene diphosphonate complexes to detect physiological changes in the bone in contrast to the anatomical changes depicted by plain radiographs and MRI.

An increased uptake of the isotope into the bone can result from many causes including infection, tumour, fractures and synovitis. This type of scanning is therefore non-specific and needs to be correlated with radiographs and clinical findings. It is useful when clinical symptoms and radiographs have proved inconclusive.

[67]Gallium citrate and [111]indium scans can be used to define sites of infection in bones and soft tissues, which appear as areas of increased uptake.

Single proton emission CT (SPECT), which provides cross-section imaging in skeletal scintigraphy, and positron emission tomography (PET) are more sensitive techniques, but have limited availability.

Arthroscopy

Arthroscopy is useful both diagnostically and therapeutically. Unlike needle biopsy, it allows a direct view of the joint and synovial fluid, and biopsy samples can be taken from multiple sites within the joint.

The joint most commonly examined by arthroscopy is the knee. The technique is often used to investigate trauma (e.g. sport injury). Most arthroscopies are carried out as day cases; the anaesthetic depending on the extent of the procedure.

Histopathology
It may sometimes be necessary to take an organ biopsy to help make a diagnosis, e.g.
- Synovial membrane and bone biopsy in suspected infection.
- Kidney biopsy in suspected SLE.
- Liver biopsy in suspected iatrogenic and autoimmune liver disease.
- Lung biopsy in suspected Wegener's granulomatosis.

Radiology & the role of imaging

The effective use of the radiology department relies on good communication between radiologists and their clinical colleagues. The overall aim must be to target investigations efficiently in order to provide answers to clinical dilemmas at minimal cost and radiation dose. The investigation of neurological problems has been transformed by the advent of CT and MRI, but these are not always locally available and CT in particular can add considerably to the radiation burden. Conversely, if a CT is likely to provide the best answer and minimise overall costs by resulting in an early discharge then it should be the investigation of choice. It is helpful to consider plain films, contrast studies, ultrasound and then CT/MRI as a hierarchy where plain films are requested as an initial investigation. This hierarchy may be circumvented if a more expensive investigation is likely to produce the definitive result. The following are important points to consider:

1. Will the investigation alter patient management? I.e. is the expected outcome clinically relevant? **Do you need it?**
2. Investigating too often or repeating investigations before there has been an adequate lapse of time to allow resolution or to allow treatment to take effect. **Do I need it now?**
3. Would an investigation that does not use ionising radiation be more appropriate, e.g. USS/MRI?
4. Failure to provide accurate clinical information and questions that you are hoping will be answered by the investigation may result in an unsatisfactory outcome. Have I explained the problem?
5. Would another technique be more appropriate? The advances in radiology mean that discussion with a radiologist may be helpful in determining the best possible test.
6. Overinvestigating: are you taking comfort in too many tests or providing reassurance to the patient in this way?

Typical effective doses from diagnostic medical exposures

Procedure	Equivalent number of CXRs	Equivalent period of background radiation
Chest (PA film)	1	3 days
Lumbar spine	65	7 months
Abdomen	50	6 months
IVU	125	14 months
Barium enema	350	3.2 years
CT head	115	1 year
CT abdomen	500	4.5 years
V/Q scan	50	6 months

Royal College of Radiologists. (1998) Guidelines for Doctors, *Making the Best Use of the Department of Clinical Radiology*, 4th edition.

Plain x-rays

Wilhelm Roentgen discovered x-rays in 1895. X-rays form part of the electromagnetic spectrum with microwaves and radiowaves lying at the low energy end, visible light in the middle and x-rays at the high energy end. They are energetic enough to ionise atoms and break molecular bonds as they penetrate tissues, and are therefore called *ionising radiation*. Diagnostic x-rays are produced when high energy electrons strike a high atomic number material. This interaction is produced within an x-ray tube. A high voltage is passed across two tungsten terminals. One terminal (cathode) is heated until it liberates free electrons. When a high voltage is applied across the terminals the electrons accelerate towards the anode at high speed. On hitting the anode target x-rays are produced.

The x-ray picture is a result of the interaction of the ionising radiation with tissues as it passes through the body. Tissues of different densities are displayed as distinct areas depending on the amount of radiation absorbed. There are 4 basic densities in conventional radiography: *gas* (air); *fat*; *soft tissue and fluid;* and *calcified structures*. Air absorbs the least amount of x-rays and therefore appears black on the radiograph, whereas calcified structures and bone absorb the most, resulting in a white density. Soft tissues and fluid have a similar absorptive capacity and therefore appear grey on a radiograph.

Digital radiology

X-ray film is exposed by light photons emitted by intensifying screens sensitive to radiation transmitted through the patient. Storage phosphor technology uses photo-stimulable phosphor screens to convert x-ray energy directly into digital signals. The increased dynamic range and image contrast of digital radiography compared with conventional film screen combinations and the facility to manipulate signal intensity after image capture reduce the number of repeat exposures. This increases efficiency and minimises patient radiation dose. Digital images can be made available on a local network for reporting by a radiologist or for review on a ward-based computer. Picture archiving and communication systems (PACS) are efficient at image production and manipulation and in the storage, retrieval and transmission of data. Initial costs are high and at present are limited to a few centres in the UK.

Chest x-ray: useful landmarks

In order to interpret a plain PA or lateral CXR some knowledge of chest anatomy and the major landmarks on the film is required. We have highlighted the major bony and soft tissue structures visible on the plain film in order to make it easier to spot abnormalities.

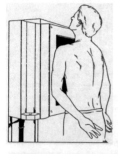

Fig. 13.1 Patient position for PA CXR.

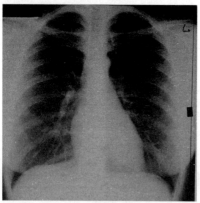

Fig. 13.2 PA CXR.

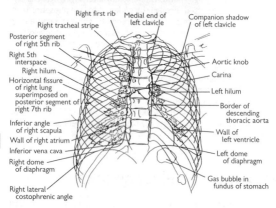

Right first rib
Right tracheal stripe
Medial end of left clavicle
Companion shadow of left clavicle
Posterior segment of right 5th rib
Right 5th interspace
Right hilum
Horizontal fissure of right lung superimposed on posterior segment of right 7th rib
Inferior angle of right scapula
Wall of right atrium
Inferior vena cava
Right dome of diaphragm
Right lateral costophrenic angle
Aortic knob
Carina
Left hilum
Border of descending thoracic aorta
Wall of left ventricle
Left dome of diaphragm
Gas bubble in fundus of stomach

498

Fig. 13.3 PA CXR landmarks.

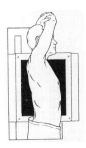

Fig. 13.4 Patient position for lateral CXR.

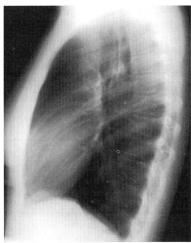

Fig. 13.5 Lateral CXR.

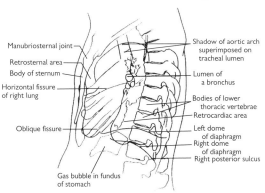

Manubriosternal joint

Retrosternal area

Body of sternum

Horizontal fissure of right lung

Oblique fissure

Gas bubble in fundus of stomach

Shadow of aortic arch superimposed on tracheal lumen

Lumen of a bronchus

Bodies of lower thoracic vertebrae

Retrocardiac area

Left dome of diaphragm

Right dome of diaphragm

Right posterior sulcus

Fig. 13.6 Lateral CXR landmarks.

Abdominal x-ray: useful landmarks

Interpretation of the AXR, like the CXR, requires experience. In order to make things slightly easier we have provided a rough guide to the various bony, soft tissue and gas shadows seen on a 'typical' AXR.

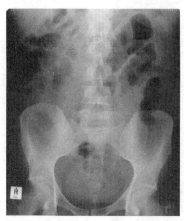

Fig. 13.7   PA AXR.

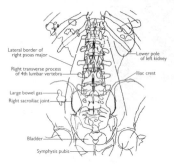

Fig. 13.8   PA AXR landmarks.

Chest radiograph

The chest film is the most widely requested, yet most easy to misinterpret, investigation. Using a logical approach will avoid most pitfalls.

Initially assess technical quality

Projection
PA *vs.* AP will determine whether assessment of cardiac size is reliable.

Posture
Erect films enable a more accurate assessment of the mediastinum since the lungs are more expanded, and allow detection of air–fluid levels, pleural thickening and comment on the size of pulmonary vasculature.

Rotation
Look for the relationship of the medial ends of the clavicles to spinous process at the same level; a common cause of unilateral transradiancy is rotation.

Degree of inspiration
Ideally 6 ribs should be seen anteriorly, and 10 ribs posteriorly. If more, this suggests hyperinflation (does the patient have asthma or COPD?). If less (e.g. poor inspiratory effort, obesity or restrictive chest disorders) there will be apparent cardiomegaly, increased basal shadowing and less commonly tracheal deviation.

The heart and mediastinum
Sequentially consider the heart, mediastinum, lungs, diaphragms, soft tissues (breast shadows) and bones. Remember to assess your review areas: the lung apices, behind the heart, under the diaphragm and the costophrenic angles.

Diaphragm: this should lie between the 5th to 7th ribs. If flattened, consider hyperinflation. In 90% of cases the right is higher than the left by 3–4 cm. Effacement of the interface between lung and diaphragm suggests pleural or pulmonary pathology. Loss of smooth contour suggests localised herniation (eventration). Peaks laterally may be due to subpulmonary effusion.

Root of neck and trachea: the upper trachea is central with slight displacement to the right inferiorly due to the oesophagus. Thickening of the paratracheal line (>5mm) may imply nodal enlargement.

Mediastinum: the mediastinum should be central. The heart is normally <50% of thoracic width. Mediastinal enlargement or widening is a non-specific finding. The silhouette sign may help but a lateral film is helpful for localisation. Based on location of mediastinal abnormality, possible pathologies include:
- Superior mediastinum: thymoma, retrosternal thyroid and lymphoma.
- Anterior mediastinum: lymphoma (HD & NHL), germ cell tumours, thymoma, retrosternal goitres and Morgagni hernias (low).
- Middle mediastinum: aortic aneurysm, bronchial carcinoma, foregut duplication cysts (including bronchogenic/oesophageal) and hiatus hernia.

Posterior mediastinum: neurogenic tumours, Bochdalek hernia, dilated oesophagus or aorta.

Enlarged lymph nodes: may be seen in any compartment.

Hila: density should be equal, left is higher than the right by 5–15 mm. If more disparity consider elevation due to fibrosis (e.g. TB, radiotherapy) or depression by lobar or segmental collapse. Hilar enlargement may be

501

vascular (e.g. pulmonary arterial or venous hypertension) or due to lymphadenopathy (e.g. sarcoidosis, lymphoma or TB). Hilar calcification is seen in silicosis, sarcoidosis and treated lymphoma.

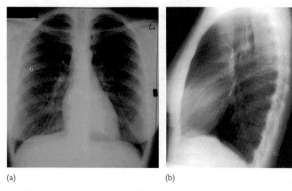

(a)   (b)

Fig. 13.9   Normal PA and lateral CXR.

Lung disease

Lung opacities may be subdivided into several basic patterns.

Alveolar (air space) shadowing—ill-defined, non-segmental and with air bronchograms. Large variety of causes:
- Fluid→pulmonary oedema (cardiogenic and non-cardiogenic).
- Fat→fat embolism.
- Haemorrhage→trauma, coagulopathies, pulmonary haemosiderosis.
- Cells→pulmonary alveolar proteinosis, sarcoidosis, alveolar cell carcinoma and infection (bacterial, fungal and viral).

Reticular (linear opacities)-associated obscuration of vessels and late appearance of chest x-ray signs:
- Collagen disorders.
- Extrinsic allergic alveolitis.
- Sarcoidosis, pneumoconiosis.
- Cryptogenic fibrosing alveolitis.
- Early left ventricular failure (LVF).
- Malignancy (lymphangitis carcinomatosis).

Nodular shadows: characterise according to their size and distribution:
- If solitary exclude tumour.
- Multiple:
  - Granulomas (TB, histoplasmosis, hydatid).
  - Immunological (Wegener's, rheumatoid arthritis).
  - Vascular (arteriovenous malformations).
  - Inhalational (PMF, Caplan's syndrome).

502

Armstrong P, Wilson AG, Dee P, Hansell DM, eds. (1997) *Imaging of Diseases of the Chest*, 2nd edition, Mosby, St Louis; Corne J et al. (1997) *Chest X-ray Made Easy*, Churchill Livingstone, Edinburgh.

Patterns of lobar collapse

Lobar collapse may be *complete* or *incomplete*. The commonest cause is obstruction of a central bronchus. The primary signs are opacification due to lack of aeration and displacement of the interlobar fissures.

Secondary signs include
- Elevation of the hemi-diaphragm (more prominent in lower lobe atelectasis than upper).
- Mediastinal displacement (tracheal displacement with upper lobe and cardiac displacement with lower lobe atelectasis).
- Hilar displacement: more prominent with upper lobe atelectasis than lower.
- Crowded vessels in the affected lobe.
- Compensatory hyperinflation of remaining lung.

Barium studies

Barium suspension is made up of small particles of barium sulphate in a solution. Due to its high atomic number it is highly visible on x-rays. The constituents of individual suspensions vary depending on the part of the GI tract being examined. The particles are coated to improve flow and aid mucosal adhesion. When made up it comprises a chalky (sometimes unpalatable!) suspension. Advantages include low cost, easy availability and good assessment of mucosal surface.

Risks are more common in the context of
- *Perforation*: if leakage occurs into the peritoneal cavity it can produce pain and hypovolaemic shock (50% mortality). Long-term sequelae include peritoneal adhesions.
- *Aspiration*: in small amounts unlikely to have any clinical significance but if pre-existing respiratory impairment or aspiration of larger amounts (i.e. more than a few mouthfuls) the patient will need physiotherapy.
- *Obscuration*: CT examination in the presence of a recent barium examination will result in a poorly diagnostic study as high density barium results in streak artefacts.
- *Barium impaction*: rarely may exacerbate obstruction if barium collects and is concentrated above a point of obstruction.

Water-soluble contrast media
These are more expensive and provide inferior coating and contrast. They include iodinated agents gastromiro and gastrograffin. Indications for their use include:
- Suspected perforation especially into the peritoneal cavity.
- Meconium ileus.
- To opacify bowel during CT examinations.

503

Risks include pulmonary oedema if aspirated and hypovolaemia, especially in children. Both are a result of hyperosmolar effects. If aspiration is likely

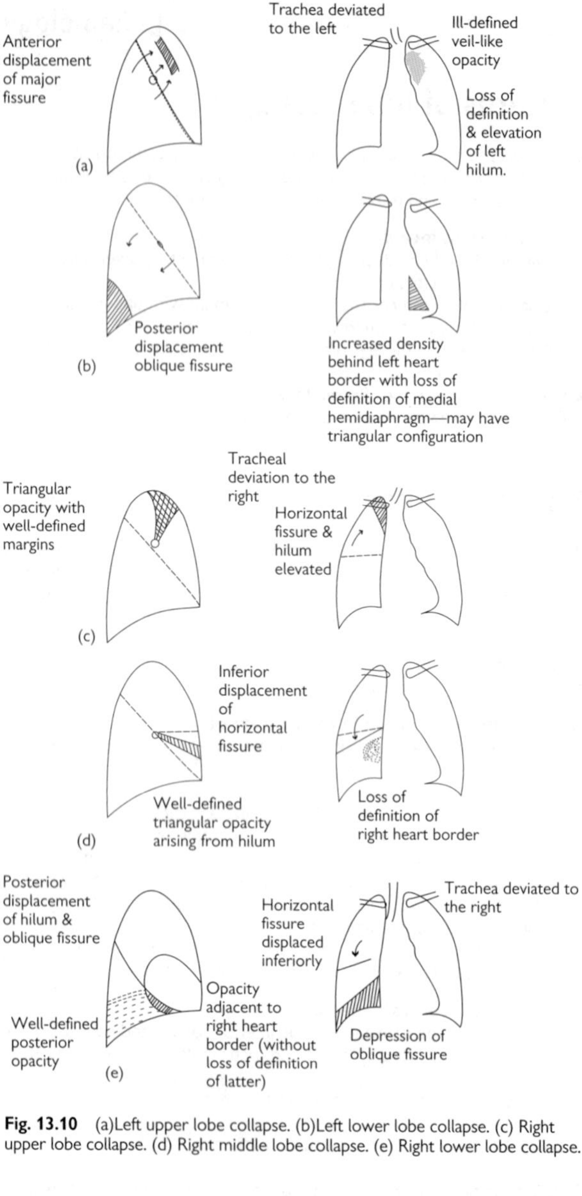

Fig. 13.10 (a)Left upper lobe collapse. (b)Left lower lobe collapse. (c) Right upper lobe collapse. (d) Right middle lobe collapse. (e) Right lower lobe collapse.

Labels within figure:

(a) Anterior displacement of major fissure. Trachea deviated to the left. Ill-defined veil-like opacity. Loss of definition & elevation of left hilum.

(b) Posterior displacement oblique fissure. Increased density behind left heart border with loss of definition of medial hemidiaphragm—may have triangular configuration.

(c) Triangular opacity with well-defined margins. Tracheal deviation to the right. Horizontal fissure & hilum elevated.

(d) Inferior displacement of horizontal fissure. Well-defined triangular opacity arising from hilum. Loss of definition of right heart border.

(e) Posterior displacement of hilum & oblique fissure. Horizontal fissure displaced inferiorly. Trachea deviated to the right. Well-defined posterior opacity. Opacity adjacent to right heart border (without loss of definition of latter). Depression of oblique fissure.

504

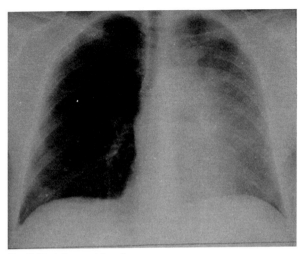

Fig. 13.11 Left upper lobe collapse.

Pharmacological agents used in barium studies.

Agent	Dose	Advantages	Disadvantages
Buscopan	20mg IV	Reduced bowel peristalsis due to smooth muscle relaxant action. Immediate onset. Short duration of action (15min).	Anticholinergic side-effects. Contraindicated with cardio-vascular disease and glaucoma
Glucagon	0.3mg IV for barium meal. 1.0mg IV for barium enema	More potent smooth muscle relaxant than buscopan. Short duration of action, no interference with small bowel transit	Contraindicated with insulinomas or phaeochrom-ocytomas, relatively expensive.
Metoclopramide	20mg PO or IV	↑ gastric peristalsis enhances barium transit during a follow-through study	Possible extra-pyramidal side-effects.

Barium swallow

Plain films do not usually demonstrate the oesophagus unless it is very distended, e.g. achalasia. They may be useful in identifying an opaque foreign body within the lumen. The barium swallow is the usual contrast examination to visualise the oesophagus. Rapid sequence films are taken with a fluoroscopy unit while the patient swallows barium (usually in the erect position). Films are taken in an AP and oblique projection (to throw the oesophagus clear of the spine) with the oesophagus distended with barium (to demonstrate its outline) and empty to show the mucosal folds.

Normal anatomy
The oesophagus commences at C5/6. There are normal indentations on its outline by the cricoid cartilage, the aortic arch, left main bronchus and left heart.

Indications
These include the assessment of dysphagia, pain, reflux disease, tracheo-oesophageal fistulae (in children) and post-operative assessment where there has been gastric or oesophageal surgery.

Contraindications
No absolute contraindications exist, but in all barium studies the quality of the study relies heavily on patient cooperation and therefore immobile patients who are unable to weight bear may only be suitable for limited studies. The post-operative oesophagus is usually assessed with gastro-miro or a non-ionic contrast.

Common disorders and patterns

Diverticulae: these include pharyngeal pouches (a midline diverticulum), traction diverticulae (due to adhesions) or pseudodiverticulae; dilated mucous glands seen in reflux or infective oesophagitis.

Luminal narrowing: strictures may be benign (e.g. oesophagitis, shown in Fig. 13.12a, scleroderma, pemphigus, corrosives or infection) or malignant.

Webs: seen with skin lesions, e.g. epidermolysis or pemphigus, graft-versus-host disease and the Plummer Vinson syndrome.

Mega-oesophagus: can be with associated obstruction as in malignant strictures or without as in achalasia, diabetic neuropathy or Chagas' disease (Fig. 13.12b–d).

Ulceration/oesophagitis: may be due to gastro-oesophageal reflux disease, infection, corrosives or iatrogenic. Findings include lack of distensibility, fold thickening and mucosal irregularity.

Oesophageal tears: spontaneous, neoplastic, post-traumatic, iatrogenic and following prolonged emesis. Look for pneumomediastinum, left pleural effusion and features of mediastinitis.

Filling defects: foreign bodies, varices (proximal due to SVC obstruction), distal (in association with portal hypertension), neoplasms which may be benign as in leiomyoma or malignant. Most commonly squamous cell carcinoma (95%).

Fold thickening: may be due to oesophagitis, varices or infiltration by lymphoma.

Air/fluid level: commonest in hiatal hernias but also seen with a pharyngeal pouch.

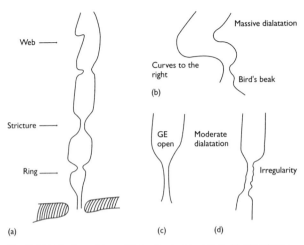

Fig. 13.12 (a) Benign strictures. Obstruction in: (b) achalasia, (c) scleroderma, and (d) cancer.

Barium meal

About 200mL of a high density (250% weight/volume), low viscosity barium is used for a double contrast study which gives good coating without obscuration of mucosal detail. An effervescent agent is given to provide adequate luminal distension. The gastric mucosa is characterised by rugae (parallel to the long axis, 3–5mm thick) and area gastricae (nodular elevations 2–3mm wide). The patient is fasted for about 6h to avoid food residue which may cause diagnostic uncertainty. The techniques for coating the stomach and projections are variable. A smooth muscle relaxant may be given as part of the routine, particularly to assess the pylorus and duodenum.

Indications
Dyspepsia, weight loss, abdominal masses, iron deficiency anaemia of uncertain cause, partial outlet obstruction and previous GI haemorrhage.

Contraindications
Complete large bowel obstruction.

Abnormal findings

507

Filling defects: these may be intrinsic or extrinsic. Carcinoma remains the commonest cause of a filling defect in an adult (irregular, shouldered with overhanging edges). If there is antral involvement there may be associated outlet obstruction. Diffuse mucosal thickening and failure to distend is seen with linitis plastica. Other causes include gastric lymphoma, polyps (histology difficult to predict) and bezoars. Smooth filling defects are seen in conjunction with leiomyomas, lipomas

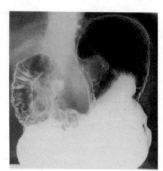

Fig. 13.13 Barium meal showing leiomyoma.

and metastases. Extrinsic indentation by pancreatic tumours or an enlarged spleen may cause an apparent filling defect.

Fold thickening (>5mm) is seen in association with hypersecretion states such as Zollinger-Ellison syndrome, gastritis and Crohn's disease. It may also be secondary to infiltration by carcinomas, lymphomas or eosinophilia.

Outlet obstruction may be diagnosed by failure of the stomach to empty <50% of the barium ingested at 4h. This may be seen in carcinomas but also by scarring caused by chronic duodenal ulceration.

Hiatal hernia: herniation of the stomach into the chest occurs via the oesophageal hiatus in the diaphragm. There are two types: in a *sliding* hernia (more common) there is incompetence of the sphincter at the cardia, often associated with reflux. Other sequelae include oesophagitis, ulceration or stricture. In a *rolling* hernia the fundus herniates through the diaphragm but the gastro-oesophageal junction remains competent.

Gastritis and ulceration: gastritis is characterised by small shallow barium pools with surrounding lucent rings due to oedema. There are features which may be used to distinguish benign from malignant ulcers on barium studies. Ulcers are seen either as a crater or as a projection from the luminal surface. Benign ulcers are commonly seen on the lesser curve with smooth radiating folds which reach the edge of the ulcer crater. Malignant lesions may have an associated mass, have a shallow crater and an irregular contour. With the ease of availability of endoscopy, the use of barium meals in diagnosing ulceration has declined. Endoscopy has the advantage of being able to diagnose gastritis more accurately, assess ulcer healing, make a histological diagnosis and more accurately assess the post-operative stomach. However, early assessment of the post-operative stomach is radiologically performed to exclude complications such as anastomotic leaks. A water-soluble contrast agent is preferred in the early post-operative phase.

Small intestine

Small bowel follow-through: the patient drinks 200–300mL of barium (with metoclopramide to speed transit time). The single contrast column is followed by films at regular intervals until the barium reaches the colon. Transit time is variable but the entire process may take 1–6h depending on adequacy of bowel preparation. Films are taken at intervals of approximately 20min initially, in the prone position which aids separation of the loops. When the barium reaches the caecum spot views of the terminal ileum are taken.

Small bowel enema (enteroclysis): this technique provides better demonstration and mucosal detail, as there is rapid infusion of a continuous column of barium directly into the jejunum. Methyl cellulose is administered following the barium to provide double contrast. This is achieved via a weighted nasogastric tube which is positioned at, or distal to, the duodendojejunal (DJ) flexure. Disadvantages include poor patient tolerance (related to intubation) and a relatively high screening dose.

Both techniques require the patient to be on a low residue diet beforehand.

Indications
The indications are the same for both techniques and include pain, diarrhoea, bleeding, partial obstruction, malabsorption, overgrowth syndromes, assessment of Crohn's disease activity and extent, and suspected masses. The small bowel enema may be preferred for assessment of recurrent Crohn's disease or complex post-operative problems but the small bowel follow-through is otherwise routinely used.

Contraindications
Complete obstruction and suspected perforation.

Normal findings
The small intestine measures ~5m and extends from the DJ flexure to the ileocaecal valve. The proximal two-fifths is the jejunum, the distal three-fifths is the ileum. Normal calibre is 3.5cm for the jejunum and 2.5cm for the ileum (up to 1cm more on enteroclysis). The valvulae conniventes are circular in configuration and ~2mm thick in the jejunum and 1mm thick in the ileum.

Abnormal findings

Dilatation is indicative of malabsorption, small bowel obstruction (SBO) or paralytic ileus. There may be accompanying effacement of the mucosal pattern. When seen with fold thickening it may be due to Crohn's, ischaemia or radiotherapy. Mucosal thickening may be due to infiltration by lymphoma or eosinophilia, adhesions, ischaemia or radiotherapy.

Strictures are seen in Crohn's disease and in lymphoma. There is usually dilatation of the bowel proximally. Crohn's disease causes skip lesions, ulceration, strictures of variable length and a high incidence of terminal ileal involvement. There may be associated ulceration, fold thickening and fistulation.

Malabsorption: radiological investigation may reveal an underlying structural abnormality. The findings in malabsorption include dilatation, fold thickening and flocculation of barium.

509

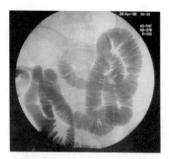

Fig. 13.14 Small bowel enema (enteroclysis).

Cholangiography

Oral cholangiograms (OCGs) were used as first line investigations when the clinical history suggested non-acute gallbladder disease. Ultrasound has largely replaced it for the initial diagnosis of gallstones but OCG remains superior in assessing the number and size of gallstones, cystic duct patency and gallbladder function. The contrast is administered 14h prior to the study. Failure to visualise the gallbladder may be indicative of pathology if contrast has been taken and absorbed. The examination is contraindicated in acute cholecystitis and is unlikely to be successful when the serum bilirubin is >34µmol/L (as the contrast media is excreted by the liver, normal hepatocyte function is required for adequate elimination).

Intravenous cholangiography

This is rarely performed but may be useful in patients with biliary symptoms post-cholecystectomy or with a non-functional gallbladder. It is contraindicated in the presence of severe hepatorenal disease, as the side effects related to the contrast media are considerable.

ERCP (endoscopic retrograde cholangiopancreatography)

The biliary and pancreatic ducts are directly filled with contrast following endoscopic cannulation and during x-ray screening. This has both a diagnostic and therapeutic role. It is particularly of value in the demonstration of ampullary lesions and to delineate the level of biliary tree obstruction in patients with obstructive jaundice. It allows sphincterotomy to be performed to facilitate the passage of stones lodged in the common bile duct.

PTC (percutaneous transhepatic cholangiography)

The biliary tree is directly injected with contrast following percutaneous puncture of the liver. This is both diagnostic in defining a level of obstruction and therapeutic in biliary duct obstruction, as it may be used as a precursor to a biliary drainage procedure or prior to insertion of a stent. Contraindications include bleeding diatheses and ascites.

Other cholangiographic techniques

- Per-operative cholangiogram in which the common bile duct (CBD) is filled with contrast during cholecystectomy to exclude the presence of CBD stones.

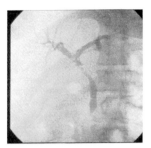

Fig. 13.15 PTC demonstrating a stricture in the common hepatic duct

- T-tube cholangiogram: after operative exploration a T-tube is left in the CBD for a post-operative contrast study to exclude the presence of retained stones.
- MRCP (magnetic resonance cholangiopancreatography): this is a non-invasive, relatively new technique where heavily T2-weighted images are obtained without contrast administration. The bile acts as an intrinsic contrast agent and stones are visualised as filling defects. The accuracy of this technique remains to be fully verified and it may replace the need for diagnostic ERCP although clearly not therapeutic ERCP.

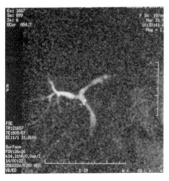

Fig. 13.16 MRCP (correlate with PTC images in same patient).

511

Barium enema

This is the technique of choice for evaluation of the large bowel. Barium is run into the colon under gravity via a tube inserted into the rectum. The column of barium is followed by air to achieve double contrast. Buscopan (a smooth muscle relaxant) may be given to minimise spasm and optimise mucosal relief. Bowel preparation prior to the examination (low residue diet and aperients) is vital to ensure that there is no faecal material which may mask mucosal abnormalities or be mistaken for small polyps. Remember the examination is uncomfortable and requires reasonably good patient cooperation and mobility. ►*Do not request this in frail or elderly patients unless there is a good clinical indication*. A rectal examination or sigmoidoscopy is essential to avoid abnormalities being missed.

Single vs. double contrast

If evaluation of the colonic mucosa is not the primary aim then a single contrast technique will suffice. This is applicable in children, where the patient is uncooperative and where gross pathology is being excluded, and in the evaluation of obstruction/volvulus or in the reduction of an intus-susception.

Indications

Change in bowel habit, iron deficiency anaemia, abdominal pain, palpable mass of suspected colonic origin, and weight loss of unknown cause.

Contraindications

Recent rectal biopsy, toxic megacolon or pseudo-membranous colitis.

Common findings

Solitary filling defect: polyps are classified according to histology. The commonest are hyperplastic (no malignant potential, adenomatous polyps are premalignant with the risk of malignancy increasing with size (<5mm = 0%, >2cm = 20–40%). Also found are adenocarcinoma (increased risk in ulcerative colitis, polyposis syndromes, villous adenoma), and less commonly metastases and lymphoma.

Multiple filling defects: polyps (polyposis syndromes or post-inflammatory pseudopolyps), pneumatosis coli, metastases and lymphoma.

Ulceration: inflammatory bowel disease (IBD), ischaemia, infection, radiation and neoplasia.

Colonic narrowing: neoplasms (apple core lesion), metastases, lymphoma, diverticular disease, IBD, ischaemia and radiation.

Dilatation: mechanical, e.g. proximal to neoplasm, volvulus or non-mechanical, post-operative ileus, metabolic and toxic megacolon.

Diminished haustration: cathartic colon, IBD and scleroderma.

Increased haustration (thumbprinting): ischaemia, haemorrhage, neoplasm and IBD.

Widening of the pre-sacral space (>1.5cm at S2): normal in up to 40% but also seen in association with IBD, neoplasms, infection and sacral/pelvic lipomatosis.

512

Colonoscopy

Remains a complementary technique and has the advantage of being both therapeutic and diagnostic (e.g. biopsy, polypectomy, etc.). In elderly patients CT with prior bowel preparation and air insufflation is less invasive and less arduous. CT colonoscopy (using 3D reconstruction of CT images and software to simulate navigation of the inside of the colon) is currently being evaluated.

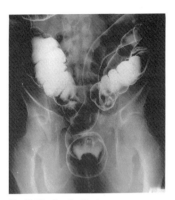

Fig. 13.17 Standard barium enema.

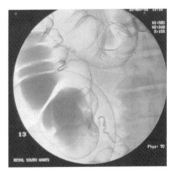

Fig. 13.18 Digital image.

Plain abdominal x-ray (AXR)

The standard plain film is a supine AXR. Erect views have largely been superseded and in the acute setting have been replaced by the erect chest to show free subphrenic air. Furthermore, chest diseases such as myocardial infarction or pneumonia may simulate an acute abdomen. If there is doubt regarding the presence of a pneumoperitoneum, consider a lateral decubitus film (displays as little as 1mL of air).

Indications
Suspected obstruction, perforation, renal colic and toxic megacolon.

Contraindications

None but where abdominal pain is non-specific and not attributable to the conditions listed above, an AXR is unlikely to be helpful.

Interpretation of the plain AXR

A normal patient will have variable amounts of gas in the stomach, small bowel and colon. You can identify the stomach, as it lies above the transverse colon, has an air/fluid level in the erect view and has rugae in its lumen. Large bowel calibre is variable; 5.5cm is considered the upper limit for the transverse colon in toxic megacolon and 9cm for the caecum in obstruction. Short fluid levels are normal. Fluid levels are abnormal when seen in dilated bowel or if numerous. If the bowel is dilated distinguish between small and large bowel by the features listed below.

	Small bowel	Large bowel
Haustrae	Absent	Present
Valvulae conniventes	Present in jejunum	Absent
Number of loops	Many	Few
Distribution of loops	Central	Peripheral
Diameter of loops	30–50mm	>50mm
Solid faeces	Absent	May be present

Causes of bowel dilatation include mechanical obstruction, paralytic ileus or a localised peritonitis (meteorism), e.g. adjacent to pancreatitis or appendicitis.

Look for extraluminal gas

Gas in the peritoneal cavity: look for air under the hemidiaphragm, outlining the falciform ligament or both sides of the bowel wall (Rigler's sign). If there is any doubt consider a lateral decubitus film. Causes include perforation (ulcer, neoplasm), post-operative, following peritoneal dialysis or tracking down from the mediastinum.

Air in the biliary tree: following sphincterotomy, gallstone ileus or following anastomosis of CBD to bowel.

Portal vein gas: pre-morbid sign in the context of bowel infarction but less sinister in neonates with NEC (necrotising enterocolitis) or following umbilical catheterisation.

Gas in an abscess: look for displacement of adjacent bowel and an air/fluid level.

Other causes include air in the urinary tract, necrotic tumours and retroperitoneal gas.

Look for any soft tissue masses or ascites: the latter is detectable on plain films if gross. There will be displacement of the ascending and descending colon from the side walls with loops of small bowel seen centrally.

Look for abdominal or pelvic calcification: first localise the site. This may require another view. The vast majority are clinically insignificant, i.e. vascular calcification, pelvic phleboliths and calcified mesenteric nodes. In the abdomen there may be pancreatic calcification (chronic pancreatitis) or hepatic calcification (old granulomas, abscesses or less commonly hepatomas and metastases from mucinous primaries).

Gallstones are less commonly calcified and may contain central lucency (e.g. Mercedes Benz sign), while renal and ureteric calculi commonly calcify. Renal tumours and cysts rarely calcify and more widespread renal calcifications may be seen in nephrocalcinosis due to a wide variety of causes. In the pelvis, ovarian calcification (less common with malignant masses and seen more often in association with benign pathologies such as dermoids) is uncommon whilst uterine calcifications due to fibroids commonly occur. Bladder wall calcifications may be seen with bladder tumours, TB and schistosomiasis. Prostatic calculi and calcifications are common and of no significance. Vas deferens calcifications are seen in patients with diabetes.

Soft tissues: look at renal outlines (normally smooth and parallel to psoas, should be between 2–3 vertebral bodies). Absence of psoas margins may indicate retroperitoneal disease and haemorrhage.

Bones of the pelvis and lumbar spine: look for osteoarthritis, metabolic bone disease (hyperparathyroidism, sickle cell anaemia), the rugger jersey spine of osteomalacia and Paget's disease (*Lumbar spine & pelvis* (p526, 528)). Bony metastases may be lytic or sclerotic.

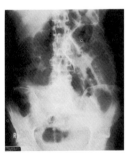

Fig. 13.19 Plain AXR showing evidence of small bowel obstruction.

Radiology of the urinary tract

Plain abdominal film

Look for any urinary tract calcification: 90% stones are radio-opaque. Other causes include hyperparathyroidism, medullary sponge kidney and renal tubular acidosis.

Renal outline: between T12 and L3 and 10–15cm. Left bigger and higher than the right.

Assess bones of spine and sacrum for bony metastases or spina bifida (may be relevant in enuresis).

515

Field S. (2001) The abdomen: the plain abdominal radiograph (Ch 45) in *A Textbook of Medical Imaging*, 4th edition, eds Grainger RG, Allison DJ, Churchill Livingstone, Edinburgh.

IVU

This provides a good overview of the urinary tract and in particular the pelvicalyceal anatomy. Fluid restriction and laxatives are no longer necessary and in particular the former is to be avoided in diabetics, renal failure and myeloma. Following the preliminary plain film, 300mg/kg of contrast media is injected IV. The film sequence is varied according to the clinical scenario. An immediate film shows the nephrogram phase and displays the renal outlines. An increasingly dense delayed nephrogram is seen in acute obstruction, acute hypotension, acute tubular necrosis (ATN) and renal vein thrombosis. A faint persistent nephrogram is seen with acute glomerulonephritis and it may be delayed in renal artery stenosis (RAS). Later films show the pelvicalyceal systems (pyelogram), ureters and bladder.

Common abnormalities

Loss of renal outline: congenital absence, ectopic kidney, tumour, abscess or post-nephrectomy (look for absent 12th rib).

Small kidney (unilateral): ischaemia (RAS), radiation or congenital hypoplasia.

Small kidney (bilateral): atheroma, papillary necrosis or glomerulonephritis.

Large kidney (unilateral): duplex, acute pyelonephritis, tumour or hydronephrosis.

Large kidney (bilateral): polycystic kidneys and infiltrative disease such as myeloma, amyloid and lymphoma.

Pelvicalyceal filling defect: smoothly marginated (clot, papilloma), irregular margins (tumour, e.g. renal cell or transitional carcinoma), intraluminal (sloughed papilla, calculus or clot), extrinsic (vascular impression or cyst), irregular renal outline (scarring, e.g. in ischaemia, TB, pyelonephritis or reflux nephropathy).

Ultrasound

May be used as an alternative or complementary examination with the IVU and may be used to:

- Demonstrate or exclude hydronephrosis especially in acute renal failure (ARF).
- Evaluate renal tumours, cysts and abscesses.
- Follow-up of transplant kidneys and chronic renal disease.
- Assess renal blood flow using Doppler.
- Serial scanning in children with recurrent urinary tract infections.
- Assess bladder morphology and volume, and the prostate.
- Provide guidance for interventional techniques, e.g. renal biopsy and nephrostomy placement.

CT and MRI

CT is more accurate for staging renal tumours, assessing retroperitoneal pathology, staging bladder and prostatic tumours and may replace IVU in some centres.

MRI is valuable in staging vascular involvement by renal carcinomas. Dedicated pelvic coils and endoluminal coils show promising results in staging bladder and prostatic carcinoma.

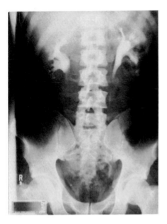

Fig. 13.20 IVU demonstrating medullary sponge kidney.

Renal cyst

Multiple renal cysts
(elongation & distortion
of calyces – polycystic
disease)

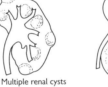

Renal tumour

Duplex kidney with
hydronephrotic
upper, moiety.
('drooping flower')

Dilatation of a
single calyk
(may be due to
vascular compression)

Fig. 13.21

517

Micturating cystourethrogram (MCUG)

Following catheterisation of the bladder, contrast is introduced. This is the
technique of choice for defining urethral anatomy and gauging the pres-
ence/degree of vesicoureteric reflux in children.

Ascending urethrography

Contrast is injected directly into the urethra in males in the assessment of urethral trauma, strictures and congenital anomalies such as hypospadias.

Retrograde pyelography

The ureters are catheterised (usually following cystoscopy in theatre) and contrast injected under x-ray screening. Of value in urothelial tumours and to define the site of obstruction, e.g. non-opaque calculi.

Angiography

A femoral approach with selective catheterisation of renal vessels. Main uses include haematuria (look for AVMs), hypertension (RAS), in transplant donors (to define anatomy) and in renal cell carcinoma (where embolisation is being contemplated).

Nephrostomy

📖 *Interventional radiology* (p531).

Breast imaging

Breast cancer is a common problem (1 in 12 women). An NHS breast screening programme is in place following the Forrest Report. Its aim is to use imaging to detect early clinically occult carcinomas. It screens women aged 50–64 years on a 3-yearly basis (the detection rate is 50 cancers for every 10,000 women screened).

Mammography

Technical factors: breast tissue has a narrow spectrum of inherent densities and in order to display these optimally a low kilovoltage (KVP) beam is used. It enhances the differential absorption of fatty, glandular and calcific tissues. Dedicated mammographic units provide low energy x-ray beams with short exposure times. The breast is compressed to minimise motion and geometric unsharpness. High resolution is paramount in order to detect microcalcification (as small as 0.1mm). The breast is a radio-sensitive organ so doses need to kept to a minimum.

Standard projections: these are the mediolateral oblique and craniocaudal views. Adequacy of the lateral oblique view may be gauged

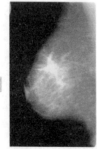

Fig. 13.22 Lateral oblique projection: shows a spiculated mass with distortion of the surrounding parenchyma and overlying skin thickening, consistent with a breast carcinoma.

by the pectoralis major muscle which should be visible to the level of the nipple, inclusion of the axillary tail, and inclusion of the inframammary fold. Additional projections such as true lateral and magnification views may be used to clarify abnormalities.

Mammographic signs: the breast parenchyma is made up of glandular tissue in a fibro-fatty stroma. Cooper's ligaments form a connective tissue network. The amount of glandular tissue decreases with age, as it is dense on mammography the suitability of the technique for detecting pathology increases with age.

Primary signs of a malignancy
- A mass with ill-defined or spiculate borders.
- Clustered, linear or irregular calcification (which may occur in the absence of a mass).
- Secondary signs include distortion of adjacent stroma, skin thickening and nipple retraction.

94% of breast carcinoma is ductal in origin.

Breast ultrasound: this largely forms a modality for assessment not diagnosis or detection. It can, however, be used to evaluate non-palpable masses, to determine internal architecture (solid vs. cystic), to assess asymmetric density and as a primary imaging modality in young women (<35 years). It is also used as a tool to guide intervention, i.e. drainage of cysts and biopsy of suspicious lesions.

MRI: MRI remains a problem-solving tool in breast imaging at present. Both MRI and ultrasound may be used to evaluate implants and their integrity but MRI is the only modality that is sensitive in the evaluation of intra-capsular implant rupture. Contrast-enhanced MRI of the breast is also a sensitive method for detection of malignancy with reported sensitivities in the region of 93%. It is especially useful to detect recurrent breast carcinoma and where conventional techniques are unable to help in the distinction from more benign lesions. Breast MRI is also being advocated for screening young patients with a family history/genetic risk of breast carcinoma.

Ultrasound

Ultrasound is a high frequency mechanical vibration produced by pizoelectric materials, which have the property of changing thickness when a voltage is applied across them. It is an important tomographic modality and has widespread applications in the abdomen, neck, pelvis and extremities. At diagnostic levels there are no known damaging sequelae to tissues and therefore it is safe for use in obstetrics providing invaluable imaging of the developing fetus. Doppler USS is based on the principle that sound reflected by a moving target has a different frequency to the incident sound wave. The frequency shift is proportional to the velocity of the flowing material. Doppler therefore not only enables detection but quantification of velocity.

Indications

USS is cheap, readily available, non-invasive and has high patient acceptability. It has a wide range of applications as listed below. There are also no radiation implications.

Contraindications

None, but remember that USS is operator- and patient-dependent and should be used as a problem-orientated modality, not as a total body survey. It cannot be used to image air-containing structures or bone. The resolution of the USS image is inversely related to the depth of penetration. Therefore image quality in obese patients is sub-optimal.

Applications

Head and neck: may be used for evaluation of the salivary glands, thyroid, lymph nodes and palpable or clinically suspected masses. Doppler is used to assess the carotid vessels and quantify degree of stenosis/occlusion.

Chest (excluding breast): the use here is limited to palpable chest wall lesions, assessment of pleural abnormalities, biopsy and drainage of pleural effusions and is occasionally of use in directing a biopsy of peripheral lung or mediastinal masses.

Abdomen & pelvis: this is the main use of USS. Useful for assessment of solid organs, e.g. liver, kidneys, spleen, gallbladder, pancreas, uterus/adnexae and bladder. A full bladder is used as an acoustic window in the pelvis. Retroperitoneal masses and lymph nodes may be visible depending on patient habitus. USS is useful for directing biopsy of solid organs/masses and for drainage of ascites, abscesses and collections.

Limbs: musculoskeletal USS has been revolutionised by advances in high frequency probes which enable characterisation of soft tissue masses, tendon-related pathology, rotator cuff lesions, masses, effusions and collections. It is also used for vascular assessment and the diagnosis of deep vein thrombosis.

Intracavitary transducers: these place the transducer as close as possible to the area of interest. They include transvaginal, transrectal, urethral, oesphageal and intravascular probes. They are usually high frequency transducers that produce detailed high resolution images. Transvaginal USS is more invasive than transabdominal scanning but is used in the

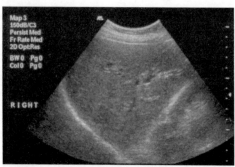

Fig. 13.23 Longitudinal USS image demonstrating dilatation of the intrahepatic ducts.

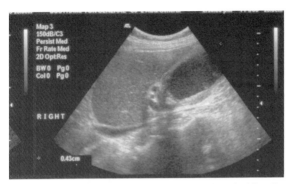

Fig. 13.24 Transverse image: showing a gallstone within the neck of the gallbladder. There is intraluminal sludge and soft tissue. This is a gallbladder carcinoma.

routine assessment of gynaecological disorders. It can also be used for infertility monitoring, egg retrieval and the exclusion of suspected ectopic pregnancy. Transrectal scanning is used for screening, assessment and biopsy of suspected prostatic pathology. Endo-anal probes may be used to assess morphology and characterise tears of the anal sphincter.

Contrast agents: ultrasound contrast agents are available as an additional tool in diagnosis, although are not yet widely used. These are microbubbles which are stable over a period of time and may be used to improve anatomical detail, assess tubal patency (hysterosalpingography), assess tumour vascularity and contrast enhancement.

Computed tomography (CT)

This technique differs from conventional radiography in that it is able to visualise a vast spectrum of absorption values and therefore tissue densities. Furthermore, being a tomographic technique, the resultant image is essentially 2D and overcomes the problem of confusing overlap of 3D structures on plain film. The image is a grey scale representation of the density of tissues (attenuation) as depicted by x-rays. Each image is made up of a matrix of squares (pixels) which collectively represent the attenuation values of tissues within that volume (voxel). With conventional CT separate exposures are made for each slice. Current scanners can acquire data in a continuous helical or spiral fashion, shortening acquisition time and reducing artefacts caused by patient movement. This improves overall throughput and increases the likelihood of a diagnostic scan, particularly in uncooperative patients. The volumetric data that is acquired may be manipulated by image processing and displayed in a variety of techniques including 3D reformats and 'virtual' endoscopy.

The attenuation values are expressed on an arbitrary scale (Hounsfield units) with water being 0, air being −1000 units and bone is +1000 units. The range of densities displayed on a particular image can be manipulated by altering the window width and level.

Prior to scanning the abdomen or pelvis dilute oral contrast is given to opacify the bowel. Intravenous contrast is given to aid the problem-solving process and differentiates vascular-enhancing lesions from surrounding tissue.

Indications

There are a wide variety as detailed below. CT is often the most diagnostic cross-sectional examination and more definitive than USS in many instances.

Contraindications

Due to the relatively high radiation dose, CT should be avoided in pregnancy. Artefact from indwelling, high density foreign material, e.g. hip prosthesis, dental amalgam and barium, may limit the diagnostic quality of the examination. Claustrophobia is less of a problem compared to MRI.

Applications

CNS/spine: CT remains the tool for primary diagnosis, pre-surgical assessment, treatment monitoring and detection of relapse in many CNS disease conditions. MRI is superior in the posterior fossa and parasellar region and for assessment in multiple sclerosis, epilepsy and tumours. Where MRI is not available it is useful for assessment of degenerative spinal and disc disease. It is superior to MRI in the assessment of head injury.

Orthopaedics/trauma: uses include diagnosis and staging of bony and soft tissue neoplasms, and assessment of vertebral, pelvic and complex

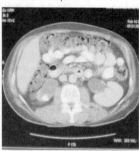

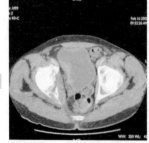

Fig. 13.25 (a) Bilateral hydronephrosis 2° to TCC lower down.

(b)TCC with pelvic side wall mass and bony destruction.

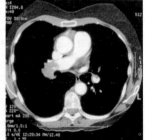

(c)CT pulmonary angiogram—shows large emolus in right main pulmonary artery.

extremity trauma (e.g. tibial plateau fractures). It is also used in the detection of loose bodies, assessment of acetabular dysplasia and providing an answer in joint instability (especially in shoulders, wrists and elbows where it may be performed as an adjunct to/in conjunction with conventional arthrography).

Oncology/radiotherapy: staging of solid tumours, treatment planning and the detection of relapse. CT is of particular value in obtaining whole body scans in oncology due to the speed and ease of use with the advent of spiral CT. CT is used for radiotherapy treatment planning to allow more precise targeting of treatment.

Chest: indications include the staging of bronchogenic carcinomas, characterisation of solitary nodules, diffuse infiltrative lung disease, widened mediastinum/mediastinal masses and pleural abnormalities. With spiral CT, pulmonary angiography has advanced the diagnosis of pulmonary emboli particularly when V/Q scanning is indeterminate or equivocal.

Abdomen: applications include the diagnosis of abdominal pathology which may be of traumatic, neoplastic, inflammatory or infective origin. CT is particularly useful for masses, pancreatic and hepatic disease, detection of the site and nature of obstructive jaundice and the assessment of abdominal trauma. It is also used in the pre-surgical assessment of abdominal aneurysms and as an aid to interventional techniques (📖p531).

Magnetic resonance imaging (MRI)

This is a non-invasive technique which displays internal structure whilst avoiding the use of ionising radiation. The nuclei of certain elements align with the magnetic force when placed in a strong magnetic field. These are usually hydrogen nuclei in water and lipid (at clinical field strengths) which resonate to produce a signal when a radiofrequency pulse is applied and display anatomical information. Further discussion of the physics is beyond the scope of this chapter.

T1-weighted images
- Contrast is due to inherent T1 relaxation.
- Provides good anatomical information.
- Fat is displayed as high signal (white).
- Distinction between cystic (black) and solid structures is possible.
- Good evaluation of marrow signal.
- The sequence of choice when evaluating enhancement, as gadolinium administration makes structures of even higher signal intensity on T1-weighted images.

523

T2-weighted images
- Technique of choice for evaluating pathology.
- Fluid is of high signal and therefore optimally displays oedema.
- Improved soft tissue contrast allows evaluation of zonal anatomy of organs such as the uterus and prostate.

MRA (magnetic resonance angiography)

MRI principles are used to exploit the properties of flowing blood. Images generated display structures containing flowing blood with suppression of all other structures. These principles can be further modified so that only vessels with flow in a specific direction (i.e. arteries *vs.* veins are visualised). MRA is currently being used in the evaluation of suspected cerebrovascular disease, renovascular disease and peripheral vascular disease.

Indications

There are a wide variety of indications as summarised below. MR is especially useful in imaging the brain, spine, peripheral limbs and joints, neck and pelvis as these structures are less prone to movement artefact. MR has limited use in the chest and increasing use in the abdomen particularly with regard to the liver, pancreas and adrenals.

Contraindications

These largely apply to patients with magnetically susceptible devices or materials whose movement or loss of function can have deleterious consequences. These include cardiac pacemakers, metallic fragments and prosthetic heart valves. Relative contraindications include pregnancy (especially the 1st trimester) and claustrophobia. MRI magnets are relatively confined and even those that are not normally claustrophobic may be provoked.

Applications

The spine: MR imaging is superior to other techniques in displaying anatomy and is the technique of choice in assessing disc disease, the post-operative back, evaluating neural compression (benign or malignant), in imaging acute myelitis, infection (such as discitis or osteomyelitis) and excluding marrow infiltration.

CNS: imaging of the CNS is used to evaluate mass lesions, hydrocephalus, white matter disease, leptomeningeal pathology, cerebrovascular disease, degenerative disorders, and visual and endocrine disorders such as pituitary dysfunction. In trauma/acute haemorrhage CT is the preferred technique.

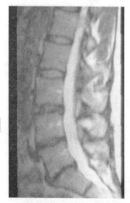

Fig. 13.26 Sagittal T2 image of the lumbar spine, showing degeneration of the lower 3 intervertebral discs.

Paediatric: the uses here include assessment of perinatal trauma/anoxic injury, congenital anomalies and developmental delay. Within the spine it is invaluable in the assessment of spinal dysraphism and progressive scoliosis.

Musculoskeletal: along with CNS disease this is a major component of the MRI workload. It has revolutionised musculoskeletal imaging and is used to characterise meniscal pathology, ligamentous injury, degeneration and the sequelae of trauma in the knee, shoulder, wrist and ankle. Further uses include imaging mass lesions, assessing the extent of infection and diagnosing early avascular necrosis.

Chest/cardiac: within the thorax MRI is useful for assessment of apical lesions such as Pancoast's tumours, chest wall and brachial plexus lesions and mediastinal masses. Cardiac applications are legion and fast evolving; they include imaging of the great vessels to exclude congenital/acquired aortic disease (including dissection) and the diagnosis of pulmonary embolus.

Abdominal/pelvic MRI: within the abdomen MR is often a problem-solving tool and can be used to more confidently characterise focal liver and pancreatic lesions as well as assess diffuse liver disease. It is also of use in evaluating indeterminate adrenal masses. Within the pelvis uses include the imaging of congenital anomalies as well as staging tumours such as cervical, prostate and rectal tumours. There have been rapid advances in techniques for imaging bowel-related pathology.

Interventional MRI: open MRI units image the patients in large bore or C-shaped units rather than the closed narrow tunnel used in conventional units. They can therefore be used for claustrophobic patients and to provide imaging guidance for interventional procedures. Disadvantages include a low magnetic field strength (0.1–0.3T *vs.* 1.5T) and a limited anatomical and spatial resolution due to their basic construct.

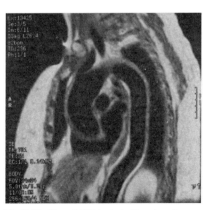

Fig. 13.27   Thoracic MRI (sagittal oblique image).

CT scanning versus MRI imaging

CT	MRI
Radiation exposure	No radiation exposure
Few contraindications other than those where radiation exposure e.g. in the young/pregnancy	Contraindicated in claustrophobic patients, those with metallic implants, pacemakers, etc.
Tolerated by most patients	Up to 10% are claustrophobic
Easy use in context of trauma or critically ill patients as imaging is rapid and coverage wide	Technically difficult in this subgroup because of longer scan time, more limited coverage and limited use of monitoring equipment
Good soft tissue contrast, but unable to display cartilage, menisci, etc.	Excellent soft tissue contrast, better than CT and shows internal structure of some organs in better detail
Susceptible to artefact from motion, bone and metal	Wide ranging artefacts include motion, CSF flow, blood flow, metallic (susceptibility) artefact
Limited to axial plane although post-processing allows some manipulation	Multiplanar imaging capability
Fast scans available	Faster sequences still slower than CT
Image formation largely influenced by attenuation of tissues	Choice of sequence determines overall weighting and image formation

Spinal imaging

Cervical spine

Trauma: obtain a cross-table lateral first (this has the highest yield) and then perform the remainder of the cervical spine series (AP and open mouth peg views), if patient mobility allows and high index of suspicion. All 7 cervical vertebral bodies should be visualised (a large number of cervicothoracic injuries are missed because of inadequate views). If not seen request a specialised lateral view (swimmers). Then *sequentially* evaluate:

Alignment: assess the following lines (Fig.13.28). They should be parallel with no step-offs.

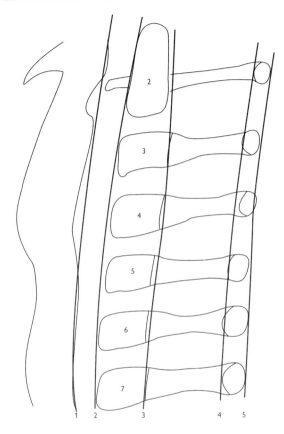

1 – Soft tissue line closely
    applied to posterior aspect of the
    airway widens at level of laryngeal
    cartilage

2 – Anterior border of vertebral bodies

3 – Posterior border of vertebral bodies

4 – Spino laminar line = posterior limit of
    spinal canal

5 – Tips of the spinous processes

Fig. 13.28

527

Bones: inspect C1 and C2. The anterior arch of C1 should be 3mm from the dens in adults (5mm in children). The vertebral bodies should be intact and they should be uniform in size and shape. Check disc spaces for any inordinate narrowing or widening which may be post-traumatic.

Cartilage:
- *Soft tissues:* look for abnormal widening or a localized bulge. 50% of patients with a bony injury will have soft tissue thickening. The soft tissues should be no more than one-third of a vertebral body until C4 and a vertebral body width thereafter.
- *The PEG views:* do not mistake a superimposed arch of C1 or the incisors as a fracture. Important points to remember are:
The lateral margins of C1 and C2 should align.
The spaces on either side of the peg should be equal (Fig. 13.28).

Remember: normal plain films do not exclude ligamentous injury.

In the routine setting cervical spine films are taken to exclude spondylosis (disc space narrowing and osteophytes) and atlantoaxial subluxation which results in long tract signs and cord compression (rheumatoid arthritis, ankylosing spondylitis, Down's syndrome).

Thoracic and lumbar spine
Degenerative disease is common with disc space narrowing, end plate sclerosis and osteophyte formation. Wedge compression fractures are common in the osteoporotic spine and need to be distinguished from the more sinister causes (absence of paraspinal mass, posterior elements spared). Multiple collapsed vertebrae are found in osteoporosis, neoplastic disease, trauma and histiocytosis X. Bone density may help narrow the differential which includes increased (sclerotic metastases, lymphoma) and decreased (acute infection, osteoporosis).

Spondylolisthesis is the subluxation of one vertebral body on another and may be degenerative or due to bilateral pars defects (spondylosis). This is a fracture/defect of the posterior elements of the vertebrae. On an oblique view the posterior elements form a Scottie dog (with the pars making up the collar). This may be a purely incidental finding, however if severe can result in neuroforaminal stenosis. Plain films are insensitive in the evaluation of disc disease. MRI is the investigation of choice for disc disease and its neurological complications.

Pelvis

Pelvic fractures are complex and there are many classification systems around. The pelvis should be regarded as being made up of three bony rings. The SI joints and pubic symphysis are part of the main bony ring. A fracture of one ring is frequently associated with a second ring fracture (Fig. 13.29).

- SI joints should be equal in width.
- The superior surfaces of the pubic rami should align. The joint width should be no more than 5mm.
- The sacral foramina should form a smooth arc.

• Acetabular fractures are subtle—look for symmetry.

Bone texture: the pelvis is a common site for metastatic involvement especially with urological malignancies, e.g. prostate (sclerotic metastases) and myeloma (multiple lytic lesions). Paget's disease of the pelvis may mimic sclerotic metastases but tends to be confined to one hemipelvis and may expand or thicken bone.

Sacroiliitis: SI joint involvement is common in the seronegative arthropathies and is usually symmetrical in conditions such as inflammatory bowel disease, ankylosing spondylitis and hyperparathyroidism. More asymmetrical change is seen in Reiter's disease and rheumatoid arthritis. It is characterised by initial erosion and widening of the joint resulting in chronic sclerosis which has a preferential involvement of the lower one-third of the joint (iliac > sacral side).

Avascular necrosis (AVN) of the femoral heads is an important finding but is often advanced when plain film findings are seen. Radiographically occult AVN may be detected on MRI or a bone scan. On plain x-ray it is characterised by sclerosis, flattening and fragmentation of the femoral head. Subchondral crescents are pathognomonic. AVN can also be a sequel of trauma, but bilateral AVN is seen in conjunction with steroid therapy, sickle cell disease and as part of Perthe's disease.

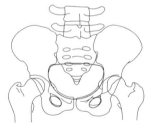

Fig. 13.29 The pelvis is made up of bony rings: the main pelvic ring and two smaller rings made up of the pubic and ishial bones.

Vascular intervention

Angiography is catheterisation of a vessel followed by subsequent opacification with a water-soluble iodine-containing contrast medium. Catheterisation is usually performed using the Seldinger technique.

529

Indications include
• Demonstration of arterial anatomy prior to surgery where this is likely to influence surgical management.
• To elucidate the nature of arterial disease, e.g. occlusions, stenoses, thrombi, aneurysms and vascular malformations.
• To identify the source of bleeding in the gastrointestinal tract.
• To demonstrate tumour circulation (often prior to embolisation).

Contrast

Volumes used are variable depending on the area being imaged. The contrast agents are iodinated, non-ionic and of low osmolarity, resulting in reduced toxicity. Nevertheless potential side effects include anaphylaxis, hypotension, urticaria and bronchospasm. Patients particularly at risk include those with a history of a previous reaction, iodine allergy and atopy. Nephrotoxicity is a potential risk and may be exacerbated by dehydration. Contrast reactions are seen in 1/1000 patients. Risk of anaphylaxis is 1/40,0000. Pre-medication with corticosteroids may reduce the incidence of reactions if contrast administration is essential, but this is not universally accepted.

Specific applications

These include pulmonary angiography (gold standard for detection of pulmonary emboli) which is highly invasive and therefore reserved for when thrombolysis or embolectomy are being considered. Cerebral angiography is useful in the diagnosis of aneurysms, AVMs, tumour vascularity and both intra- and extracranial vascular disease. Renal angiography is selectively performed to diagnose renal artery stenosis and prior to embolisation of tumours.

DSA **(digital subtraction angiography)** is a technique whereby there is subtraction of the contrast-containing shadows from the initial plain films (mask) resulting in an image containing opacified structures only. The resulting images may be digitised and manipulated. The overall advantage is smaller doses of contrast and smaller catheters may be used.

Therapeutic embolisation is used to selectively occlude arteries by introducing a variety of materials via a catheter. Materials used include metallic coil, gelatin foam and cyanoacrylate glue. This technique is used at active bleeding sites, and to reduce tumour vascularity pre-operatively in resectable tumours.

Vascular catheterisation is also used to selectively infuse vessels as with thrombolytic treatment or rarely with cytotoxics. Vascular stenting is of increasing use in coronary and peripheral vascular disease. IVC filters are percutaneously placed via the femoral vein in the treatment of patients with recurrent pulmonary emboli despite anticoagulation or where anti-coagulation is contraindicated.

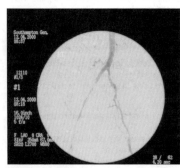

Fig. 13.30   Femoral angiogram.

Interventional radiology

Interventional radiology is a sub-speciality where a variety of imaging modalities are used to guide percutaneous procedures. This may obviate alternative surgical procedures and consequently result in lower morbidity. Interventional procedures are usually carried out under local anaesthesia and on an outpatient basis, thereby considerably reducing bed occupancy. There is a huge range of procedures that are currently performed. The following is a limited list of some of them.

Percutaneous biopsy: biopsy needle placement may be done under fluoroscopy, CT, MRI and ultrasound. This provides non-operative confirmation of suspected malignancy and with the aid of a tissue diagnosis it is possible to accurately plan treatment. For histology a 14–18G needle is used. With a fine aspiration needle (20–22G) material may be obtained for cytology. Using imaging guidance, there is avoidance of damage to vital structures such as blood vessels, solid organs and bowel loops. With chest biopsy there is a small risk of pneumothorax.

Percutaneous drainage: with image guidance, surgical intervention may be avoided by accurate placement of a drainage catheter. Calibre varies from 8 to 14F depending on the nature of the underlying fluid. Regular irrigation of the catheter may be necessary to ensure successful drainage. Successful resolution may be impeded in the more complex and multiloculated collections.

Drainage of the urinary system can be via double J stents which are placed into an obstructed collecting system with the distal catheter tip lying in the bladder. More short-term drainage is achieved via a percutaneous nephrostomy. Here the obstructed kidney is punctured under fluoroscopic or ultrasound guidance and a catheter placed in the

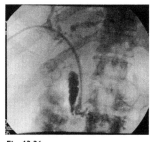

Fig. 13.31

renal calyx (preferably lower pole). This is the technique of choice in the acutely obstructed or infected kidney.

Biliary system drainage: surgical outcome in patients with malignant bile duct obstruction is often poor. This may be due to carcinoma of the pancreas or cholangiocarcinoma. Biliary stenting alleviates obstruction and improves quality of life. Stenting may be performed at ERCP or percutaneously via antegrade puncture through the liver (PTC to delineate the anatomy being performed first). Other GI interventions include stenting/balloon dilatation of oesophageal strictures and percutaneous gastrostomy insertion.

TIPS **(transjugular intrahepatic portosystemic stent shunt)** is a procedure whereby a connection is made between the hepatic and portal veins to reduce portal pressure in patients with portal hypertension. The mortality is considerably lower than in acute shunt surgery, particularly in the context of an acute variceal bleed which has failed to respond to sclerotherapy.

Hands

There are specific patterns that may be seen in the hand as an indicator of the underlying disorder. Some patterns are pathognomonic whereas others are more non-specific.

1. Generalised osteopenia: osteoporosis, multiple myeloma and rheumatoid arthritis.
2. Coarsening of the trabecular pattern is common in haemoglobinopathies especially thalassaemia and Gaucher's disease.
3. Periosteal reaction: (i) HPOA (hypertrophic pulmonary osteoarthropathy) associations include carcinoma of the bronchus, inflammatory bowel disease and coeliac disease, (ii) thyroid acropachy, most common on the radial side of the thumbs, and (iii) juvenile chronic arthritis seen in about 25%.
4. Carpal abnormalities include short metacarpals (Turner's syndrome, pseudo- and pseudopseudohypoparathyroidism), carpal fusion (inflammatory arthritis, RA & JCA, post-trauma), and look for syndactyly and polydactyly.
5. Soft tissue changes, e.g. increase in soft tissue thickness/size seen in acromegaly, localised increase seen in gouty tophi, nodes as in OA, soft tissue calcification seen in CREST and scleroderma.
6. Joint disease: the hand x-ray above all may help in sorting out the type of arthropathy and aid rheumatological management. The ABCS approach is invaluable *(see below).*

Trauma

Two views are essential for ensuring no subtle injuries are missed. On a PA view the spaces between the carpal bones and the carpometacarpal articulations should be roughly equal (1–2mm). If a dislocation is present then there is obliteration/overlap. Common injuries include Bennett's fracture, a first metacarpal base injury extending into the joint surface with dislocation at the carpometacarpal joint. Scaphoid fractures are the most common (75–90%) of carpal injuries. Because of the blood supply there is a potential risk of osteonecrosis of the proximal pole.

A: Alignment	Subluxation/dislocation common in rheumatoid arthritis and SLE.
B: Bone	Osteoporosis: mineralisation is usually normal except in acute RA.
	Erosions:
	–Aggressive (i.e. no sclerosis of margins) seen in RA and psoriasis.
	–Non-aggressive (with sclerotic margins) seen in gout; inflammatory erosions are marginal (OA erosions are central); distinguish from subperiosteal resorption (radial border, seen in hyperparathyroidism).
	Bone production: periosteal new bone formation, psoriasis, Reiter's syndrome:
	– Ankylosis (bony bridging) in inflammatory arthropathies.
	– Overhanging cortex (typical of gout).
	– Osteophyte formation, OA.
C: Cartilage	Joint space has uniform narrowing in all arthritis except OA which is eccentric
	Wide joint space in early arthritis, gout and PVNS.
S: Soft tissues	*Swelling*
	Symmetric around joint space commonest in RA.
	Asymmetric usually due to osteophytes and therefore commonest in OA.
	Lumpy bumpy soft tissue swelling: gouty tophi.
	Diffuse swelling of digits: psoriasis, Reiter's.
	Calcification
	Soft tissues: gouty tophi.
	Cartilage: pseudogout, pyrophosphate arthropathy.
	Subcutaneous tissue: scleroderma.

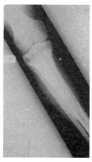

Fig. 13.32 Paget's disease.

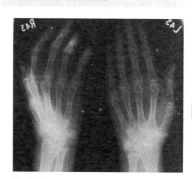

Fig. 13.33 Rheumatoid hands.

Skull x-ray

Indications
The main indication is acute trauma although they are of limited use. Occasionally the SXR is obtained as part of a skeletal survey in evaluation of metabolic bone disease, endocrine disorders and in the assessment of metastatic disease.

Contraindications
None, but if there is suspicion of underlying intracranial injury plain films are unnecessary (*see below*).

Normal findings
The bones of the skull vault have an inner and outer table of compact bone with spongy diploe between the two. Sutures are visible even after fusion and should not be mistaken for fractures. Blood vessels may cause impressions, as can small lucencies in the inner table near the vertex caused by normal arachnoid granulations which can be mistaken for small lytic lesions.

Trauma: skull x-rays are basic, widely available and yet potentially yield the least information in the context of trauma. The presence or absence of a skull fracture does not correlate with the presence or extent of any intracranial injury. Up to 50% of films may be technically unsatisfactory due to factors such as poor patient cooperation. With the advent of CT this is the technique of choice for evaluation in acute injury and neurological deficit. It allows a firm diagnosis to be made and excludes other alternate diagnoses.

Fractures and associated findings: basic radiographs include a lateral projection (obtained with a horizontal beam) and a further tangential projection, depending on the site of injury.

Findings include
- A linear fracture: well-defined margins, no branching and no sclerosis (*cf.* vascular markings or sutures which have an undulating course and sclerotic margins).
- A depressed fracture: increased density due to overlapping bone; those that are depressed by >5mm may lacerate the dura or cause parenchymal injury and therefore need elevation.
- A fluid level/pneumocephalus: implies an associated basal skull fracture or dural tear.

Note: Pineal displacement is an inconstant finding and is not a reliable method of assessing the presence of intracranial injury.

Abnormal findings
Look for intracranial calcification then examine the pituitary fossa, review bony density and look for focal areas of lysis and sclerosis.
- *Intracranial calcification*: the majority is normal and of no clinical significance. However it may be of pathological significance; causes include primary tumours such as meningiomas, craniopharyngiomas, arteriovenous malformations, tuberose sclerosis and infections such as toxoplasmosis.

- *Raised intracranial pressure*: in practice plain film changes are only seen if the condition is long standing. These include sutural widening (diastasis) and erosion of the lamina dura of the pituitary fossa.
- *Enlargement of the pituitary fossa* (normal dimensions: height 6–11mm, length 9–16mm). Expansion will result in a double floor, loss of the lamina dura and elevation/destruction of the clinoid processes. The vast majority of the lesions will be pituitary adenomas; other causes include meningiomas and aneurysms.
- *Bone lysis*: may be diffuse as in metastasis or myeloma. Large areas of bone destruction are seen in histiocytosis X and in the active phase of Paget's disease (osteoporosis circumscripta).
- *Bone sclerosis*: may be localised as in meningiomas, depressed skull fractures or generalised as in Paget's sclerotic metastases, myeloma and fluorosis.
- *Sutural widening*: may be due to raised intracranial pressure, infiltration by malignancy (neuroblastoma or lymphoma) or defective ossification as in rickets.

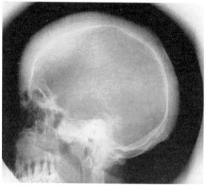

Fig. 13.34 Lateral SXR showing 'hair on end' appearance in thalassaemia major.

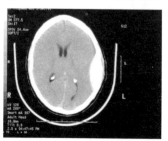

Fig. 13.35 CT brain demonstrating an acute extradural haematoma.

Reference section

List of abbreviations:

AP	anteroposterior
AXR	abdominal x-ray
CT	computed tomography
CXR	chest x-ray
IVU	intravenous urogram
MRI	magnetic resonance imaging
PA	posteroanterior
USS	ultrasound scan
V/Q	ventilation perfusion scan

Management of adverse reactions to intravascular contrast agents

Symptoms	Treatment
Nausea/vomiting	Reassurance
Urticaria	Antihistamine chlorpheniramine maleate 10–20mg by slow IV injection (0.2mg/kg body weight paediatric dose)
Angio-oedema	Adrenaline(epinephrine) 0.5–1mL 1:10,000 IV
Bronchospasm	IV hydrocortisone 100mg
Hypotension	β2-agonist by nebuliser
	O₂, IV access and IV fluids

Order of appearance of ossification centres of the elbow

The order of appearance is more important than the absolute age of appearance which varies widely. Remember 'CRITOE'.

Approximate average age (years)	
Capitellum	1
Radial head	3–6
Internal (medial) epicondyle	4
Trochlea	8
Olecranon	9
External (lateral) epicondyle	10

Epiphyseal plate fractures: the Salter Harris classification (SALTR)

- **Type I**-epiphyseal slip separates it from physis (5–6%). S = slip of physis.
- **Type II**-fracture line extends into metaphysis (50–75%). A = above physis.

- **TYPE III**-the epiphysis is vertically split, i.e. the equivalent of an intra-articular fracture (8%). L = lower than physis.
- **TYPE IV**-fracture involves the metaphysis, epiphysis and physis (8–12%). T = through physis.
- **TYPE V**-crush injury with vascular compromise, i.e. poor prognosis for growth (1%). R = rammed physis.

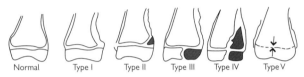

Normal   Type I   Type II   Type III   Type IV   Type V

Fig. 13.36   The Salter Harris classification.

Chapter 14

Nuclear medicine

Introduction to nuclear medicine

Nuclear medicine techniques use a carrier molecule, selected to target the organ/tissue of interest, tagged with a gamma-emitting radioisotope. The labelled drug (radiopharmaceutical) is given PO or IV. Its distribution is then mapped *in vivo* using a gamma camera or, for non-imaging tests, *in vitro* using a radiation counter.

Nuclear medicine procedures detect the earliest physiological response to disease processes, generally before structural changes have taken place. Scintigraphy is often more sensitive than conventional radiology in early disease. Specificity varies depending on the radiopharmaceutical used and characterisation of abnormalities relies upon pattern recognition within a particular clinical setting. Anatomical detail is poor compared with conventional radiology, although tomographic cameras generate high resolution 3D images.

Nuclear medicine procedures are non-invasive and allow the whole body to be imaged during a single examination. Absorbed radiation doses depend on the radiopharmaceutical used but are usually in the same range as diagnostic radiology. Pregnancy is an absolute contraindication to nuclear medicine examinations except where likely clinical benefit far outweighs potential risk—e.g. lung perfusion imaging. Some radiopharmaceuticals are excreted in breast milk and additional precautions may be advisable for lactating women.

Diagnostic radiopharmaceuticals are used in tracer quantities and toxicity is negligible. Individual hypersensitivity reactions are rare.

Specific information required when requesting nuclear medicine tests includes
- Patient identification details.
- Examination requested.
- Relevant clinical history including results of other investigations.
- Pregnancy/lactation details where relevant.
- Special needs—visual/hearing/learning difficulties; needle phobia.

Bone scintigraphy: bone scan

Indications
- Tumour staging—e.g. to assess skeletal metastases.
- Bone pain.
- Trauma—when radiographs unhelpful.
- Prosthetic loosening, e.g. THR.
- Infection.
- Avascular necrosis (AVN).
- Paget's to assess extent.

Patient preparation
Should be well hydrated and continent.

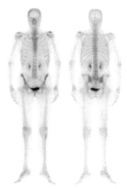

Fig. 14.1 Normal whole body ^{99m}Tc phosphate bone scan.

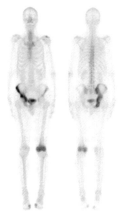

Fig. 14.2 Paget's disease—right hemipelvis and distal femur.

Procedure
Inject ^{99m}Tc-phosphate complex IV. For suspected AVN or sepsis, image immediately to assess vascularity. Otherwise, image 2–4h later. Whole body views are required for metastatic screening. Tomography improves anatomical definition and detection of small lesions, e.g. osteoid osteoma.

Results
- Radiopharmaceutical uptake reflects osteoblastic activity.
- Focal ↑ uptake in sclerotic metastases, trauma or infection.
- Diffuse ↑ uptake associated with advanced metastases, Paget's and metabolic bone disease.
- ↓ uptake in acute AVN and lytic bone metastases.

541

Interpretation

Sensitive but non-specific. Interpretation relies on pattern recognition in the clinical setting.

Advantages

Sensitive—detects early changes in bone physiology, often before abnormal plain radiographs, e.g. occult trauma, metastases and sepsis.

Pitfalls

False −ves in multiple myeloma (plain skeletal radiology is the preferred imaging technique). Artefacts due to urine contamination.

Reticuloendothelial system: bone marrow scintigraphy

Indications

- Suspected malignant marrow infiltration.
- Equivocal conventional bone imaging.
- Osteomyelitis (rarely used).

Patient preparation

None.

Procedure

- ^{99m}Tc nanocolloid injected IV.
- Whole body gamma camera imaging at 30–45min.

Results

Normal marrow distribution in thoracic cage, spine, pelvis and proximal long bones. Homogeneous uptake in liver and spleen.

Interpretation

- Focal or generalised ↓ skeletal uptake indicates marrow replacement or infiltration with marrow displacement to distal femora and humeri.
- Heterogeneous hepatic uptake is abnormal but non-specific.

Advantages

Non-invasive. Avoids sampling errors compared with bone marrow biopsy.

Pitfalls

False −ves in early malignancy.

Smith FW. (1998) The skeletal system, in: *Practical Nuclear Medicine*, 2nd edition, eds Sharp, Gemmel & Smith, Oxford University Press, Oxford.

Brain imaging

Indications

- Dementia characterisation.
- Epilepsy for localisation of epileptogenic focus.

Patient preparation

Secure venous access under resting conditions. Allow the patient to relax before injection of the radiopharmaceutical. Ensure that the patient can cooperate with the imaging procedure.

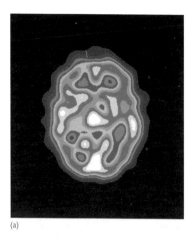

(a)

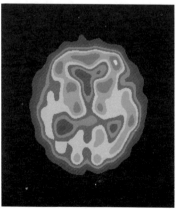

(b)

Fig. 14.3 ^{99m}Tc HMPAO brain imaging. Transaxial tomographic slices: (a) normal and (b) dementia.

Procedure
^{99m}Tc HMPAO (exametazine) injected IV in quiet, darkened room, with patient's eyes closed. Tomographic brain imaging undertaken immediately and again 4h later.

Results
Cortical grey matter uptake is proportional to blood flow.

Interpretation
Characteristic patterns of abnormal uptake recognised in different dementias. ↓ uptake at epileptogenic focus on interictal scans—often changing to ↑ uptake on ictal imaging.

Advantages
Abnormalities on functional imaging should pre-date structural atrophy on anatomical imaging.

Pitfalls
Tomographic image analysis degraded by movement artefact and asymmetric positioning. Data processing is operator-dependent.

Brain receptor imaging

Indications
Movement disorders: distinguishes Parkinson's syndrome (PS) from benign essential tremor.

Patient preparation
Block thyroid using potassium iodate/iodide.

▶▶Multiple potential drug interactions—stop:
- Amphetamine.
- Benztropine.
- Biperidin.
- Citalopram.
- Cocaine.
- Fluoxetine.
- Fluvoxamine.
- Mazindol.
- Methylphenidate.
- Orphenadrine.
- Phentermine.
- Procyclidine.
- Sertraline.

Procedure
^{123}I-labelled ioflupane injected IV. Tomographic gamma camera imaging 3–6h later.

Results
Intense, symmetric uptake in basal ganglia receptors—striatum, caudate and putamen.

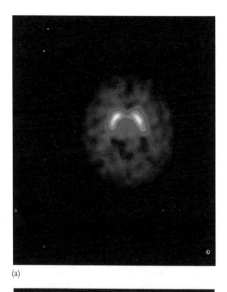

(a)

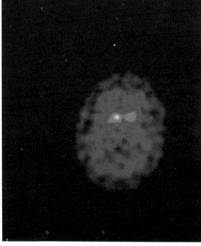

(b)

Fig. 14.4 ^{123}I ioflupane brain receptor imaging: (a) normal dopamine receptors and (b) in Parkinson's disease.

Interpretation
↓ basal ganglia uptake in PS.

Advantages
Sensitive and specific for PS.

Pitfalls
Drug interactions (*above*).

Booij J, Harbraken JBA, Bergmans P et al. (1998) Imaging of dopamine transporters with I-123 FP CIT in healthy controls and patients with Parkinson's disease. *J Nucl Med* **40**, 1091–1097; Benamer H et al. (2000) Accurate differentiation of parkinsonism and essential tremor using visual assessment of ^123I FP CIT spect imaging. The ^123I FP CIT Study Group Writing Committee. *Movement Disorders* **15**, 503–510.

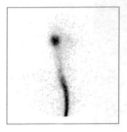

Reservoir

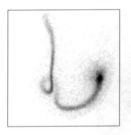

Thorax

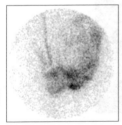

Free activity in periotoneal cavity

Fig. 14.5 Patent ventriculoperitoneal shunt showing reservoir, shunt and free activity within the peritoneal cavity.

CSF shunt patency

Indications
Suspected VP shunt obstruction.

Patient preparation
None.

Procedure
Inject ^{99m}Tc -DTPA or ^{111}In DTPA into shunt reservoir using strict aseptic technique. Image head and abdomen immediately and 30–60min post-injection.

Results
Normally, rapid reservoir emptying and shunt visualisation within 2–3min of injection. Free activity within abdominal cavity by 30min. (Fig 14.5).

Interpretation
Delayed clearance implies obstruction—level usually at reservoir/proximal shunt or due to intra-abdominal kinking.

Advantages
Sensitive, simple, rapid results.

Pitfalls
Infection risk.

Gastrointestinal bleeding: labelled red cell imaging

Indications
Helps localise source of active GI haemorrhage when other techniques (e.g. endoscopy or angiography) have failed.

Patient preparation
No recent contrast barium studies.

Procedure
Label red cells (*in vitro* or *in vivo*) using ^{99m}Tc pertechnetate. Abdominal gamma camera blood pool imaging immediately and at intervals for up to 36h post-injection or until bleeding source is identified.

Results
Activity normally restricted to vascular compartment.

547

Interpretation
Any activity in gut lumen implies active haemorrhage. Serial images helpful.

Advantages
More sensitive and less invasive than angiography for intermittent bleeding.

Pitfalls
- Poor red cell label—degrades image quality.
- Limits of detection—0.5mL/min blood loss.

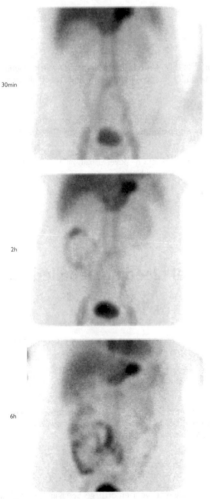

30min

2h

6h

Fig. 14.6 Anterior abdominal images showing increasing red cell haemorrhage into the distal ileum.

Meckel's scan: ectopic gastric mucosa localisation

Indications
Unexplained abdominal pain or GI haemorrhage—after endoscopy/contrast radiology.

Patient preparation
- Starve for 4h.
- H_2 antagonist administration may improve specificity.
- No recent barium studies.

Procedure
Inject ^{99m}Tc pertechnetate IV. Immediate and serial abdominal imaging over 1h.

Results
Normal uptake in gastric mucosa.

Interpretation
Focal abnormal uptake appearing at the same time as the stomach implies ectopic gastric mucosa (Meckel's diverticulum) or, occasionally, duplication cyst. Commonest site—RIF.

Advantages
Non-invasive.

Pitfalls
False +ves due to activity in renal tract—lateral images usually help.

Hepatobiliary scintigraphy

Indications
- Acute cholecystitis.
- Trauma.
- Post-operative leak detection.
- Bile duct/stent patency.
- Gallbladder emptying.
- Bile reflux.
- Neonatal biliary atresia.

Patient preparation
- Adults: starve for 6h.
- Neonates: phenobarbitone 5mg/kg/day PO for 3 days prior to study (enzyme induction).

Procedure
- Adults: IV injection ^{99m}Tc-labelled iminodiacetic acid complex (IDA). Gamma camera imaging over 1h.

- Neonates: IV injection ^{99m}Tc IDA. Immediate dynamic imaging for 5min then serial static images for up to 36h, or until activity reaches small bowel lumen.

Results
Gallbladder and biliary tree normally shown with tracer excretion via common bile duct into duodenum by 30min post-injection. Cholecystokinin 0.5u/kg IV sometimes administered to stimulate gall-bladder emptying.

Interpretation
- Acute cholecystitis: absent gallbladder.
- Obstruction, leak or reflux assessed visually.
- Neonates: passage of activity into gut lumen excludes biliary atresia. Quantification of T0 to T10 min images improves specificity for atresia diagnosis.

Advantages
Non-invasive. Straightforward pattern recognition.

Pitfalls
- Delayed IDA excretion in severe jaundice: bilirubin >300μmol/L.

Splenunculus detection: heat-damaged red cell imaging

Indications
Recurrent thrombocytopenia post-splenectomy.

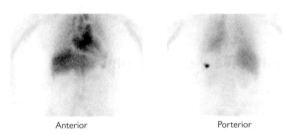

Anterior   Porterior

Fig. 14.7   Post-splenectomy. Intense uptake in splenunculus lying in splenic bed.

Patient preparation
None required.

Procedure
Obtain venous blood sample. Separate red cells and radiolabel using ^{99m}Tc pertechnetate. Heat to 39.5°C for 30min. Cool and reinject IV. Image anterior abdomen 30min later.

Results & interpretation
Damaged red cells taken up by splenic remnants.

Advantages
Investigation of choice for detection of splenunculus.

Pitfalls
Enlarged left lobe of liver may obscure small splenic remnant.

Hepatosplenic scintigraphy

Indications
Liver space-occupying lesions—now largely replaced by ultrasound, CT or MRI.

Patient preparation
None.

Procedure
^{99m}Tc colloid injected IV. Abdominal gamma camera images 30min post-injection.

Results
Normal, homogeneous liver and spleen uptake.

Interpretation
Focal ↓ uptake in space-occupying lesions. ↑ spleen and bone activity in portal hypertension. Focal ↑ uptake in caudate lobe pathognomonic of Budd-Chiari syndrome.

Advantages
Cheap.

Pitfalls
Non-specific. Largely superseded by anatomical imaging.

Gastric emptying studies

Indications
Altered GI motility—delayed or accelerated gastric emptying.

Patient preparation
Starved for 4h. Stop drugs likely to influence GI motility, e.g. opiates, domperidone.

Procedure

Milk study

Give radiolabelled milk drink orally. Image anterior abdomen immediately and at 10min intervals for 1h. Generate computer-derived clearance curves to calculate emptying half-time. Delayed thoracic image helpful to exclude lung aspiration if clearance significantly delayed.

Dual isotope method

Give ^{99m}Tc-labelled standard meal with ^{111}In-labelled water. Anterior abdomen gamma camera imaging as before using dual isotope settings. Generate solid and liquid phase clearance curves.

Results

Normal gastric emptying half-time (milk = 20min). Normal range for solids is centre-specific, depending on standard meal composition.

Interpretation

Visual image evaluation and half-time calculation.

Advantages

Non-invasive and quantitative.

Pitfalls

Vomiting during study invalidates emptying time calculations.

Thyroid scintigraphy

Indications

- Characterisation of thyrotoxicosis—diffuse toxic goitre (Graves' disease), toxic multinodular goitre (Plummer's disease).
- Autonomous nodule.
- Acute thyroiditis.

Patient preparation

Thyroxine and iodine-rich preparations, e.g. iodine supplements, contrast media, amiodarone, will block tracer uptake by the thyroid for up to 9 months. T4 should be withdrawn for 6 weeks; T3 for 2 weeks. Antithyroid drugs can be continued.

Procedure

Inject ^{99m}Tc pertechnetate IV. Image after 15–30min. Include anterior thorax views if retrosternal extension is suspected. Neck palpation essential to assess function in discrete thyroid nodules.

Results

- Uptake reflects function of the thyroid iodine trap.
- Diffuse increased uptake in Graves' disease.
- Heterogeneous uptake with suppressed background activity indicates toxic multinodular change.

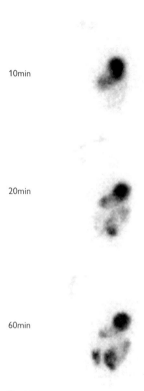

10min

20min

60min

Fig. 14.8

- Solitary autonomous nodules show intense increased uptake with complete suppression of the remainder of the gland.
- Acute thyroiditis is characterised by absent tracer uptake.

Interpretation
Sensitive and specific for hyperthyroidism.

Advantages

553

Simple, cheap and non-invasive. Essential to planning therapy in hyperthyroidism.

Pitfalls
Anatomical definition inferior to ultrasound, CT, etc. Superseded by ultrasound-guided FNA for diagnosis of thyroid mass lesions.

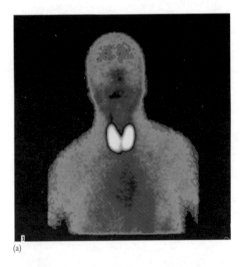

(a)

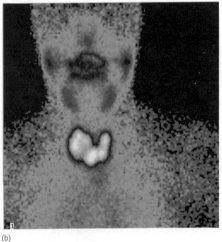

(b)

Fig. 14.9 Thyroid scintigraphy: (a) in Graves' disease and (b) in toxic multinodular goitre.

Parathyroid scintigraphy

Indications
Localisation of parathyroid adenoma in proven hyperparathyroidism.

Patient preparation
Withdraw thyroxine or iodine-containing compounds (📖*Thyroid imaging* (p553)).

Procedure
Two radiopharmaceuticals given IV: *either* ^{123}I iodide followed by ^{99m}Tc sestamibi *or* ^{99m}Tc pertechnetate followed by ^{210}thallous chloride. Image anterior neck and mediastinum after each administration.

Results
Normal thyroid concentrates ^{123}I, ^{99m}Tc pertechnetate, ^{99m}Tc sestamibi and ^{201}TL whereas parathyroid only concentrates ^{99m}Tc sestamibi and ^{201}TL. Computer-assisted image subtraction:

[(thyroid + parathyroid) – thyroid] identifies abnormal parathyroid tissue.

Interpretation
Parathyroid adenoma shown as hyperfunctioning nodule(s).

Advantages
Good when other imaging fails, particularly for ectopic adenomas and after unsuccessful neck exploration.

Pitfalls
Multinodular thyroid prevents subtraction analysis. False −ves in multiple parathyroid adenomas or hyperplasia. Many surgeons still prefer intra operative blue dye.

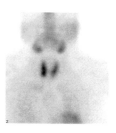

^{123}I $\qquad\qquad\qquad$ ^{99m}Tc sestamibi

Fig. 14.10

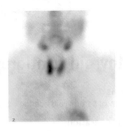

Fig. 14.11

MIBG (meta iodobenzylguanidine) imaging

Indications
- Localisation, staging and response monitoring of neuroectodermal tumours.
- Phaeochromocytoma (imaging investigation of choice).
- Neuroblastoma.
- Carcinoid tumours.
- Medullary thyroid cancer.

Patient preparation
- Multiple known and theoretical drug interactions. Stop for >48h:
    - Antidepressants: tricyclics, tetracyclics, MAOIS, serotonin re-uptake inhibitors.
    - Phenothiazines.
    - Labetolol*.
    - L-dopa, dopamine agonists.
    - Sympathomimetics—including OTC nasal decongestants.
- Block thyroid—potassium iodate/iodide; perchlorate.

Procedure
Inject ^{123}I mIBG slowly IV with blood pressure monitoring. Image posterior abdomen at 5min to identify renal outlines, then whole body imaging at 18–24h. Tomographic imaging may improve tumour localisation—not always required.

Results
Physiological uptake at 24h in salivary glands, myocardium, liver and normal adrenals with gut and renal excretion.

Interpretation
- Intense ↑ uptake in phaeochromocytomas, with suppressed activity in the contralateral, normal adrenal and myocardium. Whole body imaging identifies extra-adrenal and metastatic disease.

*No interaction with any other α or β blocker or antihypertensive.

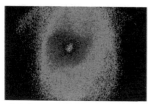

Anterior

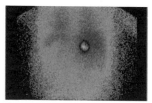

Posterior
(a)

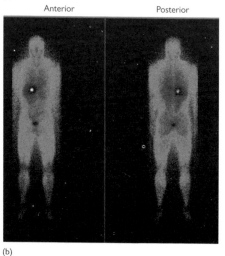

(b)

Fig. 14.12 ^{123}I mIBG scan: (a) right intra-adrenal phaeochromocytoma; (b) whole body scan—right intra-adrenal phaeochromocytoma. Excludes multi-focal, ectopic and malignant tumour.

- Diffuse bone marrow uptake common in stage IV neuroblastoma.

Advantages
Sensitive, non-invasive tumour localisation pre-operatively excludes multi-focal and extra-adrenal tumours. Non-invasive treatment response monitoring in neuroblastoma—avoids sampling errors compared with bone marrow biopsy.

Pitfalls
Drug interactions causing false –ve results. Dilated renal pelvis sometimes confused with tumour uptake. Check with 5min renal image if in doubt.

Somatostatin scintigraphy

Indications
Localise and stage neuroendocrine tumours (NETs), e.g. carcinoid, insulinoma, gastrinoma, phaeochromocytoma and medullary thyroid cancer.

Patient preparation
None required. Prophylactic laxatives at time of radiopharmaceutical administration accelerate gut clearance and improve image quality.

Fig. 14.13 Whole body ^{111}In octeotide scan showing neuroectodermal tumour with hepatic metastases.

Procedure
Inject ^{111}In-labelled somatostatin analogue (octreotide or lanreotide) IV. Whole body gamma camera imaging at 24 ± 48h, with tomography if necessary.

Results
Normal uptake in thyroid, liver, spleen, kidneys and RE system with gut and renal excretion.

Interpretation
↑ uptake in tumours expressing surface somatostatin receptors. Tomography improves detection of small pancreatic and intra-hepatic tumours.

Advantages
Tumour uptake predicts symptom response to somatostatin analogue therapy. Image co-registration with CT or MRI improves localisation of occult pancreatic NETs.

Pitfalls
Interpretation often hindered by gut excretion.

Radioiodine thyroid cancer imaging

Indications
Routine differentiated follicular thyroid cancer follow-up, after surgery and ^{131}I thyroid remnant ablation.

Patient preparation
Need high TSH drive to stimulate ^{131}I uptake—stop T3/T4 replacement for minimum of 2 (T3) or 6 weeks (T4) or give recombinant TSH. Avoid iodine administration, IV contrast media, amiodarone (📖*Thyroid imaging* (p553)).

Procedure
Give PO/IV ^{131}I sodium iodide. Whole body gamma camera imaging 2–7 days later.

Results
Physiological uptake in salivary glands. Occasional stomach and GI retention. Renal excretion.

Interpretation
Abnormal uptake indicates functioning thyroid metastasis. Anatomical markers improve localisation.

559

Advantages
Detects residual tumour and identifies patients likely to benefit from ^{131}I therapy.

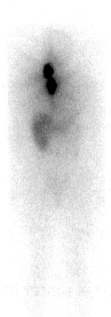

Fig. 14.14 Anterior whole body ^{131}I image showing local tumour recurrence in thyroid bed and mediastinum.

Pitfalls
False −ves without significant TSH drive—aim for TSH >50 mU/L; undifferentiated and papillary tumours may be ^{131}I negative.

Sentinel node imaging

Indications
Pre-operative assessment in breast cancer and melanoma. May have applications in head and neck, vulval and penile cancer staging.

Patient preparation
None required. Usually undertaken within 24h of planned surgery.

Procedure
Intradermal, subcutaneous or intratumoural injection of ^{99m}Tc-labelled nanocolloid. Gamma camera imaging of draining lymph nodes to identify sentinel node. Where surgery is undertaken within 24h, an intra-operative gamma probe can be used to identify the sentinel node for staging excision biopsy.

Results
Sentinel node usually identifiable 15min to 2h post-injection, depending on the primary tumour location and injection technique used.

Interpretation
The sentinel node is the first lymph node identified on gamma imaging or the node with the highest radioactive count rate using the gamma probe.

Advantages
Accurate sentinel node identification avoids block node dissection, where this is undertaken solely for tumour staging.

Pitfalls
May fail if local lymphatic channels have been disrupted by previous surgery.

Myocardial perfusion imaging (MPI)

Indications
In ischaemic heart disease.
1. Pre-angiography:
   - When conventional stress testing fails, e.g. bundle branch block.
   - Left ventricular hypertrophy.
   - Atypical chest pain.
   - Recurrent chest pain post-intervention. Good prognostic indicator.
2. Post-angiography:
   - Assess functional significance of known stenoses.
   - Identify critical vascular territory for intervention.

Patient preparation
- Stop β-blockers 24h prior to stress study.
- Sometimes helpful to withdraw all anti-anginal medication.
- Assess optimal stress technique for individual patient, i.e. exercise or pharmacological.
- Attach 12-lead ECG.
- Insert IV cannula.
- Check baseline blood pressure.

Procedure
2-part investigation comparing myocardial perfusion during stress and at rest.
- *Stress test:* treadmill or bicycle exercise to >85% maximum predicted heart rate *or* adenosine 140μg/kg/min IVI for 6min—sometimes with submaximal exercise **or**
  Dobutamine 5–40μg/kg/min in 5μg/kg/min increments over 18min.
- Inject radiopharmaceutical (^{201}Tl, ^{99m}Tc MIBI (methoxyisobutylisonitrile) or ^{99m}Tc tetrofosmin) at peak stress.
- Tomographic imaging immediately (^{201}Tl) or 15–60min post-injection (^{99m}Tc compounds).
- *Rest study:* Delayed image >4h after stress injection [^{201}Tl] or second radiopharmaceutical injection under resting conditions [^{99m}Tc MIBI, ^{99m}Tc tetrofosmin, ^{201}Tl (2nd injection may improve sensitivity)].
  Tomographic imaging as before.

Results
Myocardial uptake reflects radiopharmaceutical delivery and myocyte function.

Interpretation
Infarction causes matched perfusion defects during stress and rest. Inducible ischaemia creates a perfusion defect at stress which re-perfuses at rest = reversible ischaemia. The severity, extent and number of reversible defects are prognostically significant. A normal MPI study implies risk of an adverse cardiac event <0.5% per annum.

Advantages
Non-invasive; relatively inexpensive compared with angiography.

Pitfalls
Less sensitive in multiple small vessel coronary disease—e.g. diabetes mellitus. Sensitivity depends on stress test quality.

Radionuclide ventriculography: MUGA scans

Indications
- LV ejection fraction measurement, e.g. unechogenic patients.
- Monitor anthracycline cardiotoxicity.

Patient preparation
None required.

Procedure
Radiolabel red cells (*in vivo* or *in vitro*) using ^{99m}Tc pertechnetate. Image patient supine in anterior and left anterior oblique projections. Camera

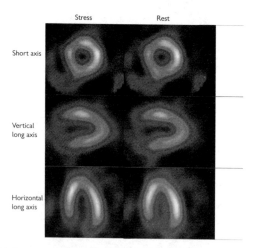

Fig. 14.15 Normal myocardial perfusion scan.

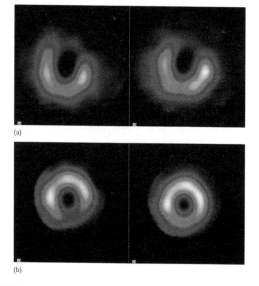

Fig. 14.16 Myocardial perfusion scan: (a) in fixed perfusion loss (anterolateral infarction), and (b) in inferior stress-induced (reversible) ischaemia .

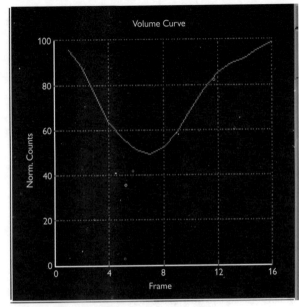

Fig. 14.17 Computer-generated ejection fraction 40%.

acquisition gated to cardiac cycle. Imaging sometimes combined with low impact exercise/pharmacologic stress to assess cardiac reserve.

Results
Visual image of 300–400 summated cardiac cycles. Computer-generated images used to assess regional wall motion and synchronous contraction. Computer-generated ejection fraction calculation. Normal LVEF 60–70%, ↓ with age.

Interpretation
LVEF used to monitor treatment response in cardiac failure, cardiomyopathy.

Advantages
Good for serial measurement during anthracycline chemotherapy. Reliable in unechogenic subjects.

Disadvantage
High radiation dose—echocardiography preferable in most patients.

Pitfalls
Cardiac dysrhythmias interfere with gating, e.g. atrial fibrillation.

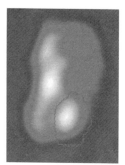

End diastole showing
LV region of interest

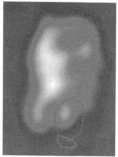

End systole showing
LV region of interest

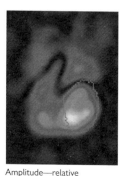

Amplitude—relative
wall motion

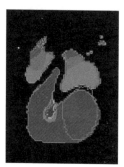

Phase—systolic timing
atria : ventricles

Fig. 14.18

Static cortical renography: DMSA imaging

Indications
- Urinary tract infection: 'gold standard' for renal scarring.
- Measurement of relative renal function.
- Renal duplication assessment.
- Ectopic kidney localisation.
- Renal trauma.
- Renal vein thrombosis.
- Pre-biopsy.

565

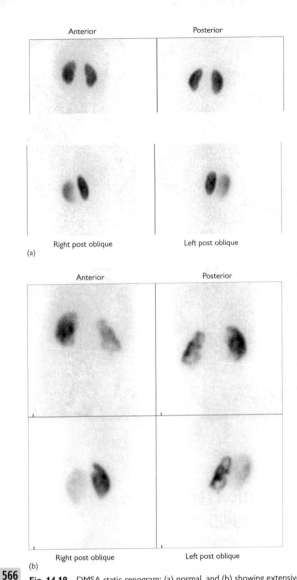

Anterior   Posterior

Right post oblique   Left post oblique

(a)

Anterior   Posterior

Right post oblique   Left post oblique

(b)

Fig. 14.19 DMSA static renogram: (a) normal, and (b) showing extensive bilateral cortical scarring.

Patient preparation
None, but avoid dehydration.

Procedure
^{99m}Tc DMSA (dimercaptosuccinic acid) injected IV. Static anterior, posterior and posterior oblique images acquired 2–4h later.

Results
Visual image evaluation, assessing integrity of cortical outlines for scarring. Quantitative computer image analysis is used to measure relative renal function, i.e. the contribution of each kidney to overall GFR.

Interpretation
Cortical scars distort renal outline. Duplication may result in non-functioning upper moiety, usually due to obstruction, or scarred lower moiety, secondary to vesicoureteric reflux. Relative renal function is usually 50:50 ± 5%.

Advantages
Sensitive for renal scarring; superior to ultrasound. Non-invasive.

Pitfalls
False +ves during or immediately after acute pyelonephritis—may give cortical defects that do not progress to scarring. Splenic impression at left upper pole may be mistaken for scarring.

Dynamic renography

Indications
- Assessment of renal drainage—discrimination between renal dilatation and outflow obstruction.
- Measurement of relative renal function.
- Loin pain.
- Post-pyeloplasty follow-up.
- Renal artery stenosis—📖*Captopril renography* (p569).

Patient preparation
Good hydration essential. Empty bladder immediately before undertaking study.

Procedure
1. Position patient supine or seated erect, with the camera behind.
2. Obtain good peripheral venous access. Bolus radiopharmaceutical injection ^{99m}Tc MAG-3 (trimercaptoacetylglycine), ^{99m}Tc DTPA (dipentaacetic acid) or ^{123}I hippuran followed by 10–20mL saline flush.
3. Image immediately acquiring real time dynamic data for 20–30min.
4. Diuretic administration is essential to distinguish dilatation from outflow obstruction.
5. Post-voiding images are always required to assess the completeness of bladder emptying and may improve drainage of the upper renal tracts in high pressure systems.

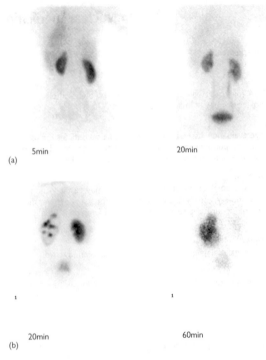

(a)　5min　　　20min

(b)　20min　　　60min

Fig. 14.20 Dynamic renogram posterior images : (a) normal, showing an early parenchymal image and later symmetrical excretion with bladder filliing. (b) outflow obstruction: early image shows left hydronephrosis secondary to per-lviureteric junction obstruction, with poor drainage at 60min.

Results
Visual inspection of renal size, perfusion, function and drainage. Quantitative computer image analysis measures relative function, transit times and generates drainage graphs.

Interpretation
Uptake and excretion of activity normally rapid. Dilated systems show progressive pooling in the renal pelvis which empties following diuretic challenge. Obstructed systems show progressive tracer accumulation with no diuretic response, often associated with ↓ function on the affected side.

Advantages
Sensitive, non-invasive, quantitative renal function assessment. Anatomical imaging, e.g. IVU better for renal morphology, stones, etc.

Pitfalls
Movement artefact, chronic renal failure and dehydration reduce data reliability. Renal drainage may be gravity dependent—always complete study with an erect image. Drainage curves invalidated by radiopharmaceutical extravasation.

Captopril renography

Indications
Diagnosis of renal artery stenosis (especially fibromuscular dysplasia) and to predict response to revascularisation.

Patient preparation
Well hydrated. Baseline blood pressure. IV access. Stop ACE inhibitors for 48h prior to test.

Procedure
- Perform standard dynamic renogram.
- Repeat renogram 1h after oral captopril 25mg single dose PO.
- Monitor blood pressure—beware hypotension.

Results
Perfusion pressure is maintained by angiotensin I/II in renal artery stenosis. Captopril reduces perfusion pressure leading to fall in relative function and delayed tracer uptake on affected side. Quantitative evaluation of R : L renal function and time to peak activity in each kidney.

Interpretation
RAS due to fibromuscular dysplasia—fall in relative renal function and delayed time to peak renal activity >10min.

Advantages
Distinguishes generalised atherosclerosis (often poor blood pressure outcome following angioplasty) from fibromuscular hyperplasia (good angioplasty response).

Pitfalls
Severe hypotension.

Lung scan: ventilation/perfusion imaging

569

Indications
- Suspected pulmonary embolism.
- Pre-operative lung function assessment.

Patient preparation
None required. Relative contraindication in right→left intracardiac shunts; caution in severe pulmonary hypertension.

Procedure
- Lie patient supine and inject ^{99m}Tc macroaggregates or albumin IV.
- Obtain gamma camera perfusion images in 4 views.
- Ventilation images are obtained in same projections by continuous breathing of ^{81m}Kr gas (same day) or using ^{99m}Tc aerosol or ^{133}xenon gas (separate day).

Results
Homogeneous, matched ventilation and perfusion patterns.

Interpretation
Four abnormal patterns recognised:
1. Segmental perfusion loss with preserved ventilation—pulmonary embolism.
2. Segmental matched perfusion and ventilation loss—pulmonary infarction/infection.
3. Segmental/subsegmental ventilation loss with preserved perfusion—infection.
4. Non-segmental, patchy, matched perfusion and ventilation LOSS—COPD.

Advantages
Quick, non-invasive. Normal scan virtually excludes PE.

Pitfalls
Specificity reduced in underlying lung disease—COPD, asthma giving indeterminate results. False +ves with tumour, bullae, vasculitides, fibrotic lung disease and old, unresolved PE.

Lung shunt studies

Indications
Suspected pulmonary AV shunting.

Patient preparation
None required.

Procedure
Inject ^{99m}Tc nanocolloid IV. Gamma camera lung, abdomen and head imaging. Calculate relative uptake in lungs, kidneys and brain. Express as fraction of cardiac output to quantify shunt fraction.

Results
Kidneys and brain not normally visible on lung perfusion imaging.

Interpretation
Abnormal extrapulmonary activity implies degree of shunting. Intensity of uptake rises with shunt severity.

(1990)The PIOPED investigators. *JAMA* **263**, 2753.

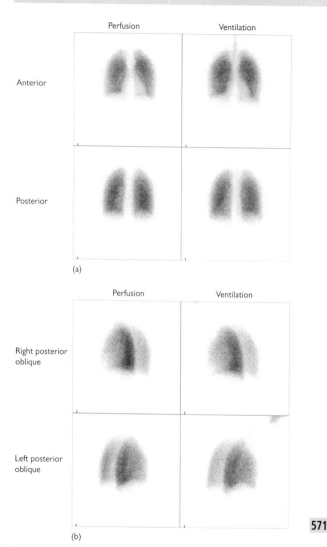

Fig. 14.21 Normal lung V/Q images.

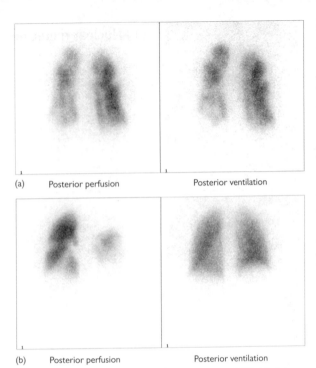

(a)   Posterior perfusion   Posterior ventilation

(b)   Posterior perfusion   Posterior ventilation

Fig. 14.22 Lung scans: (a) showing matched, non-segmental V/Q defects in COPD; and (b) showing segmental V/Q mismatch—extensive bilateral pulmonary thromboembolism and unmatched perfusion loss.

Advantages
Non-invasive, quantitative. Can be used to monitor response to intervention.

Pitfalls
Injection extravasation invalidates shunt calculation.

Lung permeability studies

572

Indications
- *Pneumocystis carinii* pneumonia (PCP)—rapid screening in high-risk patients with normal CXR.

• Monitor treatment response in cryptogenic fibrosing alveolitis.

Patient preparation
None required.

Procedure
Patient breathes ^{99m}Tc DTPA aerosol. Gamma camera images of thorax over 1h. Computer data analysis generates lung clearance curves reflecting integrity of alveolar cell barrier.

Results
Clearance curves used to calculate permeability index. Individual results compared with centre-defined normal range.

Interpretation
Accelerated clearance in PCP which ↓ with successful treatment.

Advantages
Non-invasive. Allows rapid PCP diagnosis.

Pitfalls
Non-specific, e.g. accelerated clearance in smokers.

Lymphoscintigraphy

Indications
Unexplained limb swelling, e.g. lymphatic hypoplasia.

Patient preparation
None required.

Procedure
[99m]Tc colloid injection subcutaneously into finger or toe webspace on affected and contralateral limb. Regional gamma camera imaging at 10min intervals over next hour.

Results
Normally rapid clearance via lymphatic channels to regional nodes.

Interpretation
Slow clearance and failed regional node uptake in hypoplastic systems or metastatic regional node infiltration, depending on clinical context.

Advantages
Technically easier than conventional (contrast) lymphography—avoids lymphatic channel cannulation.

Pitfalls
Lymphatic drainage may be disrupted by surgery or radiotherapy.

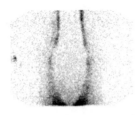

Feet/ankles

Pelvis/abdomen

Fig. 14.23 Normal lymphoscintograms.

Positron emission tomography (PET)

Indications
- Oncology: tumour localisation; staging; assess treatment response, detect relapse.
- Cardiology: myocardial hibernation.
- Neurology: cerebral blood flow; localise epileptogenic focus.

Patient preparation
Depends on pharmaceutical used and study undertaken. Commonest tracer is ^{18}F fluorodeoxyglucose (^{18}F- FDG). Uptake influenced by plasma glucose levels, insulin administered on sliding scale for maximal uptake (optional).

Procedure
Fast for 6h. Tracer given IV in restful environment. Tomographic imaging using dedicated PET scanner or modified gamma camera.

Results
Normal uptake in metabolically active tissues—brain, myocardium, liver, renal excretion.

Interpretation
- Oncology: image co-registration with anatomical imaging essential. Abnormal focal ^{18}F FDG uptake implies residual, viable tumour.
- Cardiology: myocardial metabolism compared with perfusion images. Poor perfusion but persisting ^{18}F FDG metabolism indicates hibernation.
- Neurology: localise epileptogenic foci.

Advantages
Sensitive for metabolically active lesions. Invaluable for distinguishing tumour recurrence from scarring/fibrosis.

Pitfalls
Limited availability. Expensive. Full potential not yet reached. False +ves in infection, post-exercise striatal muscle uptake.

Gallium scintigraphy

Indications
- PUO and infection localisation, especially in AIDS.
- Lymphoma follow-up.
- Sarcoidosis follow-up.

Patient preparation
None.

Procedure
Inject ^{67}Ga citrate IV. Gamma camera imaging at 48–96h with tomography. Non-specific gut retention reduced by laxative administration.

Results
Normal uptake in lacrimal glands, nasal mucosa, blood pool, liver, spleen, testes, female perineum, breast.

Interpretation
- Focal lymph node uptake in lymphoma and sarcoid distinguishes active disease from post-therapy scarring/fibrosis.
- In AIDS, ↑ lung uptake indicates infection—PCP, CMV, mycobacterium—chest radiograph correlation essential.
- ↑ activity in inflammatory bowel disease and focal sepsis; largely superseded by WBC imaging.

Advantages
Excellent, non-invasive marker of disease activity in lymphoma—but likely to be superseded by PET.

Pitfalls
Poor specificity. High radiation dose often difficult to justify when alternative techniques are available.

Dacroscintigraphy

Indications
Epiphora.

Patient preparation
None required.

Procedure
1–2 drops ^{99m}Tc-labelled DTPA or pertechnetate instilled into outer canthus of each eye. Immediate dynamic gamma camera imaging for 20min with delayed static scans as required.

Results
Normal rapid radiopharmaceutical clearance through nasolacrimal apparatus.

Interpretation
Delayed clearance implies obstruction—level of dysfunction usually identified, i.e. punctum, lacrimal sac, nasolacrimal duct.

Advantages
Non-invasive. Avoids nasolacrimal duct cannulation (compared with dacrocystography).

Pitfalls
Obstructed systems result in excess radiolabelled tears on cheek altering drainage times.

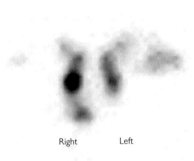

Right   Left

Fig. 14.24 Dacroscintigram (lacrimal drainage) showing normal lacrimal drainage on the right and, on the left, obstructed drainage at the proximal nasolacrimal duct.

Labelled leucocyte imaging

Indications
- Sepsis localisation.
- Inflammatory bowel disease to help determine extent and severity.

Patient preparation
None. Avoid recent barium contrast radiology.

Procedure

Obtain 40–60mL blood sample. Separate white cell layer and radiolabel *in vitro* using ^{99m}Tc exametazine (HMPAO) or ^{111}In oxine. Re-inject labelled cells IV. Image 1 and 3h later (inflammatory bowel disease) or 2, 4 and 24h for intra-abdominal sepsis/osteomyelitis. ^{99m}Tc exametazine (HMPAO) preferred for routine imaging and inflammatory bowel disease—lower radiation dose and earlier result than ^{111}In oxine label.

Results

Physiological uptake in reticuloendothelial system. Variable GI and renal excretion, depending on radiopharmaceutical used.

Interpretation

Focal ↑ uptake indicates sepsis. Diffuse ↑ gut uptake reflects extent and activity of inflammatory bowel disease.

Advantages

Very sensitive in inflammatory bowel disease. Non-invasive, useful in sick patients, e.g. acute exacerbation of inflammatory bowel disease.

Pitfalls

- *False −ves*: leucopenia and poor white cell label, perihepatic and peri-splenic collections obscured by normal liver and spleen uptake.
- *False +ves*: physiological gut and renal activity.
- Damaged white cells during labelling causing lung sequestration.
- Reserve ^{111}In oxine for low grade bone sepsis localisation.

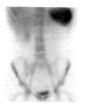
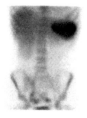

Fig. 14.25 Labelled leucocyte imaging: (a) normal, and (b) acute inflammatory bowel disease—intense uptake in small and large bowel loops (Crohn's disease).

Glomerular filtration rate measurement

Indications
Accurate GFR to monitor renal failure, cytotoxic chemotherapy, immuno-suppression, e.g. cyclosporin.

Patient preparation
Well hydrated.

Procedure
- IV injection of ^{51}Cr EDTA or ^{99m}Tc DTPA.
- Venous sampling 2 and 4h later.
- Count plasma sample radioactivity in gamma counter. Correct for height and weight.

Results
Normal GFR = 125mL/min.

Interpretation
↓ values in CRF.

Advantages
More reliable and reproducible than creatinine clearance—avoids need for urine collection.

Pitfalls
Accuracy depends on good injection technique—avoid *any* extravasation. Unreliable results in severe peripheral oedema.

Urea breath test

Indications
Helicobacter pylori detection—diagnosis and confirmation of eradication.

Patient preparation
Stop antibiotics, H_2 antagonists and, proton pump inhibitors for 2–4 weeks.

Procedure
Patient swallows urea drink labelled with ^{13}carbon (stable isotope) or ^{14}carbon (radioactive isotope). Breath samples (CO_2) collected over next 30min. Labelled CO_2 measured by mass spectroscopy (^{13}C) or liquid scintillation counting (^{14}C).

Results
Normal range varies according to local protocol.

Interpretation
Increased exhaled CO_2 levels imply abnormal urea breakdown by urease-producing bacteria in stomach, e.g. *H. pylori*.

Advantages

Very sensitive marker of active *H. pylori* infection (📖*Serology* (p268)). Non-invasive (📖*Endoscopy* (p346)) and avoids sampling errors. Good for non-invasive monitoring of recurrent symptoms.

Pitfalls

Occasional false +ves in oral *H. pylori* infection.

B_{12} absorption studies

Indications

Vitamin B_{12} malabsorption; pernicious anaemia.

Patient preparation

Investigate before initiating B_{12} therapy where possible. Otherwise, avoid B_{12} supplements for 1 month prior to investigation.

Procedure

Two techniques are available:
1. Administer ^{57}cobalt-B_{12} PO. Measure retention using gamma camera or whole body counter at 7 days. Normal retention >50%.
2. Give 1mg IM B_{12} then PO. Collect all urine for 24h. Measure ^{57}CO-B_{12} excretion. Normal excretion 14–40%. If normal results, B_{12} malabsorption is excluded. If abnormal, repeat whole procedure using ^{57}Co-B_{12} and 100mg intrinsic factor PO. Calculate retention/excretion ratio for ^{57}Co-B_{12} + IF versus ^{57}Co-B_{12} alone.

Results

Retention method
Normal ratio ^{57}Co-B_{12} + IF: ^{57}Co-B_{12} + IF <1.8.

Urinary method
Normal ratio ^{57}Co-B_{12} +IF: ^{57}Co-B_{12} + IF = 0.7–1.2.

Interpretation

- ↓ ^{57}Co-B_{12} levels indicate B_{12} malabsorption.
- Intrinsic factor corrects B_{12} absorption in pernicious anaemia, i.e. ^{57}Co-B_{12} + IF: to ^{57}Co-B_{12} ratio rises.

Advantages

Non-invasive. Only available technique.

Pitfalls

Urine excretion method—incomplete urine collection invalidates result. Severe GI atrophy—may invalidate IF response.

Ferrokinetic studies

Indications
- Unexplained, refractory anaemia.
- Abnormal iron metabolism.

Patient preparation
None.

Procedure
- Inject ^{59}Fe-labelled transferrin IV.
- Measure activity over liver, spleen, sacrum and heart using gamma probe daily for 14 days.
- Measure blood ^{59}Fe clearance daily for 14 days.
- Calculate plasma iron clearance, plasma iron turnover (μmol/L/day) and iron utilisation.
- Organ ^{59}Fe uptake/clearance curve identifies extramedullary haemopoiesis.

Results
- Normal plasma iron clearance half-time = 60–120min.
- Normal iron utilisation at 14 days = 80%.
- Normal iron turnover = 70–140 μmol/L/day.

Interpretation
- Haemolysis—↑ plasma iron turnover, utilisation and marrow activity.
- Myelofibrosis—↑ splenic uptake compared with marrow.
- Aplasia—prolonged plasma iron clearance, low utilisation and hepatic accumulation.

Advantages
Only technique available for iron metabolism.

Pitfalls
Lengthy and labour-intensive. Consistent probe positioning essential for accurate organ uptake curves.

Red cell survival studies

Indications
- Haemolytic anaemia (to confirm ↓ RBC survival, i.e. active haemolysis).
- Localise abnormal red cell sequestration.
- Predict response to splenectomy.

Patient preparation
None. Avoid blood transfusion during study.

Procedure
Label patient's red cells with ^{51}Cr chromate. Re-inject cells and measure blood activity over 14 days using gamma counter. Measure activity over liver, spleen and heart using gamma probe daily for 14 days.

Results
- Normal red cell half-life >24 days.

- Equal fall in heart, liver and spleen counts with time.

Interpretation
Short red cell life confirms abnormal destruction. Ratio of counts in liver : spleen indicates site of red cell destruction.

Advantages
Only available technique.

Pitfalls
Lengthy and labour-intensive. Sensitivity reduced by blood transfusion during 14-day measurement period. Consistent probe positioning essential for accurate organ sequestration curves.

Red cell volume/plasma volume measurement

Indications
Polycythaemia, to distinguish between true polycythaemia ($\uparrow$ RBC mass) from apparent polycythaemia ($\downarrow$ plasma volume).

Patient preparation
Avoid recent therapeutic venesection. Less sensitive in patients already receiving myelosuppressive therapy.

Procedure
- Block thyroid using potassium iodide/iodate.
- Obtain 10mL venous blood.
- Separate plasma and red cells.
- Radiolabel red cells using ^{99m}Tc/^{51}Cr and plasma using ^{125}I albumin.
- Re-inject radiolabelled blood.
- Obtain venous samples at 15 and 30min.
- Count activity in blood samples compared with known standards using gamma counter to establish plasma and red cell volumes.

Results
Compare measured red cell mass and plasma volume with predicted values for height and weight.

Interpretation
Distinguish relative polycythaemia (due to $\downarrow$ plasma volume) from genuine elevation of red cell mass.

Advantages
Only technique available.

Pitfalls
Recent venesection or myelosuppressive therapy reduces test reliability. Plasma volume measurement unreliable in severe peripheral oedema.

Bile salt deconjugation studies

Indications
Bacterial overgrowth; bile salt malabsorption.

Patient preparation
Starve overnight. Avoid antibiotics for 1 month before study.

Procedure
Give oral ^{14}Ca-labelled glycocholic acid in water. Count $^{14}CO_2$ activity in breath samples over 6h using beta liquid scintillation counter.

Results
Glycocholate is deconjugated into ^{14}C glycine and cholic acid by small intestine bacteria releasing expired $^{14}CO_2$. Correct result for age-related variations in endogenous $^{14}CO_2$ production.

Interpretation
↑ $^{14}CO_2$ levels imply bacterial colonisation or bile salt malabsorption.

Advantages
Accurate. Only available test.

Pitfalls
False −ves unusual.

Chapter 15

Normal ranges

Index

Index

Index

Index